Massachusetts
General
Hospital

MANUAL OF
ORAL AND
MAXILLOFACIAL
SURGERY

Massachusetts General Hospital

MANUAL OF ORAL AND MAXILLOFACIAL SURGERY

R. BRUCE DONOFF, D.M.D., M.D.

Professor and Chairman, Department of Oral
and Maxillofacial Surgery, Harvard School of
Dental Medicine; Chief of Service, Department
of Oral and Maxillofacial Surgery, Massachusetts
General Hospital, Boston, Massachusetts

with 35 illustrations

THE C. V. MOSBY COMPANY

ST. LOUIS • WASHINGTON, D.C. • TORONTO 1987

MOSBY

A TRADITION OF PUBLISHING EXCELLENCE

Acquisitions editor: Donna Saya Sokolowski
Manuscript editor: George B. Stericker, Jr.
Book design: Liz Fett
Production: Ginny Douglas

Printed in the United States of America

The C. V. Mosby Company
11830 Westline Industrial Drive, St. Louis, Missouri 63146

Library of Congress Cataloging-in-Publication Data

Massachusetts General Hospital manual of oral and
    maxillofacial surgery.

    Prepared by members of the Oral and Maxillofacial
Surgery Service of the Massachusetts General Hospital.
    Includes bibliographies and index.
    1. Mouth—Surgery. 2. Maxilla—Surgery. 3. Face—
Surgery.   4. Massachusetts General Hospital. Oral
and Maxillofacial Surgery Service. I. Donoff, R. Bruce.
II. Massachusetts General Hospital. Oral and Maxillo-
facial Surgery Service. [DNLM: 1. Dentistry, Operative—
handbooks. 2. Surgery, Oral—handbooks. WU 39 M414]
RK529.M37 1987   617′.52059   87-1639
ISBN 0-8016-1415-5

TSI/MV/D 9 8 7 6 5 4 3 2 1 01/B/002

List of Contributors

MEREDITH AUGUST, D.M.D., M.D.
Clinical Fellow, Department of Oral and Maxillofacial Surgery, Harvard School of Dental Medicine; Senior Resident, Oral and Maxillofacial Surgery Service, Massachusetts General Hospital, Boston

CHARLES N. BERTOLAMI, D.D.S., D.MSC.
Assistant Professor, Department of Oral and Maxillofacial Surgery, Harvard School of Dental Medicine; Associate Visiting Surgeon, Oral and Maxillofacial Surgery Service, Massachusetts General Hospital, Boston

ROBERT CHUONG, D.M.D., M.D.
Private practice; formerly Clinical Associate, Oral and Maxillofacial Surgery Service, Massachusetts General Hospital; formerly Instructor, Department of Oral and Maxillofacial Surgery, Harvard School of Dental Medicine, Boston

R. BRUCE DONOFF, D.M.D., M.D.
Professor and Chairman, Department of Oral and Maxillofacial Surgery, Harvard School of Dental Medicine; Chief, Oral and Maxillofacial Surgery Service, Massachusetts General Hospital, Boston

RAY ENGLISH, Jr., D.M.D.
Private practice; formerly Senior Resident, Oral and Maxillofacial Surgery Service, Massachusetts General Hospital; formerly Clinical Fellow, Department of Oral and Maxillofacial Surgery, Harvard School of Dental Medicine, Boston

DAVID A. KEITH, B.D.S., F.D.S.R.C.S., D.M.D.
Associate Professor, Department of Oral and Maxillofacial Surgery, Harvard School of Dental Medicine; Associate Visiting Surgeon, Oral and Maxillofacial Surgery Service, Massachusetts General Hospital, Boston

JOHN P. KELLY, D.M.D., M.D.
Assistant Professor, Department of Oral and Maxillofacial Surgery, Harvard School of Dental Medicine; Associate Visiting Surgeon, Oral and Maxillofacial Surgery Service, Massachusetts General Hospital, Boston

EDWARD B. SELDIN, D.M.D., M.D.

Assistant Professor, Department of Oral and Maxillofacial Surgery, Harvard School of Dental Medicine; Visiting Surgeon, Oral and Maxillofacial Surgery Service, Massachusetts General Hospital, Boston

WILLIE L. STEPHENS, D.D.S.

Instructor, Department of Oral and Maxillofacial Surgery, Harvard School of Dental Medicine, Assistant in Oral and Maxillofacial Surgery, Oral and Maxillofacial Surgery Service, Massachusetts General Hospital, Boston

JOSEPH W. WILKES, III, D.M.D., M.D.

Instructor, Department of Oral and Maxillofacial Surgery, Harvard School of Dental Medicine; Assistant in Oral and Maxillofacial Surgery, Oral and Maxillofacial Surgery Service, Massachusetts General Hospital, Boston

To my father,
the most self-educated man I've ever known.
Books were his joy,
new knowledge his excitement.

Preface

In the past 20 years, oral and maxillofacial surgery has made significant progress in the diagnosis and treatment of pathology, malformation, and injury involving the oral and perioral structures. The *Massachusetts General Hospital Manual of Oral and Maxillofacial Surgery* contains the essentials for diagnosis, treatment, and management of the oral and maxillofacial surgery patient. Manuals in other specialties have proved to be invaluable to students and house staff. This manual seeks to fill the need for a concise reference in our specialty. It should be of value to other members of the dental and medical profession as well.

The manual was prepared by members of the Oral and Maxillofacial Surgery Service of the MGH and reflects our methods and judgment in management of selected problems. No attempt has been made to be all-inclusive. There are no substitutes for textbooks, journals, and hands-on experience. The development of good doctors and surgeons should be a continuing preoccupation of educator-clinicians. Without thought, there is little learning. Without reading, there is little to think about. Without discussion, it is difficult to distinguish between good and bad thinking. This manual is designed to be available for students, house staff, oral and maxillofacial surgeons, and other medical professionals.

My thanks to Ms. Darlene Warfel Cooke and Ms. Donna Sokolowski and to the editorial staff of The C.V. Mosby Co. for their assistance and guidance. Special thanks to all my colleagues who contributed to this work and the superb secretarial staff of our hospital service. Last, but by no means least, thanks to my wife, Mady, for putting up with another extra.

R. Bruce Donoff
Boston, Mass., 1986

Contents

Massachusetts
General
Hospital

MANUAL OF
ORAL AND
MAXILLOFACIAL
SURGERY

SECTION I
Algorithms

KNOWN DIABETIC PATIENT UNDERGOING ELECTIVE SURGERY

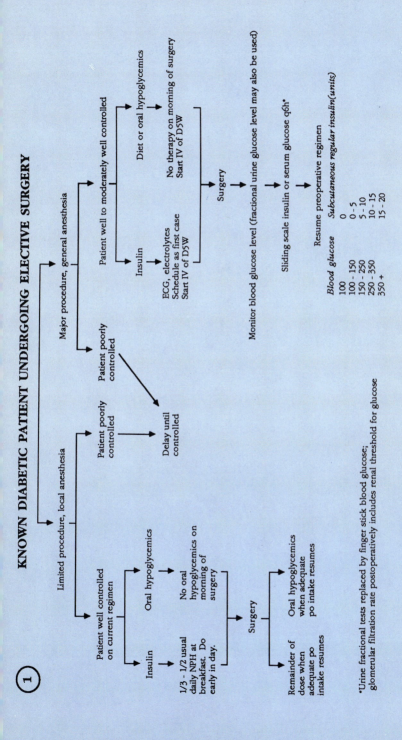

(1)

Limited procedure, local anesthesia

Major procedure, general anesthesia

Limited procedure, local anesthesia:

Patient well controlled on current regimen

- Insulin → 1/3 – 1/2 usual daily NPH at breakfast. Do early in day.
- Oral hypoglycemics → No oral hypoglycemics on morning of surgery

Surgery

- Remainder of dose when adequate po intake resumes
- Oral hypoglycemics when adequate po intake resumes

Patient poorly controlled → Delay until controlled

Major procedure, general anesthesia:

Patient well to moderately well controlled

- Insulin → ECG, electrolytes; Schedule as first case; Start IV of D5W
- Diet or oral hypoglycemics → No therapy on morning of surgery; Start IV of D5W

Patient poorly controlled → Delay until controlled

Surgery → Monitor blood glucose level (fractional urine glucose level may also be used) → Sliding scale insulin or serum glucose q6h* →

Resume preoperative regimen

Blood glucose	Subcutaneous regular insulin(units)
100	0
100 – 150	0 – 5
150 – 250	5 – 10
250 – 350	10 – 15
350 +	15 – 20

*Urine fractional tests replaced by finger stick blood glucose; glomerular filtration rate postoperatively includes renal threshold for glucose

STEROID COVERAGE

Patient taking glucocorticoids or with 2 wk history
of steroid intake within preceding 2 yr

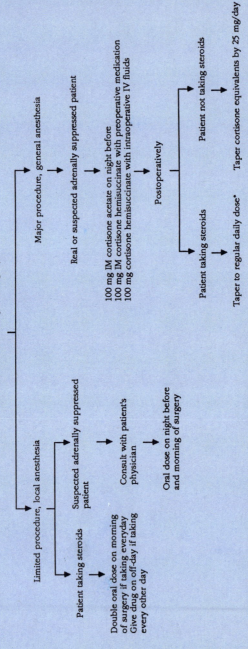

Limited procedure, local anesthesia

Patient taking steroids

Double oral dose on morning
of surgery if taking everyday
Give drug on off-day if taking
every other day

Suspected adrenally suppressed
patient

Consult with patient's
physician

Oral dose on night before
and morning of surgery

Major procedure, general anesthesia

Real or suspected adrenally suppressed patient

100 mg IM cortisone acetate on night before
100 mg IM cortisone hemisuccinate with preoperative medication
100 mg cortisone hemisuccinate with intraoperative IV fluids

Postoperatively

Patient taking steroids

Taper to regular daily dose*

Patient not taking steroids

Taper cortisone equivalents by 25 mg/day

*Approximate equivalent doses (mg) for glucocorticoids

USP name	mg
Hydrocortisone	20.0
Cortisone	25.0
Prednisone	5.0
Prednisolone	5.0
Dexamethasone	0.75

2

BLEEDING DISORDERS

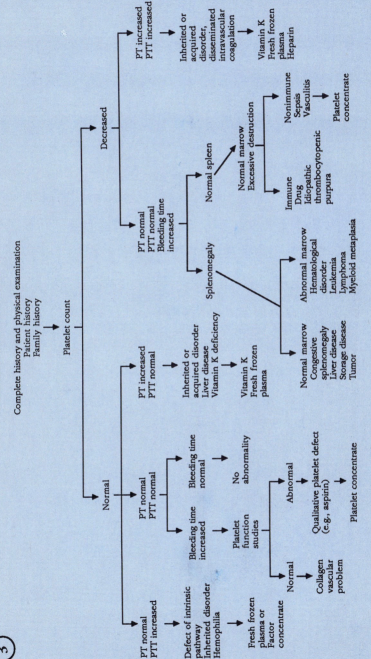

Complete history and physical examination
Patient history
Family history

→ Platelet count

Normal

PT normal
PTT increased

Defect of intrinsic
pathway
Inherited disorder
Hemophilia

→ Fresh frozen
plasma or
Factor
concentrate

PT normal
PTT normal

Bleeding time
increased → Platelet function studies

Bleeding time
normal → No abnormality

Normal → Collagen vascular problem

Abnormal → Qualitative platelet defect (e.g., aspirin) → Platelet concentrate

PT increased
PTT normal

Inherited or
acquired disorder
Liver disease
Vitamin K deficiency

→ Vitamin K
Fresh frozen
plasma

Normal marrow
Congestive
splenomegaly
Liver disease
Storage disease
Tumor

Abnormal marrow
Hematological
disorder
Leukemia
Lymphoma
Myeloid metaplasia

Decreased

PT normal
PTT normal
Bleeding time
increased

Splenomegaly

Normal spleen

Normal marrow
Excessive destruction

Immune
Drug
Idiopathic
thrombocytopenic
purpura

Nonimmune
Sepsis
Vasculitis → Platelet
concentrate

PT increased
PTT increased

Inherited or
acquired
disorder,
disseminated
intravascular
coagulation

→ Vitamin K
Fresh frozen
plasma
Heparin

③

PAROTID ENLARGEMENT

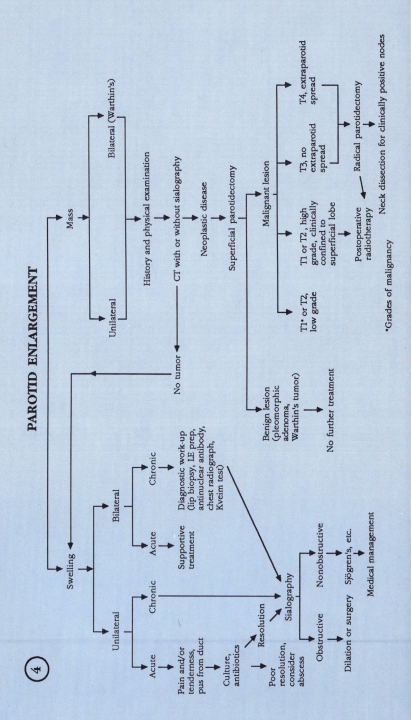

Mass

Unilateral   Bilateral (Warthin's)

History and physical examination

CT with or without sialography

Neoplastic disease

No tumor

Superficial parotidectomy

Benign lesion (pleomorphic adenoma, Warthin's tumor) → No further treatment

Malignant lesion

T1* or T2, low grade

T1 or T2, high grade, clinically confined to superficial lobe

T3, no extraparotid spread

T4, extraparotid spread

Postoperative radiotherapy

Radical parotidectomy

Neck dissection for clinically positive nodes

*Grades of malignancy

Swelling

Unilateral   Bilateral

Acute   Chronic   Acute   Chronic

Pain and/or tenderness, pus from duct

Culture, antibiotics

Resolution

Poor resolution, consider abscess

Supportive treatment

Diagnostic work-up (lip biopsy, LE prep, antinuclear antibody, chest radiograph, Kveim test)

Sialography

Obstructive   Nonobstructive

Dilation or surgery   Sjögren's, etc.

Medical management

④

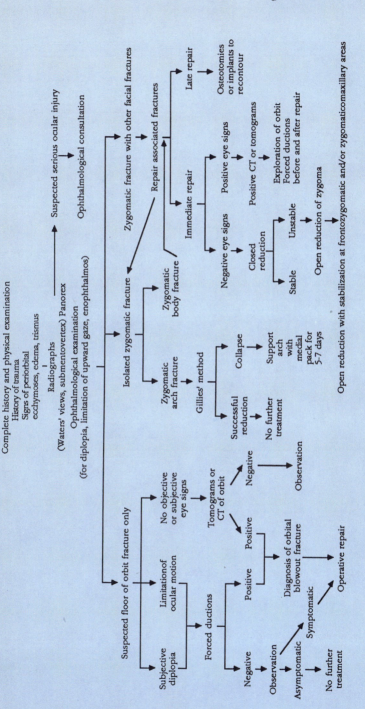

ZYGOMATIC COMPLEX FRACTURES

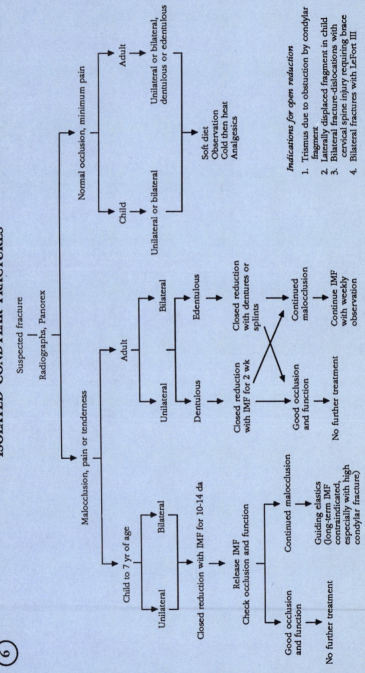

ISOLATED CONDYLAR FRACTURES

Suspected fracture
|
Radiographs, Panorex

Malocclusion, pain or tenderness

Child to 7 yr of age
- Unilateral
- Bilateral

Closed reduction with IMF for 10-14 da

Release IMF
Check occlusion and function

- Good occlusion and function → No further treatment
- Continued malocclusion → Guiding elastics (long-term IMF contraindicated, especially with high condylar fracture)

Adult
- Unilateral — Dentulous
- Bilateral — Edentulous

Closed reduction with IMF for 2 wk (Dentulous)
Closed reduction with dentures or splints (Edentulous)

- Good occlusion and function → No further treatment
- Continued malocclusion → Continue IMF with weekly observation

Normal occlusion, minimum pain

Child
- Unilateral or bilateral

Adult
- Unilateral or bilateral, dentulous or edentulous

Soft diet
Observation
Cold then heat
Analgesics

Indications for open reduction

1. Trismus due to obstuction by condylar fragment
2. Laterally displaced fragment in child
3. Bilateral fracture-dislocations with cervical spine injury requiring brace
4. Bilateral fractures with LeFort III

⑥

MIDFACE TRAUMA

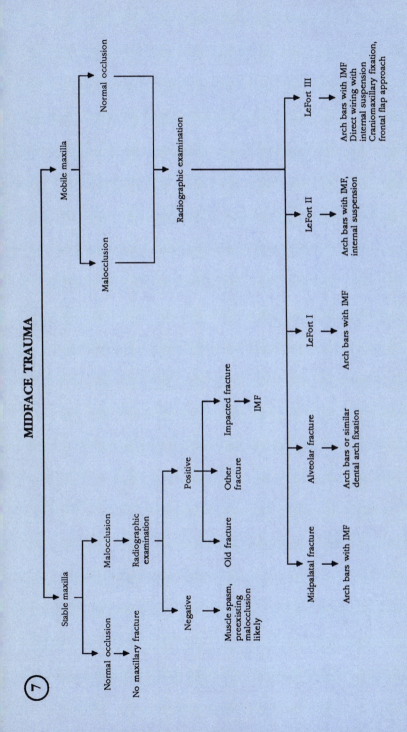

ORTHOGNATHIC SURGERY FOR VERTICAL DISCREPANCY

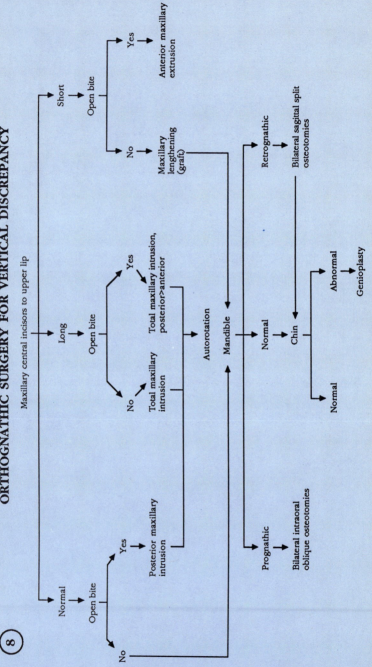

ORTHOGNATHIC SURGERY FOR HORIZONTAL DISCREPANCY

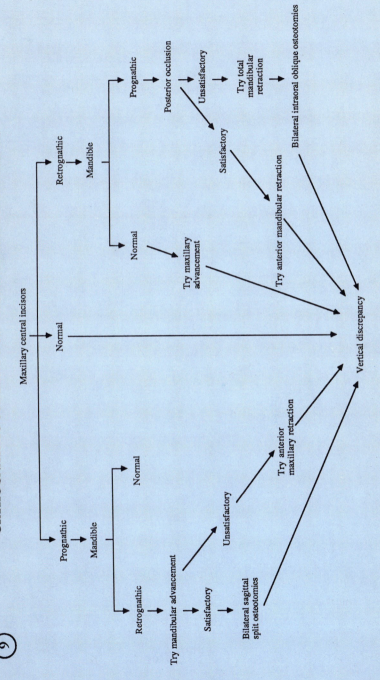

MANDIBULAR RECONSTRUCTION

Defect result of

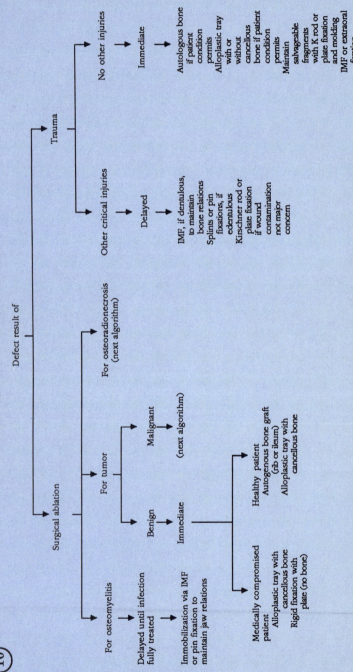

Surgical ablation

For osteomyelitis
→ Delayed until infection fully treated
→ Immobilization via IMF or pin fixation to maintain jaw relations

For tumor
- Benign → Immediate
  - Healthy patient
    Autogenous bone graft (rib or ileum)
    Alloplastic tray with cancellous bone
  - Medically compromised patient
    Alloplastic tray with cancellous bone
    Rigid fixation with plate (no bone)
- Malignant
  (next algorithm)

For osteoradionecrosis (next algorithm)

Trauma

Other critical injuries
→ Delayed
→ IMF, if dentulous, to maintain bone relations
Splints or pin fixations, if edentulous
Kirschner rod or plate fixation if wound contamination not major concern

No other injuries
→ Immediate
→ Autologous bone if patient condition permits
Alloplastic tray with or without cancellous bone if patient condition permits
Maintain salvageable fragments with K rod or plate fixation and molding
IMF or extraoral fixation

⑩

MANDIBULAR RECONSTRUCTION FOR MALIGNANCIES

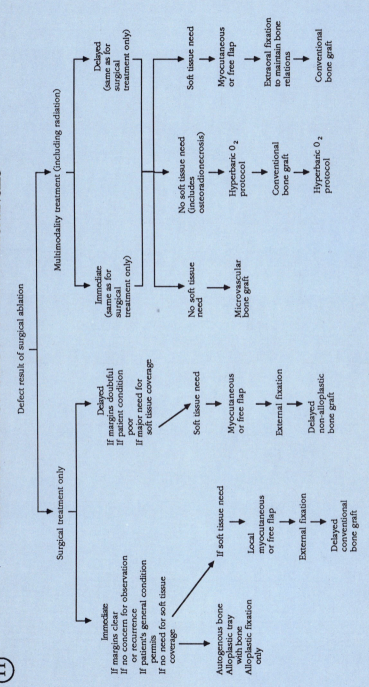

Defect result of surgical ablation

Surgical treatment only

Immediate
If margins clear
If no concern for observation or recurrence
If patient's general condition permits
If no need for soft tissue coverage

Autogenous bone
Alloplastic tray with bone
Alloplastic fixation only

If soft tissue need → Local myocutaneous or free flap → External fixation → Delayed conventional bone graft

Delayed
If margins doubtful
If patient condition poor
If major need for soft tissue coverage

Soft tissue need → Myocutaneous or free flap → External fixation → Delayed non-alloplastic bone graft

Multimodality treatment (including radiation)

Immediate (same as for surgical treatment only)

No soft tissue need → Microvascular bone graft

No soft tissue need (includes osteoradionecrosis) → Hyperbaric O_2 protocol → Conventional bone graft → Hyperbaric O_2 protocol

Delayed (same as for surgical treatment only)

Soft tissue need → Myocutaneous or free flap → Extraoral fixation to maintain bone relations → Conventional bone graft

11

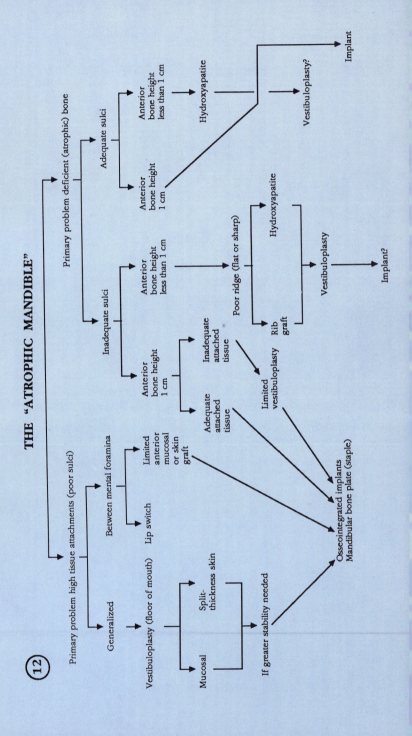

THE "ATROPHIC MANDIBLE"

FACIAL PAIN

(13)

Complete history and physical examination
Determine location, character, trigger points, duration and frequency of attacks
Psychological status
Sites of radiation
Percuss teeth, examine TMJs and sinuses
Perform nerve blocks, radiographs, consultations

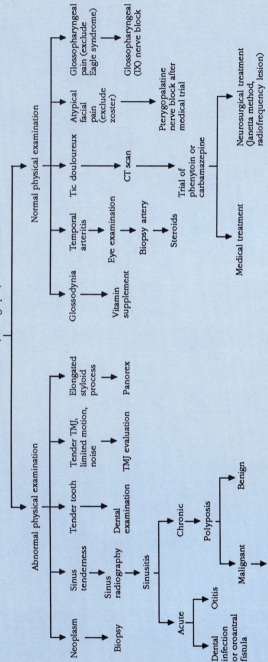

Abnormal physical examination

- Neoplasm → Biopsy
- Sinus tenderness → Sinus radiography → Sinusitis
  - Chronic → Polyposis
    - Benign
    - Malignant → CT to look for bone destruction
  - Acute
    - Dental infection or oroantral fistula
    - Otitis
- Tender tooth → Dental examination
- Tender TMJ, limited motion, noise → TMJ evaluation
- Elongated styloid process → Panorex

Normal physical examination

- Glossodynia → Vitamin supplement
- Temporal arteritis → Eye examination → Biopsy artery → Steroids
- Tic douloureux → CT scan → Trial of phenytoin or carbamazepine
  - Neurosurgical treatment (Janetta method, radiofrequency lesion)
  - Medical treatment
- Atypical facial pain (exclude zoster) → Pterygopalatine nerve block after medical trial
- Glossopharyngeal pain (exclude Eagle syndrome) → Glossopharyngeal (IX) nerve block

NERVE INJURY

(14)

Indications for microsurgery

1. Peripheral dysesthesia confirmed by diagnostic nerve blocks
2. Known or highly suspicious nerve injury with acute anesthesia and/or pain
3. No improvement at monthly sensory examinations over 6 mo
4. Continued deterioration at monthly sensory examination
5. Sudden halt in improvement at monthly sensory examination
6. Immediate microsurgical reconstruction of nerve resected during ablative surgery

Clinical neurosensory examination

Noninvasive

A. Pin pressure nociception—mediated by small-diameter nerve fibers with and without myelin (A-delta and C)
B. Two-point detection—primarily tests for quantity of larger myelinated axons innervating pacinian corpuscles
C. Directional stroke determination mediated by specific receptors innervated by larger myelinated nerve fibers (A-delta and B)—tests for rapidly adapting mechano-receptors
D. Weinstein-Semmes static light pressure—same as C but tests slowly adapting mechano-receptors
E. Examination for Tinel's sign—shooting sensation distally or pain directly when palpating over surgical site or lingual alveolus

Invasive

A. Diagnostic nerve blocks—failure of peripheral block to alleviate pain suggests psychological, sympathetic, or central origin to dysesthesia despite original cause (deafferentation)
B. Somatosensory evoked potentials—noninvasive technique, experimental

Injury noted at surgery

1. Lingual nerve or inferior alveolar nerve torn
2. IAN torn at sagittal split osteotomy
3. IAN avulsed with malformed root structure

Intraoperatively

A. Repair immediately with tendon transfer technique using smallest absorbable suture available

or

B. Repair under magnification with 9-0 or 10-0 suture if possible

Postoperatively

A. Document and map sensory loss and recovery
B. Follow monthly
C. If pain a problem with sensory return, use analgesics and/or Dilantin 300mg/day

(15)

SUSPICION OF NERVE INJURY AT SURGERY

Basic observations

1. Persistence of paresthesia less in inferior alveolar than in lingual
2. Anesthesia (poor sign)
3. Deterioration suggests need for surgery
4. Sudden halt in improvement suggests need for surgery

Postoperative observations

1. Area of sensory loss
2. Subjective symptoms

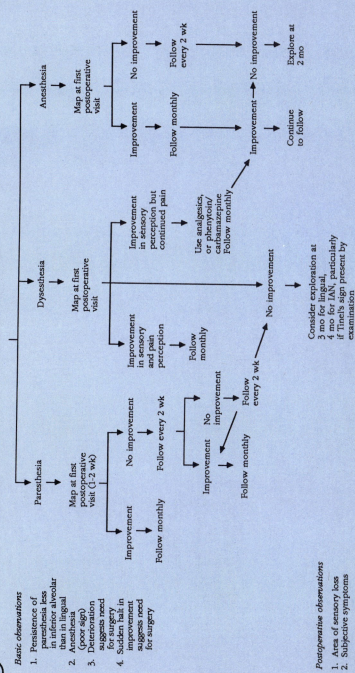

Paresthesia → Map at first postoperative visit (1-2 wk)

Improvement → Follow monthly

No improvement → Follow every 2 wk → Improvement → Follow monthly; No improvement → Follow every 2 wk

No improvement → Consider exploration at 3 mo for lingual, 4 mo for IAN, particularly if Tinel's sign present by examination

Dysesthesia → Map at first postoperative visit

Improvement in sensory and pain perception → Follow monthly

Improvement in sensory perception but continued pain → Use analgesics, or phenytoin/carbamazepine; Follow monthly → Improvement → Continue to follow; No improvement → Explore at 2 mo

Anesthesia → Map at first postoperative visit

Improvement → Follow monthly

No improvement → Follow every 2 wk

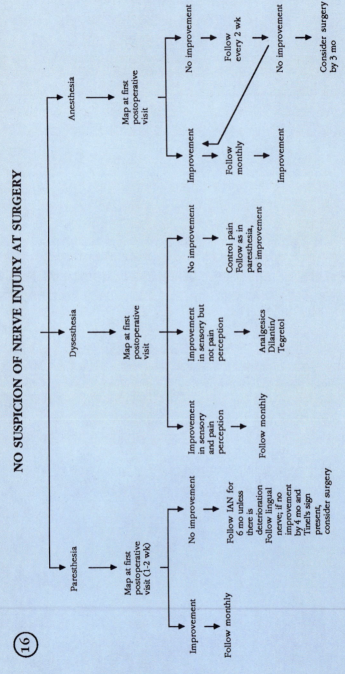

NO SUSPICION OF NERVE INJURY AT SURGERY

(16)

Paresthesia

Map at first postoperative visit (1-2 wk)

- Improvement
  - Follow monthly

- No improvement
  - Follow IAN for 6 mo unless there is deterioration
    Follow lingual nerve; if no improvement by 4 mo and Tinel's sign present, consider surgery

Dysesthesia

Map at first postoperative visit

- Improvement in sensory and pain perception
  - Follow monthly

- Improvement in sensory but not pain perception
  - Analgesics
    Dilantin/ Tegretol

- No improvement
  - Control pain
    Follow as in paresthesia, no improvement

Anesthesia

Map at first postoperative visit

- Improvement
  - Follow monthly
    - Improvement

- No improvement
  - Follow every 2 wk
    - No improvement
      - Consider surgery by 3 mo

Postoperative observations

1. Area of sensory loss
2. Subjective symptoms

Hospital Procedures

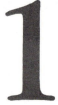

RULES AND REGULATIONS

I. Medical records
   A. The chief of service or department shall be responsible for ensuring that an adequate medical record is established for every patient rendered care by that service or department.
   B. All clinical entries must be dated and authenticated.
   C. Notes sufficient to document the progress of the patient shall be entered in the medical record.
   D. The medical record shall contain evidence of the patient's informed consent for any procedure or treatment that is appropriate.
   E. Reports of ancillary services requiring doctor interpretation shall be authenticated by the interpreting doctor and filed in the medical record.
   F. Reports of clinical laboratory examinations shall be filed in the medical record.
   G. The entire contents of the medical record shall be legible.
   H. The use of abbreviations shall be limited to those approved by the medical staff.
   I. All consultation requests shall be written in the medical record and indicate the name of the doctor requesting the consultation and the reason for consultation.
   J. All medical records are the property of the hospital. They shall not be removed except by a court order or subpoena.
   K. All diagnoses and procedures shall be recorded in the face sheet and/or discharge summary without the use of abbreviations or symbols.
II. Admission records
   A. The inpatient record shall include the following:
      1. Identification data
      2. Chief complaint
      3. Personal and family history
      4. History of present illness
      5. Physical examination
      6. Report of special examination (e.g., clinical and radiological examination)

7. Consultant's notes
8. Provisional or working diagnosis
9. Medical and surgical treatment
10. Gross and microscopic findings
11. Progress notes
12. Final diagnosis
13. Condition on discharge
14. Discharge summary
15. In the event of death and autopsy, a final autopsy report of the gross and microscopic diagnosis. The complete autopsy protocol shall be retained on file in the pathology department.

B. Within 24 hr of admission, the patient's history, physical examination, summary of findings, provisional diagnosis, and diagnostic or treatment plan must be recorded.

C. The responsible doctor shall review and authenticate the admission history, physical examination, therapeutic treatment plan, and summary or shall enter an appropriate admission note of his own.

III. Operative records

A. Immediately after surgery, a brief operative note shall be dictated, authenticated, and entered in the medical record. It shall contain a description of the finding, the technical procedures used, the specimens removed, the postoperative diagnosis, and the name of the primary surgeon and any assistants (Fig. 1-1).

Name of patient:	Date:	Hospital number:
Service and floor:	Surgeon:	Assistants:

Preoperative diagnosis:

Postoperative diagnosis:

Name of operation:

Procedures
1. Description of surgical approach:
2. Findings:
3. Technical procedures used:
4. Specimens removed:
5. Type of closure and sutures used:
6. Drains placed if any:
7. Estimated blood loss and replacement:

Fig. 1-1 Operative report.

B. All use of anesthetic agents shall be fully recorded and authenticated. A postanesthesia note in the medical record will describe the presence or absence of anesthesia-related complications and be authenticated by the anesthesiologist.

C. Reports of pathology examinations shall be authenticated promptly and filed in the medical record.

IV. Discharge records

A. In all cases a concise discharge summary, either written or dictated, shall be prepared within 15 da following discharge

B. The clinical resumé shall recapitulate the reason for hospitalization, the significant finding(s), the procedures performed and treatment rendered, the condition of the patient on discharge, and special instructions given to the patient and/or family.

DOCTOR'S ORDERS

I. General requirements

A. Clear, concise, and complete orders are essential to safe patient care. They ensure optimum communication and expeditious implementation of the patient care plan

B. The following guidelines are designed to assist the house officer in the preparation of a written plan of care. A complete set of orders must include

    1. Medication orders only

       a. Medications

          (1) Complete name

          (2) Metric dose

          (3) Frequency

          (4) Route

          (5) Parameters (when appropriate)

       b. IV orders

    2. All other orders

       a. Diagnosis (upon admission)

       b. Condition (upon admission)

       c. Allergies (upon admission)

       d. Activity

       e. Diet

       f. Diagnostic studies, including radiographs

       g. Vital sign frequency

       h. Wound care

       i. Respiratory orders, including O_2

       j. Special equipment

          (1) Cardiac monitor

          (2) Wire cutter at bedside

C. Additional requirements

    1. Written orders must be dated and signed.

    2. All verbal orders must be signed by the doctor within 24 hr.

3. There shall be automatic termination of all narcotic orders at noon of the third day following the order.
4. There shall be automatic termination of all antibiotic orders at noon of the tenth day following the order.
5. IV orders must be rewritten daily.
6. IV orders and narcotic orders must be specific. "Same IV" or "Renew pain med" is not acceptable.
7. Orders must be written in indelible blue or black ink.
8. The most current page must be used for new orders.
9. Abbreviations must be limited to those in the accepted list.
10. Deletion of errors is legally prohibited. If an error occurs, a line must be drawn through the incorrect entry and must be initialed and dated.
11. All orders must be flagged on the front of the order book.
12. Stat orders must be brought to the attention of the nurse.
13. When diagnostic studies are ordered, clinical indication should be included to assist in the preparation of a requisition.
14. Medication doses must be specified (a dosage range is not acceptable).
15. Verbal or telephone orders may be taken by a registered nurse from a doctor who is unable to write the order because of unusual circumstances; the order can be for a single dose of medication, with one repeat of the order. The nurse must read it back for verification and sign it with the doctor's name and the nurse's own name and licensure status. The prescribing doctor shall sign these orders as soon as possible and within 24 hr.

II. Intravenous orders
   A. IV orders must be completely rewritten daily.
   B. They must be specific.
   C. A written order is required for a "heparin lock."

III. Discharge orders
   A. The discharge plan must be communicated to the nursing staff well in advance to allow time for teaching appropriate referrals and for coordination of patient care.
   B. Orders for discharge must be written.
   C. When at all possible, discharge plans should enable the patient to leave the hospital by 11 am.

INFORMED CONSENT (Fig. 1-2)

I. Communication and consent
   A. A doctor performing a medical or surgical procedure on a patient must obtain the patient's informed consent to the procedure. This is essential to good medical practice (and is also required by law).

DATE:

PATIENT:

UNIT NO:

PROCEDURE:

Patient Identification Stamp

I have explained to the patient the nature of his/her condition, the nature of the procedure, and the benefits to be reasonably expected compared with alternative approaches.

I have discussed the likelihood of major risks or complications of this procedure including (if applicable) but not limited to loss of limb function, brain damage, paralysis, hemorrhage; infection, drug reactions, blood clots and loss of life. I have also indicated that with any procedure there is always the possibility of an unexpected complication.

Additional comments (if any):

All questions were answered and the patient consents to the procedure.

_____ M.D.

Dr. _____
has explained the above to me
and I consent to the procedure.

_____

Signature

If signature cannot be obtained, indicate reason in comments section above.

Fig. 1-2 Surgical consent form.

B. Informed consent involves effective communication in which the doctor must provide enough information for the patient to make a judgment on the proposed treatment. Specifically, the doctor must disclose in a reasonable manner all significant medical information that he possesses or reasonably should possess as a practitioner in that specialty and is pertinent to an intelligent decision by the patient. This information should include
   1. The nature of the patient's condition
   2. The proposed treatment and possible alternatives (including no treatment)
   3. The benefits of the proposed treatment and alternatives
   4. The nature and probability of risks of the proposed treatment and alternatives
   5. The inability of the doctor to predict results and the irreversibility of the procedure
C. The information that must be provided will vary according to the patient's intelligence, experience, age, and other factors. Information that the doctor reasonably believes is already known to the patient (e.g., the risk of infection associated with any surgical procedure) need not be disclosed.

II. Documentation
   A. Procedures requiring documentation of consent
      1. The doctor must document, on the approved hospital form, consent for all therapeutic and diagnostic procedures for which disclosure of significant medical information, including major risks involved, would assist the patient in making an intelligent decision as to whether to undergo the procedure. Such procedures will vary from institution to institution but will include (though not necessarily be limited to) the following:
         a. Any operation performed under general or local anesthesia, including paracentesis, thoracentesis, and arthrocentesis; this will include biopsies and excisions but may not include simple extractions
         b. Cardiac catheterizations and angiography
         c. All endoscopies, excluding sigmoidoscopy and proctoscopy without biopsy
         d. Invasive diagnostic and therapeutic radiologic procedures
         e. Extracorporeal and peritoneal dialysis
         f. Radiation therapy
         g. Invasive cancer chemotherapy
         h. Electroconvulsive therapy
         i. Administration of general or regional anesthesia
         j. Insertion of centrally placed venous lines
      2. Except in an emergency, when the patient's well-being would be seriously endangered, these procedures require the doctor to obtain the patient's informed consent, docu-

mented on the proper form and including the patient's signature.

B. Securing the patient's consent

1. Although the best practice is for the person performing the procedure to obtain and document the informed consent, another licensed doctor who is also a member of the group responsible for administering care to the patient may obtain the consent and complete and file the form, indicating on the form the name of the doctor for whom the consent has been obtained. If a surrogate obtains the informed consent, the doctor with ultimate responsibility is to countersign the form.

2. The consent may be obtained and the form completed in a doctor's office, but the form must ultimately be placed in the hospital record.

C. Concessions for patients who are physically incapable of signing or are mentally incompetent to sign a consent form

1. If the patient is physically unable to sign the form, after full discussion with and consent by him, the doctor may sign the form, which must include a written note indicating the reason for the absence of the patient's signature.

2. If the patient does not have the mental capacity to consent, the doctor should so document with an appropriate note on the form, and a family member or close friend may sign on the patient's behalf.

D. Selection of consent form

1. The standard hospital form should be used for documenting consent.

2. It is also desirable that a written note be placed on the chart indicating that consent has been obtained.

Commonly Used Medications

2

MEDICATIONS FOR AFFECTIVE DISORDERS

I. Affective disorders include the following:
   - A. Depression
     1. Reactive—usually a specific cause, and usually self-limited
     2. Endogenous—no precipitating cause; tricyclic antidepressant therapy is often used
     3. Drug induced (e.g., alcohol, barbiturates, and some antihypertensives)—dosage is often reduced or the drug may be discontinued
   - B. Manic depression
     1. Manic form—often responds to lithium
     2. Depressed form (endogenous)—may respond to electroshock and antidepressants
     3. Circular (bipolar) form—usually responsive to lithium with or without initial antidepressant therapy
   - C. Phobias, anxiety-panic attacks. These frequently accompany depression, often a specific situation; tricyclic antidepressant (TCA) therapy (especially imipramine) or a monoamine oxidase inhibitor (MAOI) can be used.
   - D. Schizoaffective disorders. These usually respond to neuroleptic drugs. They may require simultaneous administration of a TCA or lithium.
II. Classes of medication used for affective disorders (along with psychotherapy) include
   - A. Tricyclic antidepressants (TCAs). These drugs inhibit neurotransmitter reuptake at the presynaptic membrane.
   - B. Monoamine oxidase inhibitors (MAOIs). These block the intracellular metabolism of biogenic amine neurotransmitters.
   - C. Lithium. This agent is used for manic illnesses.
   - D. Stimulants (e.g., amphetamines). These are sometimes used for short periods in depression refractory to other modalities, but there is considerable disagreement over their efficacy.

Tricyclic antidepressants (Table 2-1)

I. Action and uses

Table 2-1 MEDICATIONS USED FOR AFFECTIVE DISORDERS

Drug	Usual dose (mg)		Adverse effects	
	Adult	Elderly	Sedation	Anticholinergic
TCAs (oral route preferred)				
Desipramine (Norpramin)	50-100 noct., maintenance	25-50 q.d., divided	+	+
Amitryptyline (Elavil)	50-160 noct., maintenance	Up to 10 t.i.d.	+++	+++
Imipramine (Tofranil)	50-150 noct., maintenance	30-40 q.d.	++	++
Doxepin (Sinequan)	25-150 q.d.		+++	+++
MAOIs				
Phenelzine (Nardil)	15-25 t.i.d.			
Antimanics				
Lithium	200-700 t.i.d.	Use with caution		

Code:
+ Moderately effective
++ Effective
+++ Strongly effective

A. The TCAs include
   1. Desipramine (Norpramin)
   2. Amitriptyline (Elavil)
   3. Imipramine (Tofranil)
   4. Doxepin (Sinequan)
B. These agents will often increase physical activity as well as elevate mood. They may also improve alertness, sleep patterns, and appetite while reducing morbid preoccupations.
C. TCAs are absorbed orally, extensively metabolized, highly bound by plasma proteins, and slowly eliminated (their half-lives range from 8-93 hr).
   1. Reduced doses are given to elderly and/or debilitated patients.
   2. The drug is initially given twice a day in increasing doses until symptoms are controlled, and then a lower maintenance dose is used daily. If insomnia is a side-effect, the dose can be given at bedtime.
D. Imipramine is often used for enuresis in children and adolescents.
E. Constant central pain syndromes frequently respond to amitriptyline, doxepin, or imipramine.

II. Adverse reactions
A. Anticholinergic activities and alpha-adrenergic blockade may induce any of the following symptoms:
   1. Flushing
   2. Sweating
   3. Xerostomia
   4. Visual disturbances
   5. Constipation (adolescents)
   6. Tachycardia
   7. Orthostatic hypotension
   8. Glaucoma
   9. Urinary retention
B. Sedation, tremor, and paradoxical anxiety have been reported.
C. Cardiac reactions include heart block and bundle branch block. A baseline ECG should be obtained before therapy and the width of the QRS complex monitored on subsequent ECGs.

III. Precautions
A. Elderly patients and those with hepatic failure metabolize the drugs slowly, so reduced doses are given or the drugs are avoided.
B. TCAs are administered with caution in any patient who has a history of
   1. Urinary retention or glaucoma
   2. Cardiac disease (congestive heart failure, angina, recent myocardial infarction, ECG changes)
C. The dose must be tapered to avoid a withdrawal syndrome.

IV. Drug interactions
   A. TCAs may interfere with antihypertensives that involve action
      on the biogenic amines (e.g., guanethidine or clonidine) and
      hypertension may return.
   B. The effects of epinephrine and vasoconstrictors in local anes-
      thetics are potentiated by TCAs. Local anesthetics without vaso-
      constrictors must be used.
   C. The anticholinergic effects of TCAs are additive when antipsy-
      chotic drugs are given simultaneously; also delirium and gastric
      hypomotility may occur. The TCA should be given 1-2 hr
      before or after the antipsychotic if the two must be used togeth-
      er.
   D. Concomitant use of MAOIs with TCAs may produce tremors,
      muscle rigidity, excitability, or death.
      1. Stop the TCA several days before giving an MAOI.
      2. Stop the MAOI 2 wk before giving a TCA.
   E. The effect of sedatives is potentiated when they are given with
      TCAs.
   F. Barbiturates increase the metabolism of TCAs (hepatic) but
      also potentiate the effects of toxic levels of TCAs in TCA over-
      dose situations.
   G. Alcohol has an increased sedative effect when used with a TCA,
      but it also potentiates the effects of toxic levels of TCAs.

Monoamine oxidase inhibitors (Table 2-1)

   I. Action and uses
      A. Phenelzine (Nardil) is most often prescribed.
      B. MAOIs are useful in the treatment of atypical depressions, anx-
         iety reactions, and amphetamine-like psychomotor stimulation.
         They are possibly also useful in migraine syndromes.
      C. After initial therapy, maintenance may be by one daily dose; but
         because of psychomotor stimulation, an MAOI should not be
         given at bedtime. Unlike TCAs, the MAOIs may be terminated
         abruptly.
  II. Adverse reactions
      A. Sedation, xerostomia, visual disturbances, constipation, and
         orthostatic hypotension are most common.
      B. Insomnia, tremors, or hypomania may reflect overdosage.
      C. Tachycardia, palpitations, and hypertension may occur togeth-
         er, so these drugs should be used cautiously in any cardiac
         patient.
      D. Coma may occur in overdosage.
 III. Precautions
      A. Strict dietary control must be followed to avoid hypertension
         induced by interaction with tyramine.
      B. Foods high in tyramine include cheese, red wines, chocolate,
         beer, yeast, meat extracts, fava beans, yogurt, herring, and pick-
         les.

IV. Drug interactions
  A. Tyramine ingested simultaneously can cause hypertension with headaches, tachycardia, nausea, vomiting, pulmonary edema, intracranial hemorrhage, unconsciousness, or syncope. Symptoms are treated with phentolamine and propranolol.
  B. Indirect-acting adrenergic drugs (e.g., amphetamines or the sympathomimetic amines in proprietary cold medicines) are potentiated and should be avoided.
  C. Direct-acting adrenergic drugs (e.g., catecholamines) appear safe since MAOIs do not strongly block the reuptake of catecholamines as do TCAs.
  D. Simultaneous use with levodopa, tryptophan, and 5-hydroxytryptamine is contraindicated. These drugs must be withdrawn at least 2-4 wk before starting an MAOI.
  E. Concomitant use of meperidine with an MAOI can produce hyperpyrexia and excitement, so meperidine must be avoided. The alternative narcotic chosen should have its dose reduced by one half to one fourth.
  F. General anesthetics may require lower doses since the CNS depressant effects are potentiated by MAOIs.
  G. The action of insulin is increased by administration with an MAOI, so hypoglycemia may result. The insulin dosage may need to be reduced.
  H. Convulsions and death have been noted experimentally when tranylcypromine was administered in the presence of disulfiram (Antabuse).

Lithium (Table 2-1)

  I. Action and uses
    A. Lithium counteracts mood changes without sedation.
    B. Administration of lithium for 3-5 da may be necessary to reach therapeutic tissue levels. Then any antipsychotic drugs can be withdrawn gradually.
    C. Lithium is indicated for
      1. Bipolar depression, when clearly diagnosed
      2. Cluster headaches
  II. Precautions
    A. Serum lithium levels must be measured every 2-3 wk.
    B. Lithium may cause irreversible morphological changes in the kidney.
      1. Renal function must be monitored with renal function tests (e.g., creatinine clearance, serum and urine osmolality).
      2. Lithium is contraindicated in known renal disease.
    C. Vomiting and diarrhea may occur, leading to dehydration and salt loss. Lithium must be discontinued, and salt and fluid given.
    D. Lithium is contraindicated if the patient has cardiac disease (e.g., sick sinus syndrome).

E. In the elderly patient, lithium may reduce renal function.

F. Lithium is generally contraindicated during the first trimester of pregnancy.

III. Drug interactions

A. When used with diuretics, lithium may be selectively absorbed because of relative dehydration and sodium potassium depletion. Close monitoring of serum lithium and electrolyte levels is necessary; the lithium dose is reduced if needed.

B. Lithium increases the serum insulin levels. Blood sugar levels need periodic monitoring in diabetes.

C. Iodine-containing medications (e.g., cough medicines, multivitamins) used with lithium are toxic to the thyroid gland and may produce hypothyroidism.

Stimulants

I. Stimulants include

A. Dextroamphetamine

B. Methylphenidate (Ritalin)—sometimes used in children for extreme hyperkinetic syndrome

II. They are not recommended for most patients with affective disorders, since they have a high potential for abuse or tolerance.

NEUROLEPTICS (Table 2-2)

I. Action and uses

A. Neuroleptic (antipsychotic) drugs are indicated in the treatment of

1. Schizophrenia (acute and chronic)—a thought disorder
2. Schizoaffective disorders
3. Organic brain syndromes with psychosis
4. Huntington's chorea
5. Intractable hiccups (chlorpromazine)
6. Ballismus
7. Nausea and vomiting (prochlorperazine)

B. Routes of administration include

1. Oral—preferred for convenience
2. Intramuscular—one fourth to one half the oral dose is used; reliable absorption and uptake; preferred in aggressive treatment of acutely psychotic patients

C. Half-lives range from 10-30 hr.

D. The maintenance dose after subsidence of the acute symptoms should be the minimum necessary to obtain a therapeutic response and allow the patient to function (usually once or twice daily).

E. Overdoses are rarely fatal in adults, and addiction does not occur.

F. Neuroleptic agents (e.g., haloperidol) are sometimes used for their sedative effect but may be poorly tolerated (especially in elderly patients). Antianxiety drugs are often more effective.

II. Adverse reactions

A. Behavioral effects include
   1. Sedation—the dose is reduced, or a single dose may be given at bedtime.
   2. Toxic psychosis—the dose is reduced; a toxic psychosis must be differentiated from an exacerbation of the underlying psychosis.
B. Extrapyramidal effects include
   1. Acute torsion dystonia (bizarre posturing, spasms, tics, dysphasia)—this occurs early in the course of (especially) parenteral therapy (e.g., prochlorperazine).
      a. Reduce the dose.
      b. Administer benztropine or an antihistamine parenterally.
   2. Akathisia (restlessness and agitation)—inability to sit still
      a. Reduce the dose.
      b. If not possible to reduce the dose, then give diazepam temporarily.
   3. Parkinsonism (tremors, rigidity, masklike facies, shuffling gait)—these occur after longer-term therapy.
      a. Reduce the dose.
      b. Alternatively, substitute a centrally acting anticholinergic drug.
   4. Tardive dyskinesia (choreiform movements, ballismus)—this is seen especially in older patients. The dose should be reduced.
C. Autonomic nervous system effects include both alpha-adrenergic and anticholinergic reactions.
   1. Orthostatic hypotension if symptoms are severe—IV fluids are given since vasopressors may pardoxically worsen the hypotension
   2. Xerostomia, tachycardia, visual disturbances, urinary retention, and constipation
D. Idiosyncratic and allergic reactions consist of
   1. Cholestatic jaundice (usually self-limited)—the drug is withdrawn
   2. Allergic reaction of the skin
   3. Photosensitivity
E. Neuroendocrine effects include delayed ovulation, amenorrhea, galactorrhea, gynecomastia, loss of libido, and weight gain.
F. Cardiac effects consist of ECG changes resembling those seen in hypokalemia (which can be ruled out by checking the serum K^+).
G. Hematological effects are as follows:
   1. Agranulocytosis may occur.
   2. Fever, cellulitis, or other evidence of infection—these warrant discontinuation of the drug and a check of the WBC count.
   3. The patient should recover after withdrawal of the drug.

Table 2-2 NEUROLEPTICS

Drug	Type	Usual dose (mg) Adult	Usual dose (mg) Elderly	Usual dose (mg) Child	Autonomic	Effects Sedation	Extrapyramidal
Fluphenazine (Prolixin)	Phenothiazine	IM (acute): 1.25-2.5 q.d., divided Oral: 2.5-3 q.d., divided	0.9-1.25 q.d., divided	NA*	+	++	++
Haloperidol (Haldol)	Butyrophenone	IM (acute): 2-5 q.4-8h. Oral: 1-4 q.d., divided	Poorly tolerated Poorly tolerated	Poorly tolerated Poorly tolerated	+	+	++
Trifluoperazine (Stelazine)	Phenothiazine	IM (acute): 2-5 to start, then 1-2 q.4-6h.	0.6-2.5 to start, then 0.3-1 q.6-8h.	1 b.i.d. if over 5 yr	+	++	++

Drug	Class	Adult dose	Pediatric dose			
Prochlorperazine Available rectally Dose for nausea and vomiting: Adult, 5-10 mg IM-p.o.-p.r. q.6h. Child, 0.1 mg/kg IM-p.o.-p.r. q.6h.	Phenothiazine	IM (acute): 10-20 q.1-4h. Oral: 15-75, divided	0.13/kg, age > 2 yr 0.4/kg, age > 2 yr	+	++	+++
Chlorpromazine (Thorazine)	Phenothiazine	IM (acute): 25-100 q.1-4h. Oral: 200-800 q.d.	25 q.1-4h. 100-400 q.d. 0.5/kg q.6-8h. 0.5/kg q.4-6h.	+++	+++	
Thioridazine (Mellaril)	Phenothiazine	Oral: 150-300 q.d., divided	50-150 q.d., divided if over 12 yr 1/kg q.d.	+++	+++	+

Code
+ Moderately effective
++ Effective
+++ Strongly effective
* Not applicable.

III. Precautions
  A. These drugs can cause inhibition of growth hormone release in children.
  B. Sleep disturbance and psychiatric syndromes may occur in the elderly and may require withdrawal of the drug.

ANALGESIC AGENTS
Opiates and opioids (Table 2-3)
  I. Action and uses
  A. The opiates are
    1. Purified alkaloids of opium
      a. Morphine
      b. Codeine
    2. Semisynthetic modifications of morphine
      a. Hydromorphone (Dilaudid)
      b. Nalbuphine (Nubain)
      c. Oxymorphone (Numorphan)
      d. Oxycodone (in Percocet and Percodan)
  B. The opioids are synthetic compounds that resemble morphine in action; they include
    1. Meperidine (Demerol)
    2. Methadone
    3. Propoxyphene (hydrochloride and napsylate)
    4. Pentazocine (Talwin)
  C. Both categories interact with the several postulated opiate receptors to produce varying degrees of analgesia, behavioral effects, and dependence.
  D. These drugs are indicated for use in
    1. Acute pain—to obtain analgesia and alter the psychological response to pain, reducing anxiety and apprehension
      a. Morphine used for severe pain; small to moderate doses for dull constant pain, large doses for intermittent sharp pain
      b. Other opiates or opioids used for mild to moderate pain
    2. Chronic pain management with opiates or opioids is questionable, since dependence may result
      a. Opiates and opioids should be withdrawn and the patient reevaluated.
      b. Consideration should be given to the nonopiates (acetaminophen, aspirin, nonsteroidal antiinflammatory agents).
      c. Antidepressants, sedatives, or antianxiety agents may possibly be needed.
      d. Nerve blocks should be considered.
      e. Pain of neoplastic disease is a special consideration, especially in terminal phases.
        (1) A nonopiate is the first choice of treatment.

(2) Opiates or opioids are used in increasing strength as required, on a fixed schedule rather than as needed, to keep the patient free of pain.

(3) The oral route is preferred for convenience. Adjusting the oral dose may compensate for the usually poor oral effectiveness of meperidine and morphine.

3. Myocardial infarction
   a. Morphine is used for analgesia.
   b. Peripheral pooling of blood may occur, decreasing venous return.
      (1) Cardiac work load is decreased.
      (2) Pulmonary edema is reduced. (Note: equipment for artificial ventilation should be available if needed.)
   c. Any resultant excessive bradycardia, hypotension, or respiratory depression can be counteracted with naloxone (Narcan).

4. Obstetrical analgesia

5. Preanesthetic medication and general anesthesia
   a. Drugs cause sedation and reduce anxiety when given as a preanesthetic medication. (Note: also consider other antianxiety agents, such as diazepam.)
   b. They are used with nitrous oxide–oxygen in a "balanced" general anesthetic technique. Equipment for artificial ventilation must be at hand.

II. Adverse reactions
   A. Respiratory depression, especially in the elderly or debilitated patient or in one with pulmonary disease, is rare in the common dose ranges. It can be reversed with intravenous naloxone administered repeatedly (since naloxone's half-life is shorter than that of the opiates).
   B. Hypotension. The drugs should be withheld from any patient in shock.
   C. Increased intracranial pressure and cardiovascular dilation may result from hypoventilation and hypercapnia, so these drugs should be withheld from the patient with head injuries or delirium tremens.
   D. Miotic drugs may mask pupillary response, an important diagnostic sign in the head injury patient.
   E. Drowsiness and altered sensorium can follow administration of opiates and/or opioids.
   F. Increased ventricular work may be noted, especially with pentazocine; this drug therefore should be used cautiously in cardiac patients.
   G. Reduced urinary output by release of ADH may be an important consideration in the patient with renal insufficiency.
   H. Increased sphincter tone can lead to biliary colic, urinary retention, and constipation.

Table 2-3 OPIATES AND OPIOIDS

	Usual dose (mg)		Effectiveness of route			Hours of analgesia (maximum/duration)	Remarks
	Adult	Child	Oral	IM	IV		
Opiates							
Morphine	IM 0.1-0.2/kg q.3-4h. IV 2.5-15 slowly (1-3/kg for general anesthetics) Oral 10-30 q.3-4h.	0.1-0.2/kg q3-4h	+	++	+++	1/4	For severe pain
Codeine	IM/oral 30-60 q4-6h	0.5/kg q.4-6h.	++	+++	NA*	1/4-6	For mild to moderate pain
Hydromorphone (Dilaudid)	IM 1-1.5 q.4-6h. IV 1-1.5 slowly Oral 2 q.4-6h.	NA	+	+++	+++	1/4-6	Potency 8× that of morphine
Nalbuphine (Nubain)	IM/IV 10 q.3-6h.	NA	NA	+++	+++	0.5/3-6	For moderate to severe pain
Oxymorphone (Numorphan)	IM 1-15 q.4-6h. IV 0.5 q.4-6h. Rectal 5	NA	NA	++	+++	0.5-1/4-6	Available rectally
Oxycodone (Percocet, Percodan)	Oral q.4-6h.	NA	+++	NA	NA	1/4-6	Usually in combination

Opioids

Meperidine (Demerol)	IM and oral 50-150 q.3-6h.	1-1.5/kg q.3-6h.	+	++	+++	0.5-1.3-6	Spasm of smooth muscle (e.g., GI tract)
Methadone	IM and oral 2.5-10, repeated when pain recurs	NA	+	++	NA	1.5	Half-life 25 hr; strict FDA regulations to its use in severe pain; detoxification possible in mild to moderate pain
Propoxyphene hydrochloride	Oral 65 q.6-8h.	NA	+++	NA	NA	1-1.5/6-8	Half the potency of codeine; 65 mg usually less effective than 650 mg aspirin or acetaminophen; frequently abused, especially with ethyl alcohol
napsylate	Oral 100 q.6-8h.	NA	+++	NA	NA		
Pentazocine (Talwin)	Oral 50 q.3-4h.	NA	+++	NA	NA	0.5-1/2-3	Potency ¼-½ that of morphine; for moderate pain; less dependence than with morphine; increased cardiac workload; injection sites rotated to avoid "sterile abscess"

Code

+ Moderately effective

++ Effective

+++ Strongly effective

* Not applicable.

III. Drug interactions and precautions
   A. Reduced doses should be used in the patient with hypothyroidism, myxedema, or hypoadrenalism.
   B. Reduced doses also should be used in any patient taking other CNS-depressing medications (barbiturates, antipsychotics, or anxiolytics).
   C. Severe adverse reactions may occur when meperidine is administered to the patient taking an MAOI. These reactions are not observed with morphine.
IV. Tolerance and dependence
   A. These vary with the individual patient.
   B. The abuse potential with morphine is greater than that with pentazocine, propoxyphene, or codeine.
      1. Dependence is unlikely with short-term use of even large doses.
      2. One must beware of undermedicating in a patient with acute severe pain.
      3. The smallest effective doses must be given.
      4. Physical dependence may develop without psychological dependence after prolonged use.
      5. Any patient with a dependency history needs careful observation.

Nonopiates (analgesic-antipyretic) (Table 2-4)

Action and uses
   A. Nonopiates do not bind to opiate receptors.
   B. The postulated mechanisms of action are
      1. Analgesic blockade of pain impulse generation peripherally
      2. Antipyretic stimulation of the hypothalamic nuclei and thermal regulatory center
      3. Antiinflammatory inhibition of prostaglandin synthesis
   C. Indications include
      1. Mild pain (e.g., headache, myalgia)
      2. Fever (the underlying cause needs to be sought)
      3. Inflammation

Aspirin

   I. Action and uses
      A. It is given for headache, neuralgia, myalgia, arthralgia, and pain affecting integumental structures.
      B. Buffered formulations improve its absorption but have little effect on its onset of action or its analgesic or dyspeptic properties. Effervescent preparations have faster absorption and less gastric irritation than does regular aspirin but alkalinize the urine, resulting in faster excretion.
   II. Adverse effects
      A. Gastrointestinal distress is reduced if aspirin is taken with food or a full glass of water.
         1. Dyspepsia and nausea

Table 2-4 NONOPIATES (ANALGESIC-ANTIPYRETIC)

Drug	Usual dose (mg) Adult	Child	$t_{1/2}$(hr)	Absorption	Remarks
Aspirin	650 q.4h.	0.25/m^2 q.4h.	3-3.5	+++	
Sodium salicylate	650 q.4h.	NA*	3-4	+++	Less effective, less GI bleeding than with aspirin
Acetaminophen	325-650 q.4h.	0.25/m^2 q.4h.	1-3	++++	Rare adverse reactions; rectal potency half oral potency
Ibuprofen (Motrin)	400 q.4h. 600 q.4h.	NA NA	4-6	++	Low incidence of adverse reactions Some GI bleeding, especially in ulcer patients
Naproxen (Naprosyn)	Doses for analgesia not well established			+++	Useful for moderate to severe postoperative pain

Code:
++ Moderately well
+++ Well
++++ Very well
* Not applicable.

2. Gastrointestinal hemorrhage—rarely life-threatening and rarely correlated with dyspepsia; caused by direct action of the gastric mucosa and platelet dysfunction; a synergistic effect occurs with alcohol to cause it; aspirin should be avoided in any patient with ulcers or a history of GI tract bleeding

B. Hypoprothrombinemia may occur with large aspirin doses taken over several days but is reversed with vitamin K. It is usually insignificant unless the patient is also taking anticoagulants. The degree of hypoprothrombinemia can be measured by a PTT test.

C. Platelet inhibition may be seen, even with the usual analgesic doses. (It is measured by bleeding time.)

D. Reversible hepatotoxicity is caused by large doses in a patient with preexisting liver disease.

E. Anaphylaxis results from common cross-sensitization with other prostaglandin inhibitors (e.g., ibuprofen). It is uncommon to find sensitization with salicylic acid and acetaminophen.

F. Tinnitus can be a result of chronic aspirin overdosage. Children should be monitored closely.

G. Preexisting renal disease may be exacerbated by the decreased glomerular filtration rate.

III. Precautions

A. Aspirin is contraindicated in any patient with a coagulopathy or in one taking anticoagulants.

B. It should be discontinued at least 1 wk before surgery to reverse its anticoagulant effect. Bleeding time must be checked.

IV. Drug interactions

A. Aspirin enhances the effects of oral hypoglycemics and decreases blood glucose levels. The dose of oral hypoglycemic must be decreased if concomitant administration is necessary.

B. Aspirin antagonizes uricosuric agents, so it is to be avoided in patients with gout.

C. Concurrent use with corticosteroids or indomethacin may increase the incidence of gastric ulceration.

D. Aspirin decreases serum protein binding of sulfonamides, increasing their toxicity.

Sodium salicylate

I. Action and uses

A. No platelet effect has been found, and there is less occult GI bleeding than seen with aspirin.

B. It does produce hypoprothrombinemia, rarely.

C. It may be tolerated by the patient hypersensitive to aspirin.

II. Precautions. Avoid in the patient on a low-sodium diet.

Acetaminophen

I. Action and uses
  A. Its analgesic and antipyretic properties are equivalent to those of aspirin. It has no antiinflammatory or antiplatelet action.
  B. It is preferred in the patient with ulcer disease, hemophilia, or aspirin allergy.
  C. It does not antagonize uricosuric agents.
  D. The rectal form is of about half the potency of the oral tablet.

II. Adverse reactions. Large doses (15 g single) may cause hepatic damage and death. Overdose is treated with acetylcysteine.

III. Drug interactions. Large doses can potentiate the action of oral anticoagulants.

Ibuprophen (Motrin)

I. Action and uses
  A. Its analgesic, antipyretic, and antiinflammatory properties are similar to those of aspirin.
  B. It is often tolerated by the patient who is intolerant of aspirin.

II. Adverse reactions. These include nausea, vomiting, diarrhea, constipation, heartburn, and epigastric pain (low incidence).

III. Precautions. There is a lower incidence of gastrointestinal bleeding than occurs with aspirin, but ibuprophen must be used with caution in any patient known to have ulcer disease.

Naproxen (Naprosyn)

I. Action and uses
  A. It has analgesic, antiinflammatory, and antipyretic actions.
  B. Its principal uses are in rheumatoid arthritis, ankylosing spondylitis, osteoarthritis, and moderate to severe postoperative pain.
  C. Approximate dose equivalences (in milligrams) are as follows:

220-330	600 (aspirin)
250	50 (indomethacin)
400	70-150 (oral meperidine)
400	>65 (propoxyphene) or 30 (codeine with aspirin)

II. Adverse reactions. There are GI effects, even though the gastric mucosa is less severely affected than with the other agents in this group. GI bleeding with naproxen is less than with aspirin.

III. Precautions. The rare ulcerative reaction can be severe, and thus caution is indicated in the patient with a history of ulcer disease.

Analgesic mixtures

I. Theoretically these provide greater pain relief, a wider range of therapeutic uses, and less severe side effects than a single agent can alone.

II. Commonly used mixtures include
   A. Codeine with aspirin (for moderate pain):
      1. Ascriptin with codeine—325 mg aspirin, 16.2 or 32.4 mg codeine phosphate
      2. Empirin with codeine—325 mg aspirin, 15 or 30 mg codeine phosphate
   B. Codeine with acetaminophen (for moderate to severe pain):
      1. Empracet with codeine—300 mg acetaminophen, 30 or 60 mg codeine phosphate
      2. Tylenol with codeine—300 mg acetaminophen, 7.5 (no. 1), 15 (no. 2), 30 (no. 3), or 60 (no. 4) mg codeine phosphate
      3. Tylenol with codeine elixir—120 mg acetaminophen and 12 mg codeine phosphate per 5 ml
   C. Oxycodone (available only in mixtures in the U.S.). Its potency and dependency potential are greater than those of codeine. It is used for moderate to severe pain:
      1. Percodan—4.5 mg oxycodone hydrochloride, 0.38 mg oxycodone terephthalate, 224 mg aspirin
      2. Percocet-5—5 mg oxycodone hydrochloride, 325 mg acetaminophen
      3. Tylox—4.5 mg oxycodone hydrochloride, 0.38 mg oxycodone terephthalate, 500 mg acetaminophen
   D. Pentazocine. Its effectiveness is comparable to that of combinations containing codeine or oxycodone—e.g., Talwin compound (pentazocine HCl, equivalent to 12.5 mg base, and 325 mg aspirin).

ANTICONVULSANTS (Table 2-5)

I. Action and uses
   A. Seizures—barbiturates, hydantoins, etc.
      1. Seizures represent a focal or generalized brain disturbance, caused by
         a. Infection, neoplasms, congenital defects, head trauma
         b. Fever, metabolic disturbances, drug withdrawal
         c. Epilepsy (recurrent pattern with sudden disturbances in consciousness accompanied by uncontrolled motor activity, unusual sensory phenomena, and inappropriate behavior)
      2. Types of seizure include
         a. Partial (benign locally, usually remain focal)
            (1) Elementary—consciousness unimpaired (e.g., jacksonian seizures)
            (2) Complex—consciousness impaired (e.g., temporal lobe epilepsy)
         b. Generalized
            (1) Absences—staring, subtle clonic movements (petit mal epilepsy)

          (2) Bilateral myoclonic without loss of consciousness
          (3) Tonic-clonic (grand mal epilepsy)
          (4) Atonic—loss of postural tone
          (5) Akinetic—relaxation of all musculature
      c. Unilateral

   3. General principles of drug therapy for seizures include the following:

      a. There should be no or only minimum adverse reactions from the medication.

      b. Therapy is individualized.

      c. Seizures may "escape" control if liver enzymes are induced over time to augment metabolism of the anticonvulsant (e.g., barbiturates). The dose may need to be increased, or another agent tried.

      d. Discontinuation of the anticonvulsant should be considered with time, since spontaneous resolution of seizure disorders may occur. The dose should be gradually reduced.

  B. Trigeminal neuralgia (tic douloureux)—carbamazepine, phenytoin

  C. Certain cardiac arrhythmias—phenytoin

II. Adverse reactions

  A. Gastrointestinal disturbances may necessitate a dose reduction.

  B. Sedation may (rarely) induce personality changes and psychoses.

  C. Ataxia may be found especially with phenytoin. Cerebellar damage is possible if the dose is not reduced.

  D. Hypersensitivity reactions may make drug discontinuance necessary, and an anticonvulsant of another class can then be tried. Skin eruptions may precede the Stevens-Johnson syndrome. Anaphylaxis is rare.

  E. Acute intermittent porphyria may be precipitated by barbiturates and phenytoin. Therefore these agents are contraindicated in this disease.

  F. Visual disturbances may occur but are reversible with decreased dose or discontinuance.

  G. Gingival hyperplasia is found especially with phenytoin use in children. If hygiene becomes a problem, gingivectomy (especially with an electrocautery) may provide temporary improvement.

  H. Lymphadenopathies, generally rare, may be caused by any of the hydantoins but are reversible with discontinuation of the drug. A few cases of lymphoma have been reported that seemed possibly to be related to hydantoin use.

  I. Megaloblastic anemias have been found especially with hydantoin and barbiturate use. They are treated with folic acid. Blood counts must be monitored, and the agent may need to be discontinued.

Table 2-5 ANTICONVULSANTS

	Usual dose (mg) Type		Common adverse reactions
	Adult	Child	
Barbiturates Phenobarbital	Oral 50-100 b.i.d. IM 200-300 q.6 h. IV (slow) 200-300 q.6 h.	Oral 15-50 b.i.d. IM 3-5/kg q.6 h. IV (slow) 3-5/kg q.6 h.	Sedation, ataxia, paradoxical hyperactivity
Hydantoins Phenytoin	Oral 100 b.i.d.-t.i.d. IV (slow) 10-15/kg (slow infusion for status epilepticus only)	Oral 1.5-2.5/kg to 1 g IV (slow) 750/m² body surface	Skin eruptions (rarely serious), gingival hyperplasia (children), hepatitis, blood dyscrasias, Stevens-Johnson (all rare); hypotension from too rapid IV administration (exceeding 50 mg/min); GI disturbances
Succinimides Ethosuximide (Zarontin)	Oral 500 q.d.	Oral 250 q.d.	Sedation, headache, depression (rare)

Benzodiazepines Diazepam (Valium)	Oral 2-10 b.i.d.-q.i.d. (2 elderly) IV (slow) 5-10 injected at 5 mg/min	Oral 0.5-1 b.i.d.–4 q.i.d. IV (slow) 0.5-1 q.2-5 min (max. 5-10 mg)	CNS depression, GI disturbances, sensitivity reactions, dependence, respiratory depression (parenteral route)
Carbamazepine (Tegretol)	Oral 400-800 b.i.d., maintenance	Oral 200-400 b.i.d., maintenance	CNS depression, nausea, vomiting, visual disturbances, confusion, dysphasia, paresthesias, dermatological reactions, aplastic anemia and thrombocytopenia (rare but may be fatal); follow blood counts and cross-sensitivity with TCAs
Valproic acid (Depakene)	Oral 5/kg b.i.d.-t.i.d.		Enhances sedative effect of phenobarbital, increases plasma phenytoin levels, interferes with platelet aggregation; GI disturbances, sedation, rare hepatic dysfunction
Acetazolamide (Diamox)	Oral 2-10/kg b.i.d.-t.i.d.		Rapid development of tolerance

Table 2-6 ANTIARRHYTHMICS

	Action	Common indications	Common adverse reactions	Remarks
Digitalis glycosides	Depress AV conduction time and refractory period, prolong atrial and ventricular refractory period	Control ventricular rate in atrial fibrillation, treat congestive heart failure	Intoxication	
Quinidine gluconate (Quinaglute) Procainamide (Pronestyl)	Depresses automaticity, prolongs refractory period	Control supraventricular and ventricular tachyarrhythmias, prevent PVCs with digitalis in atrial fibrillation	Gastrointestinal disturbances, AV block	Quinidine increases serum digoxin levels and can be given IM with less severe local reactions
Disopyramide (Norpace)	Depresses automaticity, prolongs refractory period, depresses myocardial contractility	Control ventricular and supraventricular tachyarrhythmias	Anticholinergic activity, gastrointestinal disturbances, AV block, hypoglycemia	Avoid in poorly compensated congestive heart failure
Lidocaine	Depresses automaticity, decreases refractory period, does not decrease conduction velocity in therapeutic doses	Control ventricular tachyarrhythmias, prophylaxis against ventricular tachycardia in acute myocardial infarction	CNS depression, convulsions	Avoid in hepatic insufficiency

	Action	Indications	Side Effects	Comments
Phenytoin	Depresses automaticity, decreases refractory period	Control digitalis-induced arrhythmias	Fatigue, gastrointestinal distress, hepatitis (rare), blood dyscrasias	Needs *slow* IV push
Bretylium	Prevents norepinephrine release at sympathetic nerve terminals	Control refractory supraventricular tachyarrhythmias	Uncommon angina	
Beta blockers (propranolol)	Block cardiac beta receptors, reduce rate and contractility, prolong AV conduction, suppress automaticity	Control supraventricular and ventricular tachyarrhythmias, atrial flutter and fibrillation	Congestive heart failure and bronchospasm	Avoid in asthma, needs slow withdrawal
Calcium channel blockers	Interfere with Ca transport at cell membrane, delay AV conduction, suppress automaticity at sinus node	Control supraventricular tachyarrhythmias	Hypotension	
Atropine	Increases sinus rate, speeds AV conduction	Control sinus bradycardia, sinoatrial arrest and block, second-degree AV block (type I)	Xerostomia, glaucoma (rare), urinary retention	
Isoproterenol	Enhances automaticity, increases contractility and rate, stimulates cardiac beta receptors	Control second- and third-degree block (propranolol-induced) and myocardial depression	Tachycardia, PVCs	

J. Severe blood dyscrasias are rare. If sore throat, fever, petechiae, epistaxis, or signs of infection develop, one must order blood studies.

K. Hepatitis also is rare. Hydantoins and valproic acid are the most common causes. Baseline liver function tests must be performed before therapy begins and repeated if symptoms of liver dysfunction occur.

L. Nephropathies, likewise, are rare and necessitate discontinuation of the agent being used.

III. Precautions. Abrupt withdrawal of anticonvulsants can precipitate seizures. The dose must be reduced gradually. Abrupt withdrawal can be done only if another anticonvulsant is to be substituted.

IV. Common drugs (by seizure type)

A. Generalized clonic-tonic (grand mal epilepsy) or elementary partial seizures—phenytoin (Dilantin), a hydantoin, or phenobarbital; acetazolamide (Diamox) or valproic acid (Depakene) may be used as adjuncts

B. Complex partial seizures (temporal lobe epilepsy)—carbamazepine (Tegretol) or phenytoin

C. Absence seizures—ethosuximide (Zarontin) or valproic acid (Depakene)

D. Status epilepticus (tonic-clonic)—vigorous emergency treatment is required; IV diazepam is given initially and may need to be repeated for control; load and maintenance doses follow with phenytoin or phenobarbital; if status persists, a general anesthetic by an anesthesiologist, with resuscitative equipment at hand, may be necessary

DIGITALIS GLYCOSIDES (Table 2-6)

I. Action and uses

A. The digitalis glycosides enhance myocardial contractility, lengthen AV nodal conduction time and refractory period, and shorten atrial and ventricular refractory periods.

B. They are indicated for

1. Treatment of congestive heart failure from coronary artery disease or hypertension, if antihypertensives do not adequately control the condition

2. Control of ventricular rate in the patient with atrial fibrillation

3. Control of supraventricular tachycardias unresponsive to other measures

C. Digitalis glycosides commonly used include

1. Digoxin

a. Onset is 5-30 min, half-life 30-40 hr, and therapeutic serum level 0.5-2.5 mg/ml.

b. It is excreted largely unchanged in the urine; therefore care is needed in any patient with renal disease. It may be necessary to reduce the dose or use liver-metabolized digitoxin.

    c. The usual dose varies. Maintenance for adults is 0.125-0.5 mg q.d. For rapid digitalization, 0.25 mg IV is given q. 4-6 h. to a total of 1 mg. A pediatric text should be consulted for children's dosages.

  2. Digitoxin

    a. Onset is 1-4 hr, and half-life 5-9 da.

    b. It is metabolized in the liver to inactive substances, which are excreted in the urine. It is useful in impaired renal function but not in hepatic dysfunction.

    c. The usual dose (in a patient who has not received digitalis for 2 wk or more) is 0.1 mg q.d. for maintenance. For rapid digitalization 0.8 mg and then 0.2 mg is given q.6-8h. in 2-3 doses. A pediatric text should be consulted for children's dosages.

II. Adverse reactions (digitalis intoxication)

  A. Therapeutic and toxic dose ranges are very close. Serum digoxin levels can be determined for the therapeutic range.

  B. Predisposing factors include alkalosis, hypercalcemia, hypokalemia, and hypoxemia.

  C. Signs include

    1. Noncardiac

      a. Gastrointestinal—nausea, vomiting, anorexia, and rarely diarrhea

      b. Neurological—fatigue, sedation, vertigo, personality changes, confusion

      c. Ophthalmological—visual disturbances, photophobia

      d. Hypersensitivity (urticaria)—rare

    2. Cardiac (may be the first evidence of intoxication)

      a. Multifocal PVCs, junctional tachycardia

      b. Sinus bradycardia, sinus arrest

      c. Paroxysmal ventricular tachycardia

  D. Treatment includes discontinuation of the glycoside and administration of potassium (if the serum K is low) and other antiarrhythmics as indicated.

III. Precautions

  A. Quinidine increases the serum digoxin level. GI disturbances and ventricular arrhythmias may result.

  B. Propranolol may need to be added if the ventricular rate in atrial fibrillation is not controlled by maximum therapeutic doses of a digitalis glycoside.

  C. Diuretics that cause hypokalemia predispose to digitalis toxicity. Potassium chloride supplements or a potassium-sparing diuretic (e.g., spironolactone) are used.

GENERAL REFERENCE

Goodman, L.S., and Gilman, A.: The pharmacologic basis of therapeutics, ed. 7, New York, 1985, The Macmillan Co.

Frequently Requested Oral Surgical Consultations

3

GENERAL CONSIDERATIONS

I. Health care providers will have occasion to request oral surgical consultation. Appropriate response depends upon determining the referring doctor's purpose for seeking the consultation.
   A. The purpose might be simply to obtain assistance in establishing a diagnosis or suggestions for managing a problem. In this case the oral surgeon is being asked for opinions and should not automatically presume to take over the patient's care.
   B. Alternatively, the referring doctor might specifically request assistance in the care of a patient (or even transfer of the patient to the oral surgeon's care). The oral surgeon will then become actively involved in managing the case.
   C. If no clear indication of the reason for the consultation exists, the referring doctor should be called to establish the purpose and ascertain the questions to be answered. Often a note in the chart or a discussion with the patient will make clear the purpose.
II. When practical, inpatient consultations should be done in the oral surgical clinic, where adequate light, instruments, and radiographic studies are readily available. If the patient is confined to the ward, a bedside consultation will require adequate lighting and assistance to hold the light for the bimanual portions of the examination. Anything less can lead to a suboptimum bedside consultation.
III. Outpatient consultations are most efficient when the referring doctor sends in any radiographs and copies of records. These should be requested in advance of the appointment when possible.

CONSULTATIVE METHOD

I. When a consultation is requested, the oral surgeon should see the patient promptly to expedite patient care.
II. The following outline of procedural care may prove useful:
   A. Purpose for the consultation—the reason for the patient's being referred must be identified.
   B. Review of the record—this will ensure that recommendations for therapy are consistent with the general stability of the

patient and the medicines currently being administered. One must carefully review the record to

1. Ascertain the patient's overall condition
2. Determine the relationship and importance of the problem to the patient's situation
3. Review orders for the patient's medical regimen

C. Patient history—one must assess the acuteness and severity of the problem.
D. Patient examination
E. Additional studies—any indicated radiographs and blood studies or other consultations should be available.
F. Response—a written note should be placed in the record and, if the problem is urgent, a call made to the referring doctor. A diagnostic opinion and recommendations for further evaluation or therapy may be included. If requested, the response should include therapeutic intervention.
G. Follow-up—one must determine whether further therapy will be needed and coordinate such care with the patient's other health care providers.

FREQUENT REASONS FOR SEEKING CONSULTATION
Patient assessment before cardiac surgery

I. Purpose
   A. The oral surgeon must identify and eliminate actual and potential sources of orofacial infection that could, through bacteremia, infect prosthetic materials implanted in the heart or great vessels. Included are valve replacements, septal repairs, and replacement of aortic or pulmonic roots. Intervention to eliminate these sources of infection is usually expected by the referring doctor.
   B. Cardiac surgery not involving prosthetic material requires no routine preoperative oral surgical consultation (e.g., coronary arterial bypass surgery).
II. Review of the patient's record. Key elements affecting oral surgical management include
   A. Hemodynamic instability. A fragile patient, especially one confined to an intensive care unit, might not be able to tolerate oral surgical manipulation before cardiac surgery to correct the instability.
   B. Unstable angina. If chest pain is steadily increasing in frequency and severity and is harder to control, it might be triggered by oral surgical procedures. When hemodynamic instability or unstable angina exists, it might be necessary to allow cardiac surgery to proceed without the (optimum) removal of potential sources of infection. In this case the risks from an unstable cardiac condition would outweigh the risk of endocarditis.
   C. Arrhythmias. If an arrhythmia is difficult to control or refractory to medication, any local anesthetic used should be free of epinephrine. An intravenous injection of epinephrine must

then be avoided if aspiration fails to reveal intravenous placement of the needle. Well-controlled arrhythmias should not
require this restriction.

D. Stable angina. Epinephrine can be used in local anesthetics if
care is taken, by aspiration, to avoid an intravascular injection.
Some practitioners believe that the anesthesia obtained is more
profound and prolonged when epinephrine is in the local anesthetic and that angina will be less likely during the procedure
because discomfort and accompanying anxiety will be less.
Oxygen and 0.3 mg trinitroglycerin sublingual tablets (TNG)
must be available should angina occur. If angina does occur,
start oxygen 5-8 L/min by nasal prongs, nasal mask, or face
mask; give one TNG sublingually and repeat in 2-3 min if the
angina is unrelieved; monitor blood pressure; obtain a 12-lead
ECG if angina persists; and call the patient's physician.

E. Anticoagulants
1. Warfarin (Coumadin)—if the prothrombin time (PT) is less
than or equal to 1½ times control, carry out the prophylaxis, restorative care, and minor oral surgical procedures as
possible. If it is greater than 1½ times control or if extensive
oral surgery is needed, check with the patient's physician
on reducing or holding the warfarin until the PT is in line. If
this is inadvisable, attempt to change from warfarin to intravenous heparin (5000 units IV loading dose, 500-1200
units/hr IV drip to keep the PTT at 37-60). Heparin is
stopped 4 hr before oral surgery and restarted immediately
afterward, switching back to warfarin over the next 1-3 da
until the PT is in the appropriate therapeutic range.
2. Heparin—manage this as above, in concert with the
patient's physician.
3. Aspirin (and other antiplatelet medications)—check the
bleeding time. If it is abnormal, consult with the patient's
physician on the possibility of eliminating the medication
for 2 wk before oral surgery. If time does not allow and oral
surgery is urgent, consider infusing 10-20 units of platelets
immediately preoperatively.

F. Heart murmurs. These will require antibiotic prophylaxis as
follows*:

---

*Adapted from a statement for health professionals by the Committee of Rheumatic
Fever and Infective Endocarditis: Prevention of bacterial endocarditis, Circulation
70:1123A, 1984. Also excerpted in J. Am. Dent. Assoc. **110**:98, 1985.

Please refer to these joint American Heart Association–American Dental Association recommendations for more complete information as to which patients and
which procedures require prophylaxis.

For dental procedures and surgery of the upper respiratory tract

1. For most patients
   Oral penicillin

   Adults: 2.0 g of penicillin-V 1 hr prior to procedure and then 1.0 g 6 hr after initial dose.

   Children less than 60 lb: 1.0 g of penicillin-V 1 hr prior to procedure and then 500 mg 6 hr after initial dose.

2. For patients allergic to penicillin (may also be selected for those receiving oral penicillin as continuous rheumatic fever prophylaxis)
   Erythromycin

   Adults: 1.0 g orally 1 hr prior to procedure and then 500 mg 6 hr after initial dose.

   Children: 20 mg/kg 1 hr prior to procedure and then 10 mg/kg 6 hr after initial dose.

3. For patients at higher risk of infective endocarditis (especially those with prosthetic heart valves) who are not allergic to penicillin
   Ampicillin plus gentamicin

   Adults: Ampicillin 1.0-2.0 g plus gentamicin 1.5 mg/kg IM or IV, both given 30 min before procedure; then penicillin-V 1.0 g (500 mg for children under 60 lb) orally 6 hr after initial dose.

   Children: Timing of doses is same as for adults. Doses are ampicillin 50 mg/kg and gentamicin 2.0 mg/kg.

4. For higher-risk patients (especially those with prosthetic heart valves) who are allergic to penicillin
   Vancomycin

   Adults: 1.0 g IV over 60 min begun 60 min before procedure; no repeat dose is necessary.

   Children: 20 mg/kg IV over 60 min, begun 60 min before procedure; no repeat dose is necessary.

For gastrointestinal and genitourinary tract surgery and instrumentation

1. For most patients
   Ampicillin plus gentamicin

   Adults: 2.0 g ampicillin IM or IV plus gentamicin 1.5 mg/kg IM or IV given 30 min before procedure. May repeat once 8 hr later.

   Children: Same timing of medications as adult schedule. Doses are ampicillin 50 mg/kg and gentamicin 2.0 mg/kg.

Note: In patients with compromised renal function, it may be necessary to modify or omit the second dose of antibiotics. IM injections may be contraindicated in patients receiving anticoagulants. Children's doses should not exceed adult doses.

For gastrointestinal and genitourinary tract surgery and instrumentation—cont'd

2. For patients allergic to penicillin *Vancomycin plus gentamicin*

   Adults: 1.0 g vancomycin IV given over 60 min plus 1.5 mg/kg gentamicin IM or IV, each given 60 min before procedure.
   Doses may be repeated once 8-12 hr later.
   Children: Timing as above. Doses are vancomycin 20 mg/kg and gentamicin 2.0 mg/kg.

3. Oral regimen for minor or repetitive procedures in low-risk patients *Amoxicillin*

   Adults: 3.0 g amoxicillin 1 hr before procedure and 1.5 g 6 hr after initial dose.
   Children: Same timing of doses: 50 mg/kg initial dose and 25 mg/kg follow-up dose.

III. Patient history. Note any complaints of swelling, foul taste, drainage, bleeding gingivae, or teeth that are sensitive to pressure or thermal change.

IV. Patient examination. Note the periodontal condition, recording any fluctuant or draining areas, carious lesions, tender or mobile teeth, and mucosal lesions and irritations.

V. Additional studies
   A. Panoramic radiograph. This is obtained to help identify lesions of the jaws. It is not generally sufficient alone for accurate periodontal and periapical examination.
   B. Full-mouth periapical series (dentulous areas). Note the periodontal condition, depth of caries, and radiolucencies, along with any indications of active infection or conditions likely to result in infection.

VI. Response
   A. If time and patient stability permit, oral hygiene should be optimized, restorable teeth restored, and nonrestorable teeth removed before cardiac surgery. Severely periodontally involved teeth should also be removed. Teeth likely to need endodontic therapy postoperatively should probably be removed, although some controversy exists over this. If permanent restorations are not possible, control caries and place temporary restorations. If cardiac surgery is not urgent, attempt to postpone it until the oral health is optimized.
   B. If the patient is unstable or needs cardiac surgery on a more urgent basis, necessary oral surgery may need to be deferred. If the physician will permit oral surgery on a fragile patient preoperatively, it should be done with continuous vital sign and ECG monitoring with local anesthesia and light intravenous sedation. The operating room is a good place for this, with an anesthesiologist doing the monitoring and sedation. An awake patient can effectively communicate when chest pain first occurs so it can be dealt with immediately. If this is not possi-

ble, any needed oral surgical care will have to wait about 6 mo after cardiac surgery. Any teeth that become symptomatic before then can be treated individually, with careful vital sign monitoring and antibiotic prophylaxis as indicated.

   C. When the patient is deemed free of orofacial sources of infection, it should be so stated in the record, clearing the patient for cardiac surgery from the oral surgical standpoint.

VII. Follow-up

   A. The patient's own dentist needs to be advised as to the results of the oral surgical consultation.

   B. If prosthetic material was used in cardiac surgery or if murmurs exist, details of prophylactic antibiotic regimens for dental care should be sent to the dentist.

Assessment after cardiac surgery

I. The general scheme is as outlined for patient assessment before cardiac surgery.

II. Often the consultation is requested because the patient has a fever and bacterial endocarditis is suspected.

   A. Signs include fever of unknown origin, diaphoresis, malaise, splinter hemorrhages of the nail beds, and sometimes hemodynamic instability. An echocardiogram may show bacterial vegetations on, or dysfunction of, a natural or prosthetic valve. Blood cultures, held for 2 wk and numbering at least 6 sets (one at each fever spike), are an additional study that, together with a careful history and examination, may give evidence to support an oral source.

   B. If such a source exists, penicillin-G 2,000,000 units IV q. 2-4 h. or vancomycin 500 mg q.6h. IV should be started. Streptomycin 1 g IM q.8h. should be added if a prosthetic valve is in place. Abscesses should be drained and offending teeth removed under such coverage.

   C. Data on antibiotic sensitivities of bacteria in the cultured blood or drainage will guide further therapy.

Assessment before radiation therapy

I. Purpose. Consultation may be sought to identify and eliminate existing and potential sources of orofacial infection in a patient due to undergo radiation therapy for head and neck cancer. Poor oral hygiene, periodontitis, and nonrestorable or abscessed teeth can cause osteomyelitis in irradiated bone, whose resistance to infection is low because of radiation-induced vascular compromise.

II. Review of the record

   A. One must note the location and area of planned irradiation. Diseased or nonrestorable teeth in this area will have to be removed at least 1 wk before irradiation to allow some healing to occur before radiation begins. Restorable teeth will also need removal if the radiation is to be directed at the periodontium.

B. Restorable teeth in other areas of the mouth will need repair before radiation therapy begins so that progression of abscesses into irradiated areas does not occur.

III. Patient history and examination
   A. Symptomatic and diseased teeth are identified.
   B. Oral hygiene habits are analyzed. In the patient who has undergone radiotherapy oral hygiene must be meticulous.

IV. Additional studies
   A. Radiographs (panoramic and periapical)
      1. One must assess for teeth in need of removal or repair based on caries or periodontal condition.
      2. One must also assess for invasion of tumor into bone, which will alter the general treatment plan.
   B. Vitality testing of questionable teeth, electrically or thermally

V. Response
   A. Careful dental prophylaxis and restoration or removal of teeth that are infected, nonrestorable, or located in the radiation field must be performed before radiation.
   B. The patient must be taught assiduous brushing and flossing techniques as well as the use of daily topical fluoride application. Gels with trays can be used.

VI. Follow-up
   A. Oral examination with prophylaxis should be scheduled every 6 mo, or more often if oral hygiene is a problem. Any teeth that become carious will need early restoration. Any prosthesis that is constructed must not irritate or abrade the mucosa. Oral examinations must include careful checks for recurrent or new lesions, with early biopsy.
   B. A neck examination should be conducted to assess for the development of adenopathy.
   C. Multidisciplinary follow-up (surgical, oral surgical, radiation, oncological) in an organized setting is advisable.

Assessment after radiation therapy

I. Purpose
   A. Any new lesions are discovered and evaluated.
   B. Symptomatic teeth or periodontal tissues in or near an irradiated field are treated.
   C. Oral mucosal irritation from irradiation is treated.

II. Review of the record
   A. One must carefully determine whether the area under study is within the irradiated field.
   B. If it is, the patient should be started on a regimen of daily antibiotics before oral surgery. This will help prevent serious infections that might ensue when oral flora is introduced into irradiated tissue.

III. Patient history, examination, and additional studies
   A. These are the same as for preradiation patients.

   B. Radiographic studies can usually be limited to the symptomatic area.
IV. Response
   A. The oral surgeon should submit any suspicious lesions to biopsy, drain abscesses, and remove nonrestorable teeth.
   B. Lesions strongly suspected of being caused by irritation from a prosthesis can be treated by removal of the prosthesis, starting saline or half-strength hydrogen peroxide rinses, and reexamining the patient in 1 wk. If unimproved, the lesion should then be biopsied.
   C. Mucosal irritations and dryness, in the absence of lesions, may be managed with artificial saliva, saline rinses, or 2% viscous lidocaine (Xylocaine) rinses. Lemon-flavored lozenges can be used to try to stimulate more salivary flow. This additional moisture may soothe the mucosa.
   D. Suggested antibiotic coverage for oral surgery in irradiated areas is
      1. Potassium penicillin 2 g p.o. 1 hr before and then 500 mg p.o. q.6h. for 5 da after
      2. In the presence of penicillin allergy, erythromycin 1 g p.o. 1 hr before and then 500 mg p.o. q.6h. for 5 da after
      3. As an alternative, IV or IM penicillin-G or clindamycin

Assessment of oral lesions

   I. Purpose. The oral surgeon is often asked to diagnose oral lesions and determine whether they are cancerous.
  II. Review of the record. One notes any history of previous lesions and their diagnoses.
 III. Patient history
   A. The acuteness or chronicity of a lesion is noted. An acute lesion, especially with a concurrent viral-type syndrome, may not require biopsy unless it persists unimproved for 1 wk or 10 da.
   B. Pain, bleeding, the presence of other lesions intra- or extraorally, and any irritation from prostheses are noted.
   C. A history of smoking, alcohol abuse, or habits traumatic to the mucosa is important.
   D. Any systemic symptoms indicative of a nutritional, infective, or allergy syndrome that might have accompanying oral lesions must be treated.
  IV. Patient examination
   A. One must accurately describe the lesion and note other lesions or irritations.
   B. The neck must be examined for adenopathy.
   C. Bimanual palpation of the floor of the mouth will reveal submaxillary or submental adenopathy.
   V. Additional studies. Lesions that cannot be explained on the basis of systemic illness and lesions that are suspicious because of their

chronicity, a smoking history, adenopathy, or the lack of obvious local irritation should be submitted to biopsy.

VI. Response
   A. The definitive diagnosis of a suspicious area is by biopsy. Any lesion observed should be biopsied if it is not clearly improving after 7-10 da of treatment.
      1. If irritation is thought to be the cause, its source is eliminated (including leaving out the prosthesis) and the lesion is biopsied if the condition does not improve in 7-10 da.
      2. To clean areas of suspected irritation, the patient must start saline or half-strength hydrogen peroxide mouth rinses q.i.d.
   B. When biopsy is done, excision with a margin of normal-appearing tissue is advisable where the size of the lesion makes this practical. Thus biopsy can be the definitive and curative procedure.

VII. Follow-up
   A. Treatment planning relative to excision, radiation, or chemotherapy is needed for lesions shown to be cancerous and incompletely removed at biopsy. A multidisciplinary approach is best, especially in a clinic organized for this purpose. All patients should be observed for healing and recurrence.
   B. Recurrence of a suspicious lesion requires biopsy.

Assessment for iatrogenic dentoalveolar trauma

I. Purpose
   A. The oral surgeon is often called to the operating room to replant avulsed teeth and repair lacerations that at times may occur when a patient is intubated for general anesthesia.
   B. Elapsed time is critical if a subluxated or avulsed tooth is to survive reduction and reimplantation.

II. Patient examination
   A. Vertical fracture of a tooth or teeth and roots fractured in the cervical half are nonrestorable. A root fractured at the cervical margin may be retained, the pulp extirpated, and the tooth later reconstructed.
   B. Any cleanly subluxated or avulsed teeth are reimplanted.

III. Response
   A. Using adequate light and suction, the oral surgeon must
      1. Stop any active bleeding.
      2. Pack the pharynx if the patient is intubated.
      3. Remove any nonsalvageable teeth.
      4. Extirpate the pulps of salvageable roots and teeth with Class III fractures, plugging the canals with cotton pellets and a temporary sealer and administering antibiotics.
      5. Reduce and splint any subluxated teeth and replant and splint avulsed teeth. Endodontics "in hand" might be necessary on avulsed teeth that have been out longer than 30

minutes. (See the section on treatment of dentoalveolar trauma.)
6. Administer antibiotics and remove the pharyngeal pack.
B. Since these cases may involve litigation, care must be taken to document in the record the exact anatomical details of the injury.

IV. Follow-up
A. The oral surgeon assesses the patient for evidence of infection or developing nonvitality of the teeth. Signs include new pain, mobility, and darkening of the teeth. The patient's dentist will also need to be alerted to watch for these signs.
B. Reduced and replanted teeth may eventually require endodontic therapy. Restorative care is usually coordinated through the patient's dentist.

Assessment before chemotherapy

I. Purpose. Many chemotherapeutic agents cause oral problems, either through a direct toxic effect on the tissues or by effects on the bone marrow (making the tissues less resistant to bleeding or infection).
A. Common oral problems in chemotherapy patients include xerostomia, angular cheilitis, mucositis (bacterial, viral, or fungal), mucosal bleeding, and odontogenic infection.
B. When the patient becomes myelosuppressed, there is a predisposition to rampant infection and uncontrollable bleeding from sources not usually problematic.

II. Patient history
A. The oral surgeon can ascertain the agent to be used and discuss with the physician the experience with oral problems from that agent. Predicted effects on blood counts need to be considered.
B. The level of the patient's prior oral care and his motivation to maintain rigorous oral hygiene must be assessed. One must determine whether any teeth have been symptomatic and whether bleeding in the oral cavity is an existing problem. A history of previous mucositis consistent with bacterial, viral, or fungal infection is important.
C. A check is made to see whether prior radiation therapy has been done.

III. Patient examination
A. Odontogenic infection is carefully sought. Deeply carious teeth must be considered as potential sources of infection.
B. The periodontal condition is carefully assessed, especially for deep pockets that cannot be kept clean. Friable tissues are noted as potential sources of bleeding. Irritating factors (e.g., sharp edges of teeth, restorations, or prostheses) can also cause bleeding. The condition of the mucosa is evaluated for ulcerations or lacerations that might break down when myelosuppression occurs.

IV. Additional studies. A Panorex and full-mouth periapical series with particular attention to depth of caries, periapical disease, and periodontal condition should be obtained.

V. Response
   A. Restorable teeth should be restored. Endodontic therapy is not contraindicated.
   B. Thorough prophylaxis should be done and home care with brushing, flossing, and topical fluoride application taught.
   C. Lips can be kept moist with lanolin or nonpetrolatum lubricants to reduce mucosal irritation.
   D. Nonrestorable teeth and hopelessly periodontally involved teeth should be removed. Ideally this will be done 10-14 da before chemotherapy to allow adequate healing before any myelosuppression occurs. If the chemotherapeutic agent causes myelosuppression late in its course, oral surgical treatment can be performed closer to the scheduled start of therapy.
   E. If prior radiation therapy has been done, treatment will proceed as described earlier.

VI. Follow-up
   A. The patient should be examined several times during the course of chemotherapy and afterward. Any oral disease that becomes manifest should be dealt with swiftly.
   B. Examination and prophylaxis should be done every 6 mo thereafter, if the WBC and platelet counts permit.

Assessment during or after chemotherapy

I. Purpose
   A. Usually the clinician requests treatment of an acute oral problem in a patient debilitated by chemotherapy or by the disease for which it is being used. The chemotherapy or the underlying disease may prevent immediate necessary treatment of the oral problem. In some cases there is no specific treatment other than to await the passing of the chemotherapy side effects.
   B. Sometimes a patient will have a fever of uncertain origin while undergoing chemotherapy. Then the oral surgeon is called upon to identify and treat any likely oral sources of the fever.

II. Patient history
   A. For mucosal lesions a prior history consistent with herpes labialis, acute necrotizing ulcerative gingivitis (ANUG), or fungal infection of the mouth should be sought.
   B. The oral surgeon must determine whether the patient is myelosuppressed and if special precautions are needed. Good hand washing and use of gowns, gloves, and masks may be necessary just to examine the patient. Such patients are often in isolation.

III. Patient examination
   A. Topical anesthetics may be required to make the patient's irri-

tated mouth comfortable during treatment. Key elements include

1. Xerostomia—thickened saliva, difficulty with speech
2. Angular cheilitis or mucositis—cracking, bleeding, exudates, broad irregular ulcerations with necrotic centers and surrounding erythema, hemorrhage
3. Mucosal bleeding—usually slow oozing; may indicate a coagulopathy, especially if spontaneous; a surgically controllable bleeding point is sought
4. ANUG—necrotic gingival papillae, bleeding, adenopathy, fetor oris
5. Candidiasis—white plaques, organisms on smears
6. Herpes labialis—crops of vesicles on the mucosa or beyond the mucocutaneous border; viral inclusion bodies on smears of cells taken from the base of a vesicle

B. Odontogenic infection may be accompanied by tenderness or mobility of the teeth involved. Often, because of polymorphonuclear leukocyte (PMN) suppression, there is no purulence.

IV. Additional studies

A. The following tests may be performed:

1. Panoramic radiograph and specific periapical films if the problem relates to the teeth
2. White blood cell count with differential
3. Bleeding time, prothrombin time, partial thromboplastin time
4. Platelet count

B. The pattern of recent WBC counts and coagulation studies should be noted to see whether there is a worsening or improving trend. This will help determine the timing of oral surgery and any necessary hematological replacement therapy.

V. Response

A. Oral hygiene needs to be optimized. If the WBCs are less than 2000, with less than 10% PMNs, prophylaxis should not be done and brushing and flossing should be discontinued. This is necessary also if the platelet count is below 25,000/mm^3 or if spontaneous bleeding is a problem. At that point the teeth and tissues should be gently cleaned with gauze or cotton swabs. Rinses of peroxide mixed 1:5 with water can be used as well. If this irritates, a solution of table salt (¼ tsp) and baking soda (¼ tsp) to one 8 oz glass of water can be used instead. The baking soda may be eliminated if it is irritating.

B. Xerostomia can be palliated by glycerine swabs, artificially sweetened gum or candy, or artificial saliva.

C. Mucositis is palliated with Kaopectate rinses, often mixed with diphenhydramine (Benadryl). Orabase, again with or without benzocaine, can be used. Viscous lidocaine (2%) is helpful but often must be mixed with water (1:2-1:5) to prevent common irritation in these patients at full strength. Dyclonine or cocaine rinses can also be tried for more refractory cases (but not in patients taking MAOIs). Systemic analgesics are sometimes necessary. Angular cheilitis can usually be palliated with lanolin or nonpetrolatum lubricants. In myelosuppressed patients, steroid-containing ointments are generally not advisable.

D. Mucosal bleeding is treated with topical thrombin soaked into sponges or a topical hemostatic (e.g., Avitene) or epsilon-aminocaproic acid if the PT or PTT is abnormal. If thrombocytopenia is present, 10-20 units of platelets is transfused. Brushing and flossing are stopped. A specific bleeding point can be treated surgically with cautery (electrocautery or silver nitrate sticks) or with a suture.

E. ANUG is treated with parenteral antibiotics, especially penicillin. Gram-negative coverage to prevent opportunistic infections, common in these patients, should be considered. Debridement can be done if the platelet count allows, but this is usually not the case.

F. Candidiasis receives a nystatin swish and swallow or vaginal suppositories held in the mouth. Nystatin ointment is often more adherent to the mucosa than is the rinse. Amphotericin B may be used systemically if systemic candidiasis has been diagnosed or is suspected or when the pharynx and esophagus are involved.

G. Herpes labialis is palliated with lubricating ointments or topical anesthetics. If healing does not occur in 10-14 da, acyclovir (Zovirax) may be required in the sick patient.

H. Odontogenic infection is treated by extraction and, if necessary, drainage. Neutropenia may result in the absence of purulence. A single extraction can usually be safely done if the WBC count is 1500 and the platelet count 25,000/mm^3; otherwise, transfusions of WBCs and platelets are necessary. Coverage with parenteral antibiotic is needed. Aqueous penicillin-G (2,000,000 units q.4h.) is usually chosen, but clindamycin can be used in penicillin-allergic patients (400-600 mg IV q.4h.).

I. In any oral infection in these patients where bacterial involvement is likely, therapy needs to include coverage for gram-negative opportunistic organisms in addition to the usual oral flora. Broad-spectrum antibiotics are used.

VI. Follow-up. Hemostasis and the development or worsening of infection need to be carefully monitored, especially after oral surgical manipulation.

Assessment of a bleeding patient

I. Purpose

A. Spontaneous oral bleeding necessitates referral to disclose a possible surgically correctable cause. Often an underlying coagulopathy is known or suspected, and only its correction results in definitive hemostasis.

B. Sometimes a patient is referred for severe bleeding following an oral surgical procedure. There may be a sense of alarm that the procedure has unmasked a coagulopathy. More often, the bleeding is from a specific surgically correctable point that was not discovered. Even so, the possibility of a coagulopathy must be borne in mind.

II. Patient history
 A. One must elicit information concerning known coagulopathies in the patient or family and must inquire whether hemostasis has been a problem for the patient.
 B. It is also necessary to determine whether anticoagulants are in use and list medications that might induce thrombocytopenia (e.g., quinidine or chemotherapy) or inhibit platelet function (e.g., aspirin).

III. Patient examination
 A. One must search for a specific bleeding point, which will usually be the result of trauma or surgery rather than a coagulopathy. The presence of slow generalized oozing from tissues often indicates a coagulopathy.
 B. If petechiae are present, thrombocytopenia is likely. Ecchymosis in untraumatized areas may indicate a problem in the extrinsic or intrinsic coagulation pathway.

IV. Additional studies
 A. In the presence of a bleeding point and without a history of coagulopathies, no additional studies are needed as long as the bleeding is effectively controlled.
 B. If a coagulopathy is suspected or if bleeding is refractory despite measures that usually provide adequate control, a bleeding time (BT), prothrombin time (PT), partial thromboplastin time (PTT), and platelet count should be obtained as a start.

V. Response
 A. Surgical bleeding. "Snaps" with the electrocautery needle or sutures with deep "bites" into tissue around the bleeding vessel can be tried if biting on a gauze or tea bag does not work. A figure-8 suture placed through the tissue around the bleeding vessel usually works. If bleeding is related to a fracture, reduction may cause it to stop. If exploration is needed to identify the source of bleeding deep in the tissues, it is usually best done in the operating room with red cell and plasma replacement available.
 B. Coagulopathies
  1. Hemophilia A—BT normal, PT normal, PTT up (Factor VIII:C down); Factor VIII levels 5-25% in mild cases, 0.25-5% in severe cases; treatment: Factor VIII replacement, specifically cryoprecipitate enriched in Factor VIII (prepared from plasma [risk of hepatitis]); epsilon-amino caproic acid can also be used prophylactically (100 mg/kg preoperatively and 100 mg/kg q.6 h. × 10 da postoperatively)

2. Von Willebrand's disease—BT up, PT normal, PTT up (impaired platelet adhesiveness) (type I, Factor VIII:vW [von Willebrand factor] down; type II, Factor VIII:vW absent); treatment: cryoprecipitate

3. Hemophilia B—BT normal, PT normal, PTT up (Factor IX down); treatment: Factor IX, fresh frozen plasma

VI. Follow-up. Close monitoring for continued recurrent bleeding is necessary. Of note is the fact that tight suturing of the injured tongue or floor of the mouth in a patient with a coagulopathy can lead to massive bleeding in the tissue planes and airway obstruction. A few relatively loosely placed sutures will approximate the tissues while allowing any low-grade oozing to come out of the wound.

GENERAL REFERENCES

American Heart Association: Prevention of bacterial endocarditis. Statement for health professionals by the Committee on Rheumatic Fever and Ineffective Endocarditis of the Council on Cardiovascular Disease in the Young, Dallas, 1984.

Braunwald, E., et al.: Harrison's principles of internal medicine, ed. 7, New York, 1985, McGraw-Hill Book Co., Inc.

Halstead, C.L., et al.: Physical evaluation of the dental patient, St. Louis, 1982, The C.V. Mosby Co.

Judge, R.D., et al.: Clinical diagnosis: a physiologic approach, ed. 4, Boston, 1982, Little, Brown & Co.

Wyngarden, J.B., and Smith, L.H.: Cecil's textbook of medicine, ed. 17, Philadelphia, 1985, W.B. Saunders Co.

Management Considerations
in the Medically
Compromised Patient

PREOPERATIVE CONSIDERATIONS

In this chapter we outline considerations that arise in providing oral surgical care for patients with a variety of medical disorders. The conditions selected for discussion were chosen because they occur frequently or because they demand significant alteration of the way in which oral surgical care is delivered. Since this is a chapter on management, we discuss initial diagnosis and treatment only sparingly and assume that we are dealing with patients who have one or more established diagnoses.

The disorders discussed in this chapter are

Cardiac dysfunction
Pulmonary dysfunction
Hypertension
Renal dysfunction
Hepatic dysfunction and alcoholism
Coagulation and bleeding disorders
Seizure disorders
Endocrine dysfunction
    Diabetes mellitus
    Thyroid dysfunction
    Adrenal dysfunction and patients taking steroids
Dysfunction of the immune system

GENERAL CONSIDERATIONS

The initial contact with any new patient should be carefully orchestrated to achieve five specific goals:

  a. Assessment of the patient's oral surgical needs
  b. Identification of potential management problems
  c. Establishment of a good working rapport with the patient
  d. Formulation of a treatment plan in light of the patient's oral and medical status
  e. Preparation of the patient for indicated procedures

Assessment of the patient's needs

A. The patient appears "on his own," or is referred by a physician or dentist, usually with a specific goal in mind:

Removal of a tooth
Alleviation of pain
Biopsy of a lesion
Treatment of an infection

B. Sometimes the patient requires a general evaluation and "treatment as necessary."

C. It is essential to recognize that in all but the most straightforward circumstances (and even in some apparently straightforward circumstances), the patient and his physician and/or dentist may have different perceptions of his condition and needs. The oral surgeon should be aware of these other perceptions.

D. Having formed an impression as to the patient's needs based on history, physical examination, radiographs, and other studies as required, the oral surgeon should be prepared to assume an active role in communicating with the other participants in the patient's management, including the patient himself, in the interest of reaching a consensus.

Identification of potential management problems

A. Few things are more important than acquiring the habit of taking a brief medical history from all patients. A reasonably complete screening history can be obtained from a well patient in less than 2 min. The further elucidation of positive findings also need not be a lengthy procedure.

B. From a practical point of view, a medical illness may predispose to either or both of two kinds of problems:

Acute physiological decompensation under stress, as may occur in the perioperative period
Failure to do well postoperatively because of infection or impaired hemostasis or wound healing

C. Circumventing such problems depends in large measure upon being aware of the potential for their occurrence and then taking adequate precautions. To this end, historical points of special significance, irrespective of the specific illness, include

1. Acuteness versus chronicity of symptoms—It is important to document the stability of the patient's medical condition. If questionning reveals a pattern of increasing symptoms, an upgrading of the patient's medical regimen may take priority over oral surgical needs. The oral and maxillofacial surgeon may play a vital role in identifying the decompensating patient and placing him in proper hands.

2. Physiological reserve of the patient—It is important also to know something about the patient's capacity for handling physical or emotional stress. Inquiry may be made into the

issue of exercise tolerance, response to anxiety-provoking situations, and response to similar surgery in the past. Such information may help determine how much to do at any one time and in what setting to do it (e.g., inpatient versus outpatient, clinic versus operating room).

3. Current medications—Some patients may be unable to state their exact diagnosis. In the absence of medical records, medications can then be a useful indication of what condition(s) the patient is being treated for.

Establishment of a good working rapport with the patient

A. Most routine oral surgical procedures are not inherently physiologically stressful; however, any surgical procedure, especially one to be performed on an awake patient, may be the psychological equivalent of an assault and thus evoke fear, anxiety, even anger. Such emotional responses are accompanied by the release of endogenous catecholamines and are therefore physiologically taxing, especially to the medically compromised patient with reduced reserve.

B. A major psychological objective is to reduce the assaultive aspect of impending surgery. Toward this end, the value of good rapport with the patient can hardly be overestimated; next to good luck, it is possibly the single most important ingredient in the uneventful management of sick patients.

C. Good rapport markedly reduces anxiety and the need for sedation by pharmacological means. There are no medications that can compensate for lack of patient confidence in the surgeon. Good rapport flows naturally from a genuine concern for the well being of the patient. Most patients can immediately sense this quality in those doctors that possess it.

D. One factor that helps reduce anxiety is attention to choice of language. The manner in which the doctor speaks to the patient should be calculated to optimize communication of essential information rather than to impress the patient with expertise. Terms that have threatening connotations should be avoided, but at the same time honesty with the patient is essential. The doctrine of informed consent demands, and most patients appreciate, a thorough explanation of a proposed surgical procedure. Taking the time to explain things fully and comprehensibly helps establish rapport and builds trust.

E. A major cause of anxiety for patients is the feeling of loss of control that comes from having to submit to invasions of privacy, not to mention physical intervention. Once again, a full explanation of proposed procedures increases the patient's feeling of participation and allows him to maintain a sense of control. Especially in performing surgery on awake patients, anything that can be done to help preserve this sense of control will make the procedure less stressful.

For instance, assure the patient that he can call for a pause during a procedure if he needs to rest.

Assure him also that you will stop immediately if he reports any pain.

Formulation of a treatment plan

A. Starting from an assessment of the patient's dental needs, the goal of the oral surgeon is to determine the appropriate treatment in light of the patient's medical status. For example, a full course of periodontal therapy, endodontics, and a "roundhouse" splint might be ideal therapy in the patient with advanced periodontal disease and no medical contraindications; but appropriate treatment for the same dental findings in the patient with infective endocarditis and facing valve replacement might be multiple extractions and full denture prostheses.

B. Having established a treatment plan, the oral surgeon then determines the best setting for carrying it out.

 1. Based upon the nature and extent of treatment and the patient's condition and state of mind, a decision is made as to whether to proceed on an inpatient or outpatient basis (if the patient is not already in the hospital when seen) and whether treatment should be carried out in an outpatient unit or in the operating room. These decisions are based, in turn, upon the requirements for anesthesia, monitoring, and postoperative care and are best made in consultation with the patient's attending physician and with an anesthesia consultant when a general anesthetic is contemplated.

 2. Patient preference is an important factor in the choice of setting and type of anesthesia. An anxious patient may express strong preference for a general anesthetic. Whereas for some medically compromised patients general anesthesia has an increased element of risk, for others a well-managed general anesthetic with careful monitoring may be safer than an anxiety-provoking procedure under local anesthesia.

 3. The need for a general anesthetic may be a contraindication to elective surgery in some compromised patients and is an important consideration in treatment planning.

 4. Again, the ability to establish a good working rapport with the patient extends the range of procedures that can be successfully performed under local anesthesia.

Preparation of the patient for indicated procedures

A. Patients frequently dread oral surgery and other manipulation of their teeth more than they fear a major procedure such as heart surgery.

B. When oral surgery must be performed before other treatment can commence (e.g., before immunosuppression for organ transplantation or before prosthetic valve replacement), the patient may be referred for evaluation and treatment with little or no explanation as to why the oral surgical consultation has been requested. The oral surgeon may be the one to inform the patient that, before he can undergo the procedure for which he was admitted, he must first submit to the removal of teeth or other oral surgical procedures. In these circumstances the quality of the relationship established with the patient during the evaluation is all important in getting the patient to accept the clinically indicated oral procedure.

SPECIFIC MEDICAL DISORDERS AND ORAL SURGICAL MANAGEMENT
Cardiac dysfunction

I. Cardiac dysfunction consists of numerous clinical entities. Problems of concern to the oral surgeon include

Angina pectoris and coronary artery occlusive disease
Congestive heart failure
Cardiac arrhythmias
Cardiac valvular disease, especially mitral and aortic
stenosis and/or regurgitation
Myocardial infarction
Infective endocarditis

II. General considerations
 A. Positioning the awake patient for surgery
  1. Under local anesthesia, the most desirable position for operating may be unsatisfactory for patient comfort.
  2. In the patient with congestive failure the so-called "cardiac position," with head and feet elevated, may be optimal. This promotes venous return from the extremities, relieves neck vein engorgement, and eases respiration.
 B. Use of sedative agents
  1. In skilled hands a sedative may be useful in the outpatient care of some cardiac patients. Oral or intravenous diazepam (Valium) and nitrous oxide–oxygen are advocated by some.
  2. However, the need for sedation for a given procedure may be taken as an indication to treat the patient in the operating room, where careful monitoring by an anesthesiologist is possible while the surgeon devotes himself fully to the operation and to verbal contact with the patient. If an unstable patient is in need of sedation, he probably should be monitored since even the most innocuous of agents may have an exaggerated effect on a failing or unstable myocardium.
 C. Need for oxygen. In many cardiac patients the use of oxygen administered by nasal prongs has much to recommend it:
  1. Breathing air with elevated proportions of oxygen is known to produce a mild euphoria not associated with its other physiological effects.
  2. Breathing oxygen allows good tissue perfusion with decreased cardiac output and heart rate.

3. Myocardial oxygenation is improved, which makes ischemia less likely.

4. Should cardiopulmonary resuscitation become necessary, an initially well-oxygenated patient is at an advantage from the standpoint of both cerebral ischemia and metabolic acidosis.

D. Local anesthesia

1. Lidocaine (Xylocaine) 2% with 1 : 100,000 epinephrine is a reasonable choice of agent for the majority of cardiac patients; however, it should not be used in patients with a history of

   Syncope
   Palpitations or ventricular arrhythmias
   Aortic stenosis with symptoms
   Angina provoked by minimum exertion or stress
   Prior adverse reactions to epinephrine

2. In these cases prilocaine 4% (Citanest) is a useful agent, as is mepivacaine 3% (Carbocaine).

E. Trinitroglycerin (TNG). In patients with frequent attacks of angina, especially those whose attacks are triggered by situational anxiety, it may be useful to administer sublingual nitroglycerin just before injection of the local anesthetic agent. Such injections frequently are the most stressful point of an outpatient oral surgery visit. Patients often are more comfortable knowing that TNG is readily available should they need it.

III. Under stressful circumstances, patients with the following conditions are the most worrisome:

A. Aortic stenosis with a history of syncope

1. Patients with tight aortic stenosis with syncope and/or angina are the single most frightening group to deal with because the chances of performing a successful resuscitation in the event of cardiac arrest are extremely poor. This is because closed-chest cardiac massage provides inadequate perfusion in the face of a stenotic valve. In aortic stenosis the heart is essentially contracting isometrically in generating an enormous transvalvular pressure gradient. This kind of pressure work, in contradistinction to volume work, requires high myocardial oxygen consumption (Fig. 4-1).

2. The following suggestions may be helpful in treating a patient with aortic stenosis:

   a. Oxygen by nasal prongs is advisable for reasons already discussed.

   b. Epinephrine-containing local anesthetics must be avoided. These patients definitely do not need the chronotropic effect of this agent.

   c. Sedation. The operating room is appropriate for patients with symptomatic aortic stenosis.

   d. Monitoring of heart rate is important, as is continuous

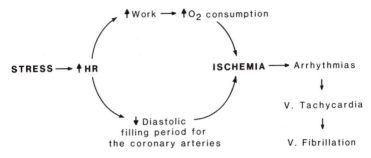

Fig. 4-1 Relationship between work and oxygen consumption. Stress increases the heart rate (*HR*), which in a diseased heart can cause ischemia by both the greater need of the coronary arteries for O_2 and the reduced time available for them to get it.

        monitoring of the ECG pattern for ST segment depression or other signs of ischemia.

    e. Intravenous propranolol (Inderal) may be indicated for the control of heart rate but must be used only in the setting of the operating room with careful monitoring.

B. Mitral stenosis or mitral regurgitation with congestive heart failure

  1. Unlike patients with aortic stenosis, this group of patients tends to decompensate more slowly and with more warning. Under stress they may develop congestive symptoms.

  2. The preemptive use of oxygen and sedation is indicated.

C. Coronary artery disease with angina or congestive heart failure. In such patients prophylactic use of nitroglycerin is important, epinephrine must be avoided, and oxygen therapy should be employed.

D. Recent myocardial infarction

  1. The conventional wisdom, backed by clinical studies, suggests that stressful surgery be avoided for 3 and preferably 6 mo after a myocardial infarction. The basis for this is that some of these patients are physiologically more stable after they have had a chance to recover from the infarction.

  2. Some of the more unstable post–myocardial infarction patients exclude themselves by having a second infarction, the likelihood of which event decreases with increasing time since the initial infarct.

  3. However, if symptomatic teeth cannot be palliated by the use of antibiotics, then emergency treatment (extraction or endodontic therapy) is indicated even in the relatively immediate postinfarction period. The operating room is the safest setting for treatment of these patients (with careful monitoring, oxygen, and sedation).

E. Unstable arrhythmias, ventricular irritability, complete heart block, Stokes-Adams attacks. The need for monitoring makes the operating room mandatory for the performance of surgery on these patients. Use of transvenous pacing during anesthesia is a controversial subject but may be indicated in some circumstances.

IV. Infective endocarditis
   A. Patients at risk of endocarditis include
      1. Those with a turbulence-producing defect
      2. Those with a murmur and unexplained fever (infective endocarditis must be presumed until excluded; a change in the character of the murmur may indicate the formation of vegetations)
   B. The onset of endocarditis may be insidious or abrupt, and the course prolonged or fulminant, depending upon the virulence of the causative organism.
   C. Untreated infective endocarditis is fatal.
   D. Defects with which endocarditis and analogous infections are associated include congenital and acquired cardiac and noncardiac lesions.
      1. Congenital lesions
         a. Ventricular septal defect
         b. Patent ductus arteriosus
         c. Bicuspid aortic valve
         d. Tetralogy of Fallot
         e. Atrial septal defect (low incidence)
         f. Prolapsing mitral valve (click murmur syndrome)
      2. Acquired lesions
         a. Rheumatic valvular lesions
         b. Syphilitic and/or atherosclerotic aortic lesions
         c. Mural thrombi adjacent to subendocardial infarction
         d. Clots in the atrial appendage in atrial fibrillation
      3. Foreign bodies
         a. Valve prostheses
         b. Indwelling catheters
         c. Vascular prostheses
         d. Pacing wires (probably *not,* since they endothelialize rapidly)
   E. *Streptococcus viridans* accounts for 70-80% of infective endocarditis.
   F. Principal manifestations include
      1. Organisms of high pathogenicity *(Staphylococcus)* may destroy the chordae and valve leaflets, leading to valvular insufficiency and fulminant congestive failure.
      2. Organisms of low pathogenicity in combination with platelets and fibrin produce vegetations associated with change in the character of the patient's murmur and with embolization.

3. Embolic phenomena may occur:
   a. Pulmonary embolization from ventricular septal defect, patent ductus, or pulmonic and tricuspid valvular lesions to the lungs leads to pulmonary infarction. The first sign of this may be hemoptysis.
   b. Systemic embolization to
      (1) Brain (stroke)
      (2) Retinal vessels (blindness or visual field defects)
      (3) Spleen (friction rub, with right upper quadrant abdominal pain)
      (4) Kidneys (hematuria, flank pain, renal infarction, glomerulonephritis)
      (5) GI tract (abdominal pain, ileus, melena)
      (6) Skin and mucous membranes (mucocutaneous petechiae, painful nodules)
      (7) Extremities (Osler's nodes, gangrene)
      (8) Coronary vessels (myocardial infarction)
      (9) Bone (osteomyelitis)
      (10) Vasa vasorum (mycotic aneurysms)
4. Persistent bacteremia produces ongoing fevers with PM temperature spikes. Chills are uncommon in infective endocarditis.
5. Filtration of bacteria and immune complexes by the reticuloendothelial system leads to
   a. Splenomegaly (usually nontender)
   b. Anemia
   c. Increased bilirubin from sequestration and destruction of RBCs, producing jaundice
   d. Immune complex nephritis, arthritis or arthralgia resembling that occurring with acute rheumatic fever, vasculitis, petechiae (Roth's spots in the eye)
G. Laboratory findings include
1. Increased WBC count and neutrophilia
2. Anemia (normocytic, normochromic)
3. Histiocytes seen on peripheral smears
4. Increased sedimentation rate
5. Increased immunoglobulins
6. Mild bilirubinemia
7. Urinalysis: proteinuria and microscopic hematuria
8. Positive blood cultures in 85% of cases (when organisms are recovered, they are found in 1 of 3 culture bottles 98% of the time)
H. Since endocardial vegetations contain anoxic slow-growing organisms, bactericidal levels of antibiotics at dilutions of 1:8 or better should be maintained for 4-6 wk. Defervescence usually occurs in 3-7 da after commencement of appropriate therapy. If symptoms recur during treatment, superinfection with a resistant organism must be ruled out.

I. Prognosis
  1. Untreated endocarditis has a fatal outcome.
  2. Treated infective endocarditis has an overall survival rate of 70%.
  3. When penicillin sensitive streptococcal organisms are cultured, survival is 90%.
  4. A poor prognosis is associated with
     a. Congestive heart failure
     b. Culture-negative endocarditis
     c. Resistant organisms
     d. Delayed treatment
     e. Prosthetic valve endocarditis (about 50% survival for plastic and metal valves, somewhat better for porcine heterografts)
J. Prophylaxis
  1. The majority of organisms implicated in infective endocarditis are constituents of the normal oral flora. It is well established that professional manipulation of the teeth, home hygiene activities, and even chewing produce transient bacteremias whose magnitude reflects the individual's state of dental and periodontal health. Equally well established is the role of transient bacteremias in the pathogenesis of endocarditis.
  2. Based on the foregoing, there are two main concerns in providing prophylaxis:

     Protection of the patient from bacteremias induced by professional manipulation
     Protection from bacteremias caused by underlying dental and periodontal disease

  3. The American Heart Association has published guidelines for prophylactic coverage for invasive dental therapy (refer to pp. 55-56). Additional copies of these guidelines can be ordered by writing to the AHA or to the journal *Circulation*. This document should be given to the dentists of patients who are at risk of endocarditis, especially those with prior episodes of endocarditis and those with prosthetic valves.
  4. Since the average patient goes to the dentist only several times a year, the antibiotics given for invasive procedures cover him only for those bacteremias that occur in the context of professional care. Equally if not more important is the protection of the at-risk patient from bacteremias that occur daily when he brushes, flosses, uses a Water Pik, or chews.
  5. Because long-term administration of antibiotics to at-risk individuals is unreasonable and probably not efficacious, the best way of protecting these patients is to reduce the magnitude of transient bacteremias by reducing dental disease as much as possible. Steps should be taken to render the at-risk

patient free of pathologically mobile teeth, and active periapical and periodontal disease should be treated either by extraction or by more conservative means consistent with the restorability of the dentition and with the patient's motivation to establish and maintain a satisfactory level of dental health. This applies particularly to patients with prosthetic valves, for whom endocarditis carries a 50-50 chance of mortality. It is similarly important for patients with prior episodes of infective endocarditis. These patients must be presumed to be uniquely susceptible and liable to have additional episodes of endocarditis.

6. The hospital-based oral surgeon should initiate a screening program for prosthetic valve and endocarditis patients in his or her institution and actively seek to confer with cardiologists, internists, or cardiac surgeons regarding the treatment of such patients.

Pulmonary dysfunction

I. General considerations

A. The respiratory apparatus, including lungs, pulmonary tree, pulmonary vasculature, and thoracic musculoskeletal system, adds oxygen to and recovers carbon dioxide from the bloodstream.

B. Carbon dioxide, produced by oxidative metabolism, forms carbonic acid and thus contributes hydrogen ion to the blood. Thus retention of carbon dioxide produces a respiratory acidosis.

C. Conversely, hyperventilation, which blows off carbon dioxide, produces a respiratory alkalosis. When hyperventilation is chronic, the resultant respiratory acidosis is normally balanced by a compensatory metabolic alkalosis, maintaining the normal pH. Therefore, the lungs, in addition to providing oxygen and recovering carbon dioxide, are intimately involved, along with the kidneys, in the maintenance of acid-base balance.

II. Diagnosis

A. The analysis of arterial blood gases (ABGs) reveals whether the respiratory apparatus is functioning properly. The interpretation of blood gases is discussed in Chapter 7.

B. In addition to ABGs, a thorough evaluation of pulmonary function includes pulmonary function tests (PFTs), which measure the mechanics of respiration (breathing), ventilation (gas exchange at the alveolar level), and oxygenation (delivery of O_2 to the hemoglobin in the blood).

1. Mechanics of respiration

a. When one takes a full breath and exhales as fully as possible, the volume of air exhaled is the vital capacity (VC) (average 4.8 L in men, 3.1 L in women). Total lung capacity includes vital capacity plus a residual volume of air that is still present in the lungs after full exhalation.

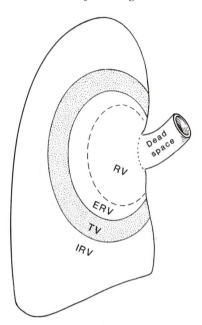

$$VC = TV + ERV + IRV$$

$$FRC = RV + ERV$$

Fig. 4-2 Vital capacity.

   b. At rest one normally inhales and exhales only a fraction of vital capacity; this volume (0.5 L) is called tidal volume. The volume of air that can be inspired above tidal volume is called inspiratory reserve volume and the volume of air that can be exhaled below tidal volume is called expiratory reserve volume. These are shown diagramatically in Fig. 4-2.

   c. Dead space volume is the volume of air in the pulmonary tree that does not come in contact with alveolar surfaces and thus does not participate in gas exchange. Residual volume plus expiratory reserve volume is called the functional residual capacity (FRC).

   d. Respiratory mechanics are measured by having the patient blow through a spirometer, which measures both volumes and flows and graphically displays these in a spirogram (Fig. 4-3).

     (1) Modern spirometers incorporate computers that allow an automatic comparison to be made between observed values and predicted values based upon age, sex, height, and weight. Some such devices will

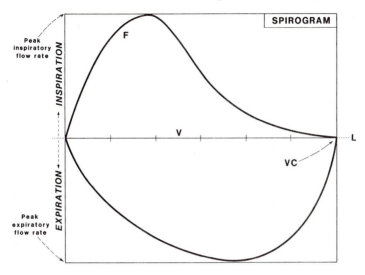

Fig. 4-3 Typical spirogram.

also print out an interpretation of differences between observed and predicted values.

(2) Parameters typically measured include

First sec VC (L)
Vital capacity (L)
First sec VC/VC%
Peak expiratory flow rate (L/sec)
Expiratory flow at 50% of VC (L/sec)
Peak inspiratory flow rate (L/sec)
Maximum breathing capacity (L/min)

(3) Different pulmonary diseases produce characteristic changes in the spirogram and parameters.

(a) Thus, for example, decreased expiratory flow at 25% of vital capacity suggests abnormality of the small airways.

(b) Parenchymal disease of the lung is associated with diminished vital capacity.

(c) Bronchitis and emphysema typically reduce expiratory peak flow and maximum breathing capacity. In emphysema, residual volume and functional residual capacity are increased in proportion to vital capacity.

2. Ventilation

a. Alveolar membranes are exposed to a mixture of freshly inspired air plus previously expired air occupying dead space in the tracheobronchial tree and pharynx.

b. Tidal volume is calculated by dividing the minute volume (measured using an expiratory spirometer) by the respiratory rate. When it is small, a larger proportion of dead space air is rebreathed and the percentage of O_2 in the mixture reaching the alveolar surface is decreased. The ratio of dead space ventilation to total ventilation (V_D/V_T) is determined by measuring expired CO_2 ($Peco_2$) and arterial CO_2 ($Paco_2$):

$$\frac{V_D}{V_T} = \frac{Paco_2 - Peco_2}{Paco_2}$$

c. Occasionally, dead space is deliberately added to increase the retention of CO_2 when a patient is hyperventilating. This is the reason for having a patient with carpopedal spasm who is hyperventilating breathe into a paper bag. Similarly, dead space may be added during mechanical ventilation by inserting a tube or rebreathing vessel into the system.

3. Oxygenation

a. Oxygen content of the blood is measured as a part of arterial blood gases. How well oxygenated the blood is when it enters the aorta, however, depends upon the percentage of pulmonary blood flow that actually circulates through the capillaries in the walls of well-ventilated alveoli.

b. Normally about 2% of cardiac output consists of blood not exposed to pulmonary exchange surfaces. This includes blood passing through the bronchial vessels and also the venous outflow from the coronary arteries. It is called the physiological shunt.

c. Various disease states lead to pathological shunting of blood and decreased oxygenation. These include a number of irreversible parenchymal diseases of the lungs plus some potentially reversible conditions (e.g., atelectasis). In atelectasis, blood flowing through the atelectatic segments contributes to the shunt but can be corrected by good pulmonary toilet and ventilatory assistance. The quantity of shunt (Q_S/Q_T) is calculable from the measured alveolar-arterial oxygen difference ($AaDO_2$) after breathing 100% oxygen long enough to reach a steady state (usually 20 min). Since this calculation is undertaken principally in the setting of intensive care, we will not elaborate further. Suffice it that even when breathing 100% oxygen the oxygenation can vary greatly as a function of the quantity of shunt present.

III. Management

A. Only the most severe respiratory compromise is a contraindication to routine outpatient oral surgical care.

B. Asthma, principally an allergic phenomenon, may also be brought on by emotional factors (e.g., stress). Thus, in at least some asthmatics, management of stress related to oral surgery is essential. Sedation agents may be useful. Establishment of a good doctor-patient relationship is very helpful. During treatment of asthmatics in the outpatient setting, oxygen should be available and it should be possible to establish an intravenous line at short notice for hydration and administration of a bronchodilator.

C. The patient with significant respiratory disease who requires general anesthesia will usually be managed on an inpatient basis. Pulmonary function tests may be important to quantify the patient's degree of compromise, and a preoperative anesthesia consultation may be advisable.

D. The presence of severe degrees of respiratory compromise is a contraindication to the use of intermaxillary fixation, since IMF increases upper airway resistance and makes pulmonary toilet difficult to maintain. Thus, alternative fixation techniques may be appropriate for both fractures and osteotomies. If IMF is unavoidable, consideration should be given to elective tracheostomy.

E. Pulmonary complications of multiple trauma, including shock lung, may delay definitive repair of facial injuries. It is therefore essential to make every effort to evaluate facial fractures acutely and to treat these as completely as possible while other members of the trauma team carry out the emergency repair of other injuries. In discussions with other members of the trauma team, the oral surgeon should be prepared to make the case for early treatment of facial injuries.

F. Under normal circumstances homeostatic control of respiratory activity is keyed to blood levels of carbon dioxide detected by sense organs in the carotid bodies. However, in patients with chronic obstructive pulmonary disease and retention of carbon dioxide the respiratory response to carbon dioxide is diminished or absent and hypoxemia becomes the stimulus to respiration. Thus, in patients with chronic obstructive disease, the sudden exposure to oxygen in high concentration may eliminate the hypoxic stimulus, leading to hypoventilation and even apnea. Therefore 100% oxygen is inappropriate for patients with COPD who are breathing spontaneously.

G. Various CNS diseases (stroke, coma, seizure disorders, brain tumors, intoxication), certain medications, and advancing age all diminish the reflex protection of the airway. The risk of aspiration increases in proportion to the degree of debilitation.

   1. In severely debilitated patients, unless appropriate measures are taken, the risk of aspiration is heightened by poor oral hygiene, increasing dental disease, and the accumulation of bacteria-laden oral debris.

2. Oral surgical consultation on such patients should stress the importance of good oral hygiene. In some instances, especially when periodontal disease is severe, prophylactic extraction of teeth may be appropriate.

Hypertension

I. Hypertension is defined as a persistent elevation of blood pressure above values normative for age measured on repeated examinations.

A. As a disease entity, hypertension denotes mainly the elevation of diastolic pressure; 90 mm Hg is considered the upper level of normal for young adults. Blood pressure tends to increase with age; thus a given elevation of diastolic pressure is considered more significant in a young person than in an older one. Diastolic pressures in the ranges of 90-110, 110-130, and over 130 define mild, moderate, and severe hypertension, respectively.

B. When diastolic pressure is normal, systolic hypertension generally denotes the loss of elasticity of arterial vessel walls as seen in atherosclerosis. It can also be seen when cardiac output is elevated above normal (as in exercise, fever, anemia, thyrotoxicosis, or the presence of large AV fistulas).

II. The principal cause of diastolic hypertension is elevated total peripheral resistance, arterioles being the major resistive element in the vascular bed. Hypertension may be asymptomatic for long periods, and early manifestations (headache, palpitations, dizziness) can be vague. Epistaxis, hematuria, and proteinuria may also occur.

III. The principal consequences of uncorrected hypertension are renal failure, accelerated cardiovascular disease (including coronary artery disease and congestive failure), and cerebral vascular disease. Examination of the retinal vessels (funduscopic) is a useful means of assessing the damage caused by hypertension. Typical changes include compression of venules by arterioles (AV nicking), segmental constriction of arterioles, flame-shaped hemorrhages, and white exudative patches. Papilledema (seen as blurring of the disc margins and due to swelling that alters the visual plane of the optic disc) is suggestive of advanced disease and is a poor prognostic sign, as is elevation of BUN because of hypertensive renal disease.

IV. The work-up for hypertension includes the following:

A. Documentation of the presence of hypertension. Since situational anxiety associated with medical visits can elevate blood pressure, the documentation of mild to moderate hypertension can be difficult, requiring multiple determinations on separate visits or during a hospital admission. Elevation of blood pressure under general anesthesia is a significant finding.

B. Attempts to identify surgically correctable causes:

Pheochromocytoma of the adrenal cortex
Renal arterial occlusion

Renal parenchymal disease
Coarctation of the aorta

C. Assessment of damage already done by the condition, especially as regards

Renal function
Cardiovascular status

V. When surgically correctable causes have been ruled out, treatment of hypertension consists of drug therapy and dietary control.
   A. Since obesity is a contributing factor, weight reduction is part of the therapy of hypertension.
   B. Sodium restriction is another dietary approach to therapy. In restricting sodium, the goal is presumably to cause a fluid volume contraction and thus a fall in cardiac output and blood pressure.
   C. Drugs used in hypertensive therapy are
      1. Diuretics (including the thiazides and aldosterone antagonists)
      2. Ganglionic-blocking agents (reduce autonomic vasoconstriction)
      3. Norepinephrine antagonists (block production or compete for receptor sites)
      4. Smooth muscle relaxants
      5. Beta-adrenergic blocking agents (work at the receptor sites [propranolol])
      6. CNS agents (work on spinal or thalamic vasomotor centers)
      7. Tranquilizers (work on the psychogenic component of hypertension)
   D. Except in mild forms of hypertension, multiple drug therapy is used both to capitalize on drug synergy and to lower the required dosage for each agent, thereby reducing undesirable side effects.
   E. Management considerations in hypertensive patients are that
      1. Mild to moderate hypertension in adults is not a contraindication to oral surgical procedures under local anesthesia.
      2. Severe hypertension, if suspected on the basis of patient evaluation for elective surgery, should be fully worked up and treated prior to elective surgery.
      3. A diastolic pressure exceeding 150 mm Hg is grounds for admission to the hospital for work-up and immediate treatment.
      4. Emergency surgery in the patient discovered to be hypertensive may be undertaken with caution. If the degree of hypertension warrants it, parenteral therapy may be instituted in conjunction with the general anesthesia as required.

5. In the patient with long-standing hypertension and associated vascular disease, adequate perfusion of brain and myocardium may require elevated blood pressure. Then "normal" blood pressure can predispose to ischemia and damage of vital organs.

6. Since psychogenic factors play a significant role in hypertension, sedative techniques may prove useful. Once again, the value of a good doctor-patient relationship cannot be emphasized too strongly as a factor in the control of such factors.

7. Some antihypertensive medications complicate the administration of general anesthesia.

   a. The issue of whether to discontinue antihypertensive medications in anticipation of elective surgery under general anesthesia engenders much discussion. The oral surgeon should present this issue to the patient's physician and also to an anesthesia consultant as much in advance of surgery as possible.

   b. Generally one would like to eliminate long-acting drugs that inhibit homeostatic cardiovascular reflexes from the patient's therapeutic regimen. However, in a severely hypertensive patient the need for control of blood pressure may preclude discontinuance of therapy.

      (1) Special care must be exercised in the case of propranolol, a beta-blocking agent that is widely used today. When this medication is stopped abruptly, blood pressure may rebound to levels exceeding those before therapy was instituted. Propranolol therefore must be withdrawn gradually. Some anesthesiologists prefer to continue propranolol in the perioperative period.

      (2) The advisability of timely anesthesia consultation can hardly be emphasized enough.

8. Preoperative evaluation of the hypertensive patient must include an assessment of renal and cardiac function. Chest radiograph, ECG, BUN, creatinine, and electrolytes are appropriate baseline studies, with further work-up as may be dictated by historical and physical findings.

9. Hemostasis requires special attention in hypertensive patients. Not only may it be more difficult to achieve intraoperatively, but there is an increased risk of postoperative bleeding if the blood pressure, well-controlled during general anesthesia, increases significantly after the patient reaches the recovery room. Postoperative orders must both stress the careful monitoring of blood pressure and specify the level of pressure above which the house officer, surgeon, and/or attending physician should be called.

10. Conversely, because of the risk of ischemia in tissues fed by

vessels adapted to high blood pressure, all parties concerned should be vigilant about hypotension.

11. The patient with both hypertension and ischemic heart disease merits special attention. Blood pressure must be high enough to perfuse myocardial tissues through partially occluded coronary vessels. However, the work required of the heart to maintain elevated pressures leads to increased myocardial oxygen consumption and augments the likelihood of ischemia. Thus, in such a patient, the range of acceptable blood pressures is much narrower than normal and careful monitoring is required.

Renal disease

I. Both the causes and the manifestations of renal disease are many and varied.

II. Renal insufficiency may be acute or chronic.

A. In the acute condition, independent of etiology, the principal manifestations are oliguria and progressive azotemia.

1. Acute renal failure may occur for reasons extrinsic to the kidneys (prerenal azotemia):

Hypotension (shock)
Congestive heart failure
Extracellular fluid volume contraction, as occurs in dehydration, blood loss, or long-term uncompensated nasogastric suction

2. Intrinsic causes of acute renal failure include

Acute glomerulonephritis
Acute vasculitis
Acute urinary tract obstruction

3. Acute renal failure is also a feature of the hepatorenal syndrome, seen in some patients with advanced liver disease and portal hypertension. The hepatorenal syndrome typically occurs following massive gastrointestinal bleeding from varices and associated therapeutic measures.

B. Chronic renal failure is associated with an irreversible loss of functioning nephrons. Decreased size of the kidneys is demonstrated by appropriate radiographic or ultrasound studies.

C. Renal disease may advance insidiously until the patient is in severe failure. The work-up of such a patient must distinguish between acute renal failure and chronic renal insufficiency.

III. Laboratory parameters in renal failure include the following:

A. Glomerular filtration rate

1. The GFR is the principal index of renal function. Normal values are 100-150 ml/min, which is the volume of plasma removed from the approximately 1250 ml of blood passing through the two kidneys per minute. (Renal blood flow is about 25% of cardiac output.) Patients with renal disease

generally remain free of symptoms until the GFR falls below 10 ml/min.

2. In clinical practice the GFR is not measured directly but is estimated by measuring the clearance of various substances from the plasma. The clearance of endogenous creatinine is considered a good indicator of glomerular function.

   a. Creatinine clearance is measured by assaying creatinine in a 24 hr collection of urine and by measuring the serum creatinine once during that period.

$$\text{Clearance} = \frac{\text{mg/ml Urine} \times \text{ml Urine/min}}{\text{mg/ml Plasma}}$$

   b. Normal creatinine clearances

     Men: 97-140 ml/min
     Women: 85-125 ml/min

3. The GFR, as approximated from creatinine clearance, is the rate of passive filtration by the glomeruli. It tells nothing about active secretion and resorption of substances by the renal tubules.

B. Blood urea nitrogen

1. The BUN is another important parameter in renal failure. However, it reflects renal function only indirectly.

   a. It rises when renal function is severely compromised, but an increase in protein degradation (e.g., as occurs with gastrointestinal bleeding) will also increase the BUN.

   b. Conversely, a BUN elevated by renal disease will fall when dietary protein is restricted but this fall need not reflect any improvement in renal function.

2. The normal BUN is 8-25 mg/100 ml. Symptoms of uremia do not generally appear until the BUN exceeds 75-100 mg/100 ml. The BUN is a measure only of renal function under steady state conditions. In these circumstances a reading of 100 suggests a GFR of less than 10 ml/min.

C. Renal tubular function

1. The renal tubules concentrate the urine and maintain normal hydration.

2. They regulate acid-base balance through active secretion of hydrogen ion and resorption of bicarbonate and other bases.

3. They also maintain normal mineral and electrolyte balance and retrieve glucose and other essential substances from the glomerular filtrate.

D. In renal failure there are disturbances of the above functions that reflect both the variety and the severity of renal disease responsible. Most of these disturbances are correctable by measures that range from dietary control to renal dialysis and renal transplantation.

E. In addition to serum creatinine, creatinine clearance, and BUN, a work-up of renal function involves determination of plasma and urine electrolytes, glucose, protein, calcium, and phosphorus as well as serum osmolarity and urine specific gravity and H^+ concentration. Microscopic examination of the urine is performed to detect RBCs, WBCs, bacteria, crystalline and amorphous solids, and tubular casts, each of which have diagnostic significance.

IV. Management considerations include the following:

A. Compensated renal disease is not a contraindication to routine oral surgery or dental care.

B. It is fair to say that the patient in acute renal failure is not a candidate for routine dental care. Dental problems arising in this setting are treated emergently, and the goal is to palliate dental pain and treat dental infection with antibiotics (incision and drainage if indicated) until the renal problem is stabilized and more definitive dental treatment can be carried out.

C. The choice of medications for the patient in renal failure must be made with reference to the mode of excretion or degradation and with consideration of possible renal toxicity. A renal route of excretion is not necessarily a contraindication to drug use, but adjustment of the dosage is called for. Such therapy should be instituted in consultation with the patient's primary physician.

D. Severe uremia may interfere with normal hemostatic mechanisms, particularly platelet function. Wound healing may also be compromised. However, the patient who has compensated renal disease (with a BUN less than 75 mg/100 ml) and who is not in negative nitrogen balance from a protein-wasting nephropathy will generally heal normally. The patient in chronic renal failure is prone to hypocalcemia and hyperphosphatemia, which, with other factors, may lead to secondary hyperparathyroidism. Osteomalacia and osteitis fibrosa may develop, and the possibility of such disorders of bone metabolism should be taken into account when a renal failure patient is being evaluated for surgery involving the facial bones.

E. Moderate renal disease, not productive of symptoms by itself, may become significant in the face of other medical problems (e.g., heart disease). Thus the patient who has a failing myocardium and also renal insufficiency may go into congestive failure at an early stage due to hypoperfusion of intrinsically damaged kidneys and resultant fluid retention. Similarly a patient prone to arrhythmias may be very sensitive to disturbances of electrolyte balance produced by renal disease, such as hypokalemia or hypercalcemia.

F. Compensated renal disease is not necessarily a contraindication to general anesthesia, but such patients deserve very careful preoperative evaluation to assess the level of renal function and to detect and correct electrolyte and other imbalances. The presence of renal disease may contraindicate some anesthetic agents and favor others. An anesthesia consultation prior to surgery is appropriate for the patient with significant renal disease.

G. Patients receiving dialysis are closely monitored by the attending physician or nephrologist. When oral surgical care is called for, it is usually necessitated by a dental emergency, and in these cases treatment is usually palliative.

   1. Simple outpatient procedures (e.g., extraction of teeth) are not generally a problem under local anesthesia, and the use of lidocaine (Xylocaine) with epinephrine is not contraindicated.

   2. Special considerations in the dialysis patient

      a. Choice of medications and regulation of dose. The medications for such a patient should be selected in consultation with the patient's physician. Penicillin is not contraindicated, but the dose will be regulated on the basis of residual renal function and the patient's frequency of dialysis. Given the difficulty of eliminating potassium by dialysis, sodium may be substituted for the more usual potassium penicillin.

      b. Anticoagulation. Since a dialysis patient is anticoagulated during dialysis runs, surgical procedures are best performed midway between runs, if possible.

      c. Elevated risk of hepatitis. It may be reasonable to institute hepatitis precautions for dialysis patients.

      d. Long-term management. When a dialysis patient is seen, it is worthwhile to discuss long-term management with the attending physician, especially as regards possible renal transplantation.

      e. The chronic dialysis patient will usually have a surgically created AV shunt (radial artery to cephalic vein) to facilitate arterial and venous cannulation during dialysis runs. These shunts are potentially infectable by transient bacteremias. Thus it is appropriate to eliminate dental foci of infection and to use prophylactic antibiotic coverage for invasive dental treatment.

H. Under favorable circumstances the renal transplant patient will maintain essentially normal renal function. Unless his donor kidney came from an identical twin or other individual with identical histocompatibility antigens, he will require chronic immunosuppressive therapy. Such therapy reduces his capacity to fight infection. Therefore it is essential that he be maintained in an optimum state of dental health. The best time for evaluating such a patient and providing for his dental needs is before the start of immunosuppression. It is worthwhile setting up a program for routine preoperative screening of prospective renal transplant patients.

Hepatic dysfunction and alcoholism

I. The liver is the largest gland in the body and performs a multiplicity of functions including the following:

   A. It secretes bile.

     1. Bile salts are essential to the emulsification and absorption of fatty substances from the intestines.

     2. Bile contains pigmented substances, bilirubin and related compounds, that are excreted conjugated to glucuronic acid. These pigments are breakdown products of hemoglobin from the lysis of RBCs.

     3. Bile contains substances deactivated, conjugated, and excreted by the liver—e.g., drugs, endogenous substances such as adrenal and gonadal steroid hormones, and toxic substances ingested as part of the diet.

   B. It plays an essential role in the metabolism of carbohydrates and fats, and it stores carbohydrate as glycogen.

   C. It is central to protein metabolism, including degradation of amino acids and formation of urea.

   D. It manufactures plasma proteins, including albumin.

   E. It produces many specialized substances (e.g., proteins active in the immune system and clotting Factors such as II, VII, IX, and X).

   F. It has a dual blood supply. In addition to arterial flow, from which it derives oxygen, the liver also receives the venous outflow from the gastrointestinal tract via the portal circulation. All substances absorbed through the GI tract must therefore traverse the liver before entering the general circulation.

II. Categories of liver disease of greatest interest to the oral and maxillofacial surgeon are hepatitis and cirrhosis.

   A. Hepatitis denotes any acute inflammatory condition of the liver. There are many kinds—ranging from hepatitis caused by toxic chemicals, such as carbon tetrachloride and chloroform, to hepatitis caused by infectious agents, including bacteria and viruses.

     1. Hepatotoxicity sets the upper limits on safe dosage for many medications, including some anesthetic agents, anticonvulsants, many antibiotics, thiazide diuretics, and oral contraceptives.

     2. Of prime concern to the oral surgeon is the patient with acute viral hepatitis or chronic active hepatitis (carrier state), because of the risk of acquiring the disease via inadvertent inoculation with contaminated instruments.

       a. There are several types of viral hepatitis—including A, B, and non-A, non-B. Hepatitis is also a feature of mononucleosis in about 5% of cases.

       b. Of the viral hepatitides, types B and non-A, non-B are the biggest concern because both can be transmitted percutaneously and because fulminant disease has a significant rate of mortality (up to 15% in some series). In addition,

10% of patients develop chronic liver disease (chronic active hepatitis) and patients with a history of hepatitis have a risk of liver cancer exceeding that of non-hepatitis patients.

3. Measures to prevent hepatitis include the following:

   a. An effective and safe vaccine for the prevention of type B hepatitis. Fears that use of this vaccine might place the recipient at risk of acquired immunodeficiency syndrome (AIDS) have been shown to be ill-founded. Many hospitals make vaccination available to at-risk personnel. Oral and maxillofacial surgeons and surgical support staff are well advised to seek vaccination if they do not already have antibodies.

   b. Hepatitis-B–specific immune globulin. This reduces the likelihood of contracting hepatitis-B after percutaneous exposure by a factor of 3 to 10. Pooled gamma globulin is not effective in type B and is only somewhat effective in non-A, non-B prophylaxis. At best, it is a poor substitute for vaccination in the prevention of hepatitis type B.

   c. Other prophylactic measures include proper isolation, proper sterilization of instruments, and proper disposal of needles and contaminated materials (drapes, sponges, and sutures). The oral and maxillofacial surgeon should be thoroughly familiar with institutional protocols for dealing with known or suspected hepatitis patients, including instructions on the proper handling, containment, and identification of laboratory specimens for the protection of other hospital personnel.

   d. It is important to bear in mind that the greatest risk of exposure to hepatitis comes not from known or suspected cases but from unknown cases. Therefore one's routine sterile technique and other practices should be fastidious enough to confer a reasonable degree of protection from any patient. Inoculation can occur via the conjunctiva, and proper eye protection tends to be underutilized.

4. Whether or not a person with an occupational risk of hepatitis elects to be vaccinated, he should be tested for antibodies, since 5-15% of the population has hepatitis-B antibodies.

   a. In the event of accidental inoculation when the status of the source is unknown, it is appropriate to test the source for hepatitis-B antigen (HBsAg), antibody (anti-HBs), and also SGPT (alanine aminotransferase) as an index of hepatocellular inflammation.

   b. Accidental inoculation from patients in the following groups merits heightened concern:

Those with acute viral hepatitis of an unknown type
Those institutionalized with Down's syndrome
Those receiving hemodialysis
Patients of (recent) Asian origin
Male homosexuals
Known drug abusers

5. Signs and symptoms of acute viral hepatitis include jaundice preceded by a variable period of other nonspecific constitutional and GI symptoms including dark urine (94% of patients), fatigue (91%), anorexia (90%), nausea (87%), and fever (76%). The onset of jaundice is usually accompanied by hepatic enlargement and right upper quadrant tenderness. Symptoms noted in the preicteric phase tend to increase in severity as the jaundice becomes manifest and to abate as the jaundice subsides.

6. Following are some management considerations in hepatitis:
   a. No elective procedure should be undertaken in a patient with acute viral hepatitis.
   b. Any emergency procedure in a patient with acute viral hepatitis should be undertaken only with full precautions, as noted above.
   c. When a choice exists, local anesthesia is preferable to general anesthesia. Many agents used for or in conjunction with general anesthesia have a degree of hepatotoxicity or are metabolized in the liver and may be poorly tolerated by the patient with acute viral hepatitis.
   d. All drugs for use by hepatitis patients should be selected with reference to possible hepatotoxicity.

B. Cirrhosis
   1. This term denotes a fibrosis disrupting the lobular architecture, on which normal hepatic function depends. If the ongoing disease process is arrested at an early stage, excellent healing may occur with preservation of normal function. When the disease process has been long standing, some healing may occur but widespread disruption of lobular architecture may prevent the return of normal liver function.
   2. Cirrhosis is seen in the 10% of patients whose viral hepatitis (type B) goes on to become chronic active hepatitis.
   3. The most common cause of cirrhosis in the United States is chronic alcoholism. Malnutrition is thought to be a contributing factor in this setting but does not independently lead to cirrhosis in the absence of alcoholism.
   4. Because of the liver's remarkable regenerative capacity and built-in redundancy, the onset of cirrhosis is insidious. Early presenting symptoms can be nonspecific and tend to be masked by the symptoms of alcoholism and malnutrition. The two primary manifestations of cirrhosis are hepatocellular dysfunction and portal hypertension.

a. Hepatocellular dysfunction

(1) Active hepatocellular disease is suggested by elevation of liver enzymes in the blood including SGOT (aspartate aminotransferase) and LDH. Alkaline phosphatase also tends to be elevated, especially when there is obstruction of biliary drainage. As hepatocellular disease progresses, serum albumin falls while globulins rise. Total protein tends to fall and the A/G ratio reverses.

(2) As noted previously, clotting Factors VII, IX, and X along with prothrombin are manufactured in the liver. The prothrombin time (PT) increases in response to decreased production of these factors; however, prolongation of the PT is a late sign of liver disease and denotes severe hepatocellular dysfunction.

(3) Carbohydrate metabolism may become disordered, with loss of glycogen stores and an increasing tendency toward hypoglycemia.

(4) Ammonia, a product of the action of bacterial deaminases on amino acids in the intestines, is normally removed from the portal circulation by the liver and converted to urea. In liver failure, ammonia accumulates in the bloodstream, leading to hyperreflexia, a characteristic tremor (asterixis or "liver flap"), and hepatic encephalopathy (marked by confusion, drowsiness, and inappropriate behavior). Uncorrected ammonia intoxication can eventually cause hepatic coma and death.

(5) The principal mode of treatment for hepatic encephalopathy is to decrease ammonia production by sharply limiting dietary intake of protein and by administering, orally or by enema, an antibiotic (e.g., neomycin) that kills intestinal bacteria but is poorly absorbed by the GI tract.

b. Portal hypertension

(1) Portal hypertension is a manifestation of advanced destruction of the hepatic lobules such that the normal flow of portal blood is partially obstructed. In this setting, portosystemic venous collaterals become dilated, shunting blood from the portal to the systemic circulation without allowing it to pass through the liver. This contributes to hepatic encephalopathy, since substances absorbed by the intestines enter the general circulation without being processed by the liver.

(2) The most significant consequence of portal hypertension is GI bleeding from esophageal varices. Such bleeding may be catastrophic in its own right; but, secondarily, the breakdown of blood in the intes-

tines leads to additional ammonia production and can precipitate hepatic encephalopathy and coma. Nasogastric suctioning, cleansing enemas, and other measures are employed to eliminate blood from the GI tract.

(3) The hypoalbuminemia that is a feature of hepatocellular dysfunction lowers the colloid osmotic pressure of blood and predisposes to edema. This tendency, coupled with portal hypertension, leads to weeping of serum from serosal surfaces in the abdomen, resulting in ascites. By a similar mechanism, pleural effusions are also seen in liver failure.

III. Alcoholism is responsible for numerous sociological and medical problems. To highlight some of these

A. Alcoholic intoxication is a major factor in the occurrence of automotive and other forms of trauma. Alcohol is a CNS depressant, adversely affecting both mentation and motor skills.

B. Chronic alcohol ingestion is a factor in the occurrence of several diseases of the nervous system, including

Wernicke-Korsakoff syndrome (encephalopathy)
Alcoholic polyneuropathy
Pellagra
Cerebellar degeneration

C. Alcohol ingestion leads to pancreatitis in some persons, which may present as an acute abdominal catastrophe with autolysis of the pancreas, pseudocyst formation, and widespread damage to the abdominal viscera.

D. Abstinence from alcohol after long periods of intoxication produces serious medical consequences jointly referred to as the alcohol withdrawal syndrome. The principal features of the syndrome are

1. Tremulousness—the earliest and most universal manifestation of alcohol withdrawal; appearing even after short periods of abstinence

2. Auditory or visual hallucinations—occurring in at least 25% of tremulous patients during alcohol withdrawal

3. Alcoholic seizures—usually of the grand mal type, usually self-limited, and tending to occur within 48 hr of the cessation of drinking; as a rule the EEGs of such patients are normal at times removed from periods of seizure activity

4. Delirium tremens (DTs)—having a fatal outcome in at least 10% of cases; the most serious feature of alcohol withdrawal

   a. Onset typically occurs several days after cessation of alcohol consumption, when other symptoms of withdrawal (tremulousness, hallucinations, and seizures) may already have resolved.

   b. Delirium tremens is variable in severity.

(1) It is mild and non–life threatening in the majority of cases. When mild, it may present as restlessness, agitation, and insomnia of several days' duration.

(2) Full-blown DTs is characterized by profound confusion and disorientation, agitation, tremors, insomnia, and symptoms of autonomic system hyperactivity and hypermetabolic state—profuse diaphoresis, tachycardia, dilated pupils, temperature elevation. Large fluid and electrolyte shifts can occur, and patients may require many liters of fluid replacement per day, along with careful monitoring of electrolytes to prevent hypotension and cardiovascular collapse. The patient may also require active cooling to prevent hyperpyrexic damage to vital organs such as the brain and kidneys.

(3) Agitation in DTs is treated with sedative agents, chlordiazepoxide (Librium) being one that is preferred. Cumulative doses up to 400 mg/da may be required, and care must be taken that the dose is tapered to prevent overmedication as the delirium resolves.

IV. Management issues in cirrhosis and alcoholism include the following:

A. A typical setting for the occurrence of delirium tremens is the alcoholic patient admitted with trauma who becomes acutely and involuntarily abstinent as a consequence of the hospitalization. Since the likelihood and severity of DTs reflect the extent and duration of alcohol consumption, a careful history of alcohol intake should be obtained. Patients tend to downplay their actual consumption, sometimes flagrantly. Furthermore, many alcoholics do not conform to the stereotype. Thus it is easy to be fooled.

B. Maxillomandibular fixation for facial fractures combines poorly with full-blown DTs in the convalescent period. Fixation is not well tolerated by the agitated and disoriented patient. Fixation may be disrupted by the seizure activity that sometimes occurs early in withdrawal, and the increased respiratory demands of the patient in a hypermetabolic state may be poorly met because of the increased upper airway resistance imposed by fixation. In the known or suspected alcoholic with a risk of DTs, there is a premium on early operative intervention so that fracture repair will not be postponed by acute withdrawal symptoms.

1. Furthermore, consideration should be given to augmented fracture fixation techniques, which allow maxillomandibular fixation to be discontinued if necessary without placing the fracture repair in jeopardy.

2. Open reduction or plating will lessen the need for intermaxillary fixation.

C. The patient with end-stage liver disease, as manifested by portal hypertension, a history of GI bleeding, and chronic elevation of the prothrombin time, is a poor candidate for elective oral and maxillofacial surgery. Malnutrition, including compromised protein metabolism frequently seen in this setting, may interfere with healing after procedures such as fracture repair.

1. The patient with a PT elevated above 18 sec (greater than 1.5× control) who requires surgery with a risk of significant blood loss (e.g., multiple extractions) will need special preoperative attention. This is a setting in which vitamin K administration is appropriate.

2. Depending upon the preoperative hematocrit, either fresh whole blood or fresh frozen plasma may be transfused preoperatively to replace deficient clotting factors. This therapy also increases the level of plasma proteins, which may reduce the tendency to form edema and also provide a measure of nutritional support. If the patient has a history of GI bleeding with multiple transfusions, the presence of unusual antibodies may make cross-matching difficult. Therefore it is appropriate to have several units of blood set up for such patients in advance of surgery, should unusual blood loss be encountered.

D. When a severely alcoholic patient is admitted with traumatic injuries or with other problems, his dietary intake is likely to improve rather suddenly in the hospital environment. In a malnourished individual deficient in thiamine, a sudden increase in carbohydrate intake may precipitate Wernicke's encephalopathy unless the deficiency is corrected. Thus, admitting orders for severe alcoholics should specify multiple vitamins including thiamine 50-200 mg IM.

E. Admitting orders for severe alcoholics should also specify the frequent recording of vital signs, with attention to onset of tremulousness, for which appropriate doses of diazepoxide (Librium) or other sedative agent should be prescribed.

F. Signs of intoxication or delirium in known or suspected alcoholics may mask or confuse the identification of other serious problems (e.g., hyper- or hypoglycemia, an expanding subdural hematoma due to head trauma [which is not uncommon in severe alcoholism]).

G. Chronic alcoholics may have a long history of repetitive facial trauma. This can complicate the physical examination of the patient and also the interpretation of radiographs. Thus, for example, a patient with evidence of a new periorbital swelling and flattening of the malar eminence may have an old untreated fracture underlying a new soft tissue injury.

1. Careful inspection of the radiograph should help in judging the age of the injury; but it is easy to be fooled, especially on suboptimum radiographs obtained from an uncooperative patient.

2. The distinction between old and new injuries is important because of their markedly different operative requirements. One may well elect not to treat an old zygomatic fracture despite some cosmetic impairment as long as ocular function has remained normal. Alternatively, if the patient, upon sober reflection, elects to have an old injury repaired, one must be ready to do the several osteotomies that this may require.

H. Patients with a history of heavy use of alcohol may detoxify barbiturates and other agents more rapidly than normal. This has a bearing on anesthesia management, because the effective dose for such agents is likely to be increased.

I. The hyperemia induced by alcohol rapidly dissipates and reduces the effectiveness of local anesthetic agents, even those containing a vasoconstrictor. Therefore larger amounts than usual may be required in performing emergency procedures on an intoxicated patient.

J. Given the current concern over informed consent, some thought is warranted on the subject of elective surgery on intoxicated patients. Intoxication compromises the validity of consent; thus there may be legal as well as medical grounds for refusing to perform elective surgery on an intoxicated individual.

Coagulation and bleeding disorders

I. Bleeding and clotting disorders may be either inherited or acquired. In the majority of instances such disorders are known to the patient. When a patient is unaware of a problem with bleeding or coagulation, it is likely to be an acquired defect of recent onset, perhaps secondary to an intercurrent medical problem or its treatment.

II. It is nearly impossible to discuss coagulation and bleeding disorders without offering a depiction of the clotting cascade (Fig. 4-4). Such diagrams suggest the complexity of the clotting mechanisms but fail to do justice to the dynamic nature of a system that can seal breaches in the vascular bed without allowing disseminated clot formation. There is little clinical utility in memorizing such a diagram, but it is worth noting that concentrates are available for the replacement of all factors whose lack produces serious bleeding and also that techniques exist for assaying specific factor deficiencies.

III. Since most patients with inherited coagulopathies have a previously established diagnosis, the management of such patients involves confirmatory factor assay and planning for replacement therapy. In most hospitals this is undertaken in consultation with a member of the hematology department and/or transfusion service.

A. The advent of agents that help stabilize clots by inhibiting fibrolysis has simplified the management of many patients with

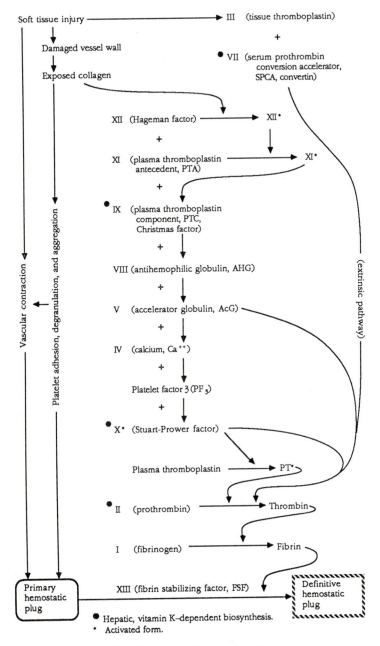

Fig. 4-4 Coagulation cascade.

inherited coagulopathies, especially classical hemophiliacs (Factor VIII deficiency, sex-linked, recessive inheritance).

B. Epsilon-aminocaproic acid (EACA)(Amicar) is such an agent, and its use has significantly reduced the requirement for Factor VIII infusion and also length of hospital stay for elective surgical procedures.

C. The clinical characteristics of the inherited coagulopathies are quite variable from patient to patient with the same disorder, and some patients will produce enough of a deficient factor to suppress clinical symptoms. Thus, for example, a patient with classical hemophilia-A might remain symptom free (no spontaneous hemorrhage) with Factor VIII levels of 3-5% and need factor replacement only in the event of trauma or for surgical procedures.

IV. A screening history on any new patient should include questions about bleeding:

> Family history of bleeding
> Unusual bleeding associated with previous surgical procedures, lacerations, or venipuncture
> Epistaxis
> Easy bruising
> Ingestion of aspirin or aspirin-containing compounds
> Anticoagulant therapy
> Liver disease or other major medical illness
> Chronic use of oral antibiotics

Since significant amounts of vitamin K are produced by the intestinal flora, chronic ingestion of broad-spectrum antibiotics, especially in the nutritionally compromised person, is known to contribute to a deficiency of vitamin K, upon which the synthesis in the liver of clotting Factors II, VII, IX, and X depends.

V. Any patient with a positive or a suggestive history deserves further evaluation, especially if he is being worked up for a significant surgical procedure. An approach to the evaluation of a patient with an undiagnosed bleeding disorder includes the following:

A. Simply referring the patient with a positive history to a hematologist is the "easy way out," and may be required as a matter of policy in some institutions. However, this approach is not consistent with a philosophy of care for the whole patient, nor is it intellectually satisfying.

   1. Ordering a large battery of tests may lead to a diagnosis but is also very wasteful.

   2. The character of bleeding noted in the past is an important aid to diagnosis.

      a. Easy bruisability, bleeding into the integument (including skin and mucous membranes), and prolonged bleeding from cuts and venipuncture sites all suggest a problem with platelets or with the blood vessels themselves (e.g., capillary fragility or a defect in vascular contraction).

    b. Spontaneous bleeding into joints (hemarthrosis) or visceral organs and muscle tissue suggests a congenital or acquired clotting factor deficiency.

B. Since organic disease is involved in acquired coagulopathies, the following should be ruled out by history and by laboratory studies as may be indicated by the historical findings:

Renal failure

Hepatic dysfunction

Leukemia and related disorders (megakaryocytes in the marrow replaced by tumor cells)

Polycythemia (excessive RBCs mechanically interfering with clot formation)

Severe infections, especially gram-negative ones (may lead to a consumption coagulopathy or disseminated intravascular coagulation [DIC])

C. In the absence of evidence of organic disease, routine screening studies consist of PT, PTT, and platelet count.

    1. If the platelet count is decreased, the causes of thrombocytopenia are sought.

Idiopathic thrombocytopenic purpura (ITP)

Hypersplenism of various etiologies with sequestration of platelets

Leukemia

Aplastic anemia

Drug reaction (thiazide diuretics, sulfonamides, antimalarial drugs, etc.)

Viral illness (thrombocytopenia a feature of mononucleosis in about 5% of cases, bone marrow biopsy may be required)

    2. If the platelet count is normal, the PT and PTT are determined.

    3. A platelet count less than 40,000 is an emergency situation because of the risk of intracranial bleeding. Medical admission is appropriate.

VI. Management of the anticoagulated patient

    A. Indications for anticoagulation include

        1. Thrombophlebitis and phlebothrombosis

        2. Embolic cerebral vascular accidents and transient ischemic attacks

        3. Prevention of mural thrombus formation following subendocardial MI

        4. Atrial fibrillation, to prevent clot formation in the atrial appendage

        5. Coronary artery bypass graft surgery

        6. Cardiac valve replacement

7. Vascular reconstruction and microvascular surgery
8. Hemodialysis for renal failure

B. Anticoagulants

1. Heparin is a naturally occurring substance found in most cells. It blocks the conversion of fibrinase to fibrin and retards the formation of thrombin from prothrombin by interfering with the activity of thromboplastin. It also decreases platelet adhesiveness. Heparin activity is assayed via the PTT or by clotting time.

   a. Heparin administered intravenously has a rapid onset of action and is rapidly metabolized. Therefore its anticoagulant effect is easy to regulate but requires close monitoring.

   b. The action of heparin is rapidly reversed by protamine sulfate.

   c. Heparin anticoagulation is used almost exclusively in a hospital setting. Given the indications for its use, it is likely that oral surgery to be performed on a heparinized patients will be of an emergency nature. The degree of urgency of the procedure must be balanced against the risk of transiently discontinuing heparin therapy. Heparin need be discontinued only an hour or so before an intended procedure if approved by the patient's physician. Patients requiring longer-term anticoagulant therapy are switched to warfarin sodium.

2. Warfarin sodium (Coumadin) is a structural analog of vitamin K and competitively inhibits the vitamin K–dependent biosynthesis of Factors II (prothrombin), VII, IX, and X in the liver.

   a. The action of warfarin is assayed via the PT. Its therapeutic range lies between 1.5 and 2 times the normal control time. Thus if control is 12 sec, the therapeutic range of warfarin is 18-24 sec.

   b. In contradistinction to heparin, warfarin (taken by mouth) is used on an outpatient basis; and many patients are chronically anticoagulated with this agent. Therefore it is not unusual for elective surgery to be performed on a patient taking warfarin. To manage such a patient successfully, it is necessary to consider the following:

      (1) The patient receiving warfarin may be anticoagulated for therapeutic or prophylactic reasons. The strength of the indication for anticoagulation will vary from patient to patient, and thus consultation with the patient's physician is appropriate to determine whether the anticoagulant therapy can be discontinued transiently and how close to normal the patient's PT is.

      (2) When a dose of warfarin is given, its peak effect

occurs approximately 48 hr later. Thus there is a latency period before an alteration in dose will have an appreciable effect. Most patients take their warfarin once a day, at bedtime.

(3) Elective oral surgery can be performed with a PT of 18 sec or less (20 sec or less in an emergency). The patient should be told to expect some oozing of blood.

(4) It is appropriate to check the patient's PT on the day of an elective procedure. When this represents a hardship for the patient, the more removed the last PT is from the time of surgery the more important it is to review the last several readings to see how much variation there has been. The greater the range of fluctuation, the more important it becomes to check the PT on the day of surgery.

(5) If the PT is 18 sec or less, no alteration in warfarin dose is called for; nor is it required to omit a dose.

(6) If the PT is substantially < 18 sec, the patient's physician should be notified so he can review the patient's status and adjust the warfarin dose as necessary.

(7) If the PT is > 18 sec, the patient should be rescheduled, warfarin discontinued 48 hr before surgery, and the PT checked once again before surgery to confirm an acceptable value for surgery and as a basis for advising the patient regarding when to resume taking the medication.

(8) After most minor procedures, and especially if there is a strong indication for anticoagulation, warfarin is appropriately restarted on the evening of surgery. It should be borne in mind, however, that the PT will probably continue to fall toward normal during the first 12-24 hr following surgery if the patient has been instructed to omit the previous one or two doses.

(9) A PT > 2 × control should be reported to the patient's physician, so he can more closely regulate warfarin administration.

(10) Although vitamin K reverses the effect of warfarin, its use should be avoided in patients with an indication for anticoagulation. Vitamin K can produce what has been termed *rebound hypercoagulability,* and it should be reserved for use in bleeding emergencies or to correct a deficiency state (e.g., malnutrition, severe liver disease).

(11) Physicians vary in their willingness to permit

manipulation of anticoagulation in their patients. The oral surgeon will need to establish an understanding about this with each physician.

3. Aspirin is occasionally used for its negative effect on platelet adhesiveness as a means of preventing platelet thrombi, which are precursors to definitive clot formation. Aspirin also decreases the hepatic biosynthesis of Factors II and VII and therefore potentiates the effects of warfarin. The patient taking warfarin is instructed to avoid all aspirin-containing medications. This can be difficult to do, owing to the large number of analgesic preparations that contain aspirin but are not conspicuously labeled as such. Occasionally a patient will have an unusual sensitivity to aspirin, and a single tablet can wipe out the adhesiveness of an entire cohort of platelets.

4. Low–molecular weight dextrans are used intravenously as anticoagulants, especially to maintain the patency of vascular grafts.

5. Elevation of the PT is a sign of severe hepatocellular disease, usually secondary to alcohol-induced cirrhosis. Alcohol also decreases both platelet count and platelet function in some persons. When aspirin-containing compounds are used for "hangover," their effect with alcohol may be additive.

VII. The following locally applied measures may be useful in the management of bleeding:

A. Fastidious suturing technique

B. Use of the smallest flaps possible consistent with good surgical technique (i.e., smallest incisions and minimal stripping of periosteum)

C. Use of absorbable gelatin sponges, oxycellulose, and other agents to provide a matrix for clot formation

D. Topical thrombin to control bleeding from denuded surfaces

E. Adhesives such as are used for attaching ostomy bags to control mucosal bleeding

F. Small pledgets of gauze or cotton tied in an embrasure space with silk suture material or dental floss to tamponade spontaneous bleeding from interdental papillae

G. Silver nitrate sticks

Seizure disorders

I. A seizure may be defined as uncontrolled motor activity, sensation, behavior, consciousness, or a combination of these produced by abnormal electrical activity in the brain.

A. The most dramatic type is grand mal, or major motor seizure. Generally a single episode in an otherwise healthy person is not a life-threatening event, especially if it is observed and supportive care can be rendered.

B. Status epilepticus, defined as repetitive seizures without intervening return of consciousness, can be life threatening, mainly because of hypoxic brain damage. It may occur secondary to

Loss of control of the thoracic respiratory muscles
Upper airway obstruction by foreign bodies (e.g., dentures or food)
Aspiration of gastric contents

II. The history of a seizure disorder should come to light during the evaluation of any new patient.
   A. The oral surgeon must document the frequency of seizures, their duration and type, any premonitory signs and postictal sequelae, any precipitating factors, and the antiseizure medications taken (including dosage).
   B. Well-controlled epileptic patients withstand routine oral surgery as well as the average patient. Anxiety may be a precipitating factor in unstable or poorly controlled epileptics but is not a major factor in well-controlled patients. Sedation may be a useful adjunct to therapy for the same indications as would apply in normal patients. However, consideration should be given to the additive effect of agents used for sedation in combination with antiseizure medications already being taken.
   C. Syncopal episodes occur in many nonepileptic patients and may be accompanied at times by short bursts of seizurelike tonic or clonic movement of the extremities. Seizure patients also experience syncope, and this may occur without provoking a seizure. However, transient hypotension and cerebral hypoxia, which account for loss of consciousness in syncope, may initiate seizure activity, especially in the poorly controlled epileptic patient.
      1. Most syncopal episodes occur after an injection of a local anesthetic agent or venipuncture. Careful observation of the patient will normally reveal premonitory signs before syncope occurs—dizziness, diaphoresis, slowing of the pulse, sudden thirst, blurring of vision.
      2. Raising the feet, lowering the head, use of spirits of ammonia, and inhalation of O_2 if rapidly available may help abort a syncopal episode and are particularly useful in epileptics.
   D. Many epileptic patients experience an aura and know when a seizure is imminent; some may be able to give warning.
III. When a seizure occurs, most of the care applied is supportive.
   A. The patient is placed in a position that minimizes the potential for physical injury from unrestrained motor activity.
   B. He is observed for airway obstruction, and measures are taken to relieve it should it occur. This is usually a simple matter of correctly positioning the head and neck so the tongue does not obstruct the pharynx. An oral airway is seldom necessary, and its use may damage the teeth. Dentures are removed whenever possible.
   C. For an isolated single seizure no medication is called for acutely.

If the patient has been taking phenytoin (Dilantin) or other assayable agents, blood may be drawn to ascertain whether the drug level is within the therapeutic range.

D. The patient's physician or neurologist should be informed so he can review the patient's therapeutic regimen.

E. After the seizure the patient may be able to go home but should be accompanied by an adult.

F. If the patient has no previous history of seizure, it is appropriate that he be conveyed to an emergency facility for evaluation. A careful description of the seizure will be helpful to any neurologist who subsequently sees him. The patient's posture, his head, eye, and limb position, and the laterality of his motor activity and character of his movements are diagnostically significant.

IV. Status epilepticus requires aggressive management.

A. The major priority is to establish an adequate airway. If this cannot be secured by positioning the patient properly or by use of an oral airway, then endotracheal intubation is called for. Endotracheal intubation has the advantage of allowing mechanical ventilation, and it also prevents aspiration of gastric contents.

B. An IV line should be established; but before infusion of any medications is started, a blood sample should be drawn for determination of antiseizure medication and serum glucose levels (hypoglycemia being a precipitating factor and one that is easily correctable). A glucose infusion (50 ml of 50% solution) can be given immediately after the blood sample is drawn.

C. Drug therapy is started.

1. Diazepam (Valium) is a rapid-acting and effective agent in all forms of epilepsy. It has less of a respiratory depressant effect than do the barbiturates, which are also used for acute management.

2. Phenytoin (Dilantin) is used but is less effective than diazepam acutely. It has the advantage of minimal respiratory depressant and sedative effect. Given the short duration of diazepam's antiseizure effect, phenytoin may be given adjunctively for long-term seizure control.

3. On occasion, general anesthesia is called for in the attempt to break status epilepticus, and it has the advantage of allowing use of muscle relaxants. This helps prevent physical exhaustion from persistent violent muscular activity. It also allows good control of respiration.

D. Especially if the patient has no prior history of seizure activity, an aggressive effort must be made to establish the cause. Typical causes or exacerbating factors include

1. Inflammatory lesions: meningitis, encephalitis (either bacterial or viral)

2. Traumatic lesions (subdural, epidural, or subarachnoid hemorrhage)

3. Electrolyte imbalances (including hyponatremia, hyperkalemia, hypocalcemia, hypomagnesemia)
4. Hypoglycemia
5. Uremia
6. Expanding intracranial tumors and other space-occupying lesions (e.g., aneurysm)
7. Increased CSF pressure
8. Inappropriate discontinuation of antiseizure medication, especially in combination with alcohol withdrawal
9. Ingestion of toxic substances

V. Some additional considerations in management of the patient with seizures follow:

   A. General anesthesia is not contraindicated. For unstable patients a hospital setting or day care unit may be the preferable site. An epileptic patient is probably less likely to have a seizure during general anesthesia than at any other time. An IV dose of phenytoin may be given intraoperatively to ensure that postanesthetic excitement does not initiate seizure activity. The preoperative evaluation of such a patient should include assay of blood levels of antiseizure medications.

   B. Intermaxillary fixation increases the risk of upper airway obstruction and aspiration of gastric contents in a fracture or osteotomy patient. If IMF is unavoidable in this setting, consideration should be given to the use of non-IMF fixation techniques when applicable.

   C. Careful monitoring of antiseizure medication blood levels is indicated. It may be worth discussing with the patient's physician a temporary increase in dosage during a period of intermaxillary fixation.

   D. When such a patient is hospitalized, there may be a real benefit in seeing that he is assigned to a multiple bed room. Surveillance by other patients can provide an added safety factor in the event of a seizure that might otherwise go unobserved in a single-bed room.

Endocrine dysfunction
Diabetes mellitus

I. Diabetes is a disease in which a defect of insulin production or secretion leads to difficulty in maintaining a normal range of serum glucose levels. Diabetics may experience hyperglycemia or hypoglycemia, both of which can have fatal consequences.

   A. This disease varies widely in severity—from mild adult onset, controllable by diet alone, to severe juvenile onset, requiring lifetime insulin injections and careful monitoring of urinary or even serum glucose levels.

   B. Brittle diabetics have metabolic disease that is unstable and difficult to regulate. They are usually thin, with juvenile onset of symptoms.

II. The complications of diabetes include retinopathy, nephropathy, neuropathy, and accelerated occlusive vascular disease. These are variable in presentation relative to the onset of symptoms of the metabolic imbalance.

III. In providing care for diabetics, one is concerned with the issue of metabolic control in the perioperative period and also with issues of wound healing and risk of infection.

A. Metabolic control

1. This is not a real problem in most adult-onset diabetics, whose condition is controlled by diet, especially for outpatient procedures under local anesthesia.

2. Diabetics taking insulin under good metabolic control generally do well in the outpatient setting as long as they are able to maintain their usual dietary habits and insulin dosage in the face of surgery.

3. Some patients must be admitted for inpatient management prior to surgery under general anesthesia.

a. The following information is important preoperatively:

(1) Answers to questions about usual insulin doses and results of urine testing give an index of the patient's education in diabetic control and his reliability, and they may also be a predictor of compliance with postoperative instructions.

(2) Fasting blood sugar obtained in the morning before ingestion of food, institution of IV, or administration of insulin establishes a baseline.

(3) A glucose tolerance test (GTT) establishes the patient's response to a known bolus of glucose and reflects the dynamics of his homeostatic mechanisms. A serum glucose determination obtained during the course of the GTT on fractional urine samples may establish the level at which glucose appears in the urine (spilling) and thereby relate urine glucose to serum glucose levels.

b. The preoperative routine includes

Writing for the ADA diet of appropriate number of calories
Keeping the patient n.p.o. after midnight
In the AM giving half the patient's usual dose of insulin and starting an IV with D5W to be run at 100 ml/hr initially

c. The intraoperative routine includes

Continuing the glucose infusion
For long cases checking the serum glucose and acetone levels intraoperatively

d. Postoperative care involves the following instructions:

(1) Continue the glucose infusion.

(2) Check serum glucose and acetone levels.

(3) After the patient has voided completely, start checking urine fractional samples for glucose and acetone.

(4) Write orders for a sliding scale indicating the amount of crystalline zinc insulin (CZI) to be given for specific urine glucose levels (with an additional 5-10 units for acetone).

10-20 units CZI	4+ urine sugar
10-15	3+
5-10	2+
0-5	1+

(5) Resume the usual AM neutral protamine Hagedorn (NPH) insulin only if the patient seems likely to begin normal dietary intake.

(6) Obtain a dietary consultation prior to discharge, especially if the surgical procedure is likely to alter the patient's ability to adhere to his usual diet.

(7) Make blood sugar determinations from a finger stick sample using reagent strips and a colorimeter. (This technology allows on-the-spot determination of blood sugar, and many diabetics utilize it at home. When available in the hospital, it makes perioperative management easier and more reliable.)

B. Other considerations in diabetic patients.

1. Wound healing. Compromise of the microvasculature and atherosclerosis may impair wound healing in some diabetics, but this is seen most significantly in the distal extremities. The soft tissues of the face and the facial skeleton, having a generally good blood supply, do not usually manifest wound-healing problems in well-controlled diabetics.

2. Infection

a. The risk of postoperative infection in a well-controlled patient is probably not greatly elevated compared to that in a normal patient undergoing the same surgery.

b. The consequences of infection may be significant in a diabetic patient in terms of the effect on diabetic control. Because of metabolic stress, insulin requirements can significantly increase. Thus in a patient who is well controlled by diet alone, a transient requirement for insulin may develop to prevent hyperglycemia and even ketoacidosis caused by an infection.

c. The diabetic patient, especially when poorly controlled, may be at risk of unusual infections not generally seen in nondiabetic patients. Mucormycosis, a systemic fungal infection occasionally seen in the head and neck, may involve the soft tissues or sinuses and spread to the CNS and cranial cavity, with fatal consequences. There is also reason to believe that the poorly controlled diabetic experiences an accelerated form of periodontal disease.

    d. Because of the detrimental effect of infection on diabetic control, a good argument can be made for the prophylactic use of antibiotics in the perioperative period.

Thyroid dysfunction

I. Thyroid hormone regulates tissue metabolism, the consumption of oxygen and nutrients (carbohydrates and lipids), and the production of heat in the maintenance of body temperature. It is required for normal development and maturation.

  A. The production and release of thyroid hormone are under the control of thyroid-stimulating hormone (TSH), secreted by the pituitary, which in turn responds to circulating thyroid hormone levels in a negative feedback loop.

  B. This feedback loop is further regulated by hypothalamic neurosecretory mechanisms, wherein a tripeptide, thyrotropin-releasing hormone (TRH), has the effect of stimulating TSH secretion by the anterior lobe of the pituitary.

II. In the absence of sufficient thyroid hormone there is cold intolerance, a general slowing of mental and physical processes, and weight gain. Symptoms of hypothyroidism are frequently nondescript and may go undiagnosed for protracted periods.

III. An excess of thyroid hormone produces a constellation of overt physical and emotional symptoms that can suggest the correct diagnosis even without confirmatory laboratory tests—tremors, nervousness, insomnia, heat intolerance, increased body temperature, muscle wasting, weight loss, tachycardia.

  A. A distinction must be made between thyrotoxicosis (which the above symptoms denote) and hyperthyroidism (which is due only to thyrotoxicosis produced by oversecretion of hormone by the thyroid gland itself). There are numerous other causes of thyrotoxicosis, including secretion of TSH by a pituitary adenoma, thyroid hormone secretion by a variety of tumors (e.g., choriocarcinoma), and inappropriate ingestion of thyroid hormone.

  B. Thyroid storm is the most severe form of thyrotoxicosis. It is a life-threatening emergency characterized by fever, diaphoresis, agitation, confusion, tachyarrythmias, heart failure, nausea, vomiting, diarrhea, gross tremors, and hyperreflexia. It can be brought on, in the face of thyrotoxicosis, by sources of metabolic stress including infection, trauma, and general anesthesia in an inadequately prepared patient.

  C. The most common form of hyperthyroidism is Graves' disease, or diffuse toxic goiter, which is caused by an abnormal immunoglobulin interacting with the TSH receptor site on the thyroid cell membrane. It is frequently accompanied by exophthalmos.

IV. Cellular metabolism is responsive to both thyroxine (T_4) and triiodothyronine (T_3). In the assessment of thyroid function, T_4 is usually measured by a radioimmunoassay. Thyroid hormone in plasma binds to proteins, including thyroxine-binding globulin (TBG), prealbumin, and albumin. A T_3 resin uptake test may also be obtained to determine whether abnormalities in the T_4 level may be due to a disturbance in protein binding (as could occur, for example, when protein metabolism is altered or when binding is altered by drugs such as salicylates and phenytoin).

V. Management considerations include the following:

A. The patient most in need of assessment of thyroid function is the one with overt physical symptoms suggestive of thyrotoxicosis or severe hypothyroidism. It is also appropriate to check the status of any patient previously treated for hyperthyroidism before attempting major elective oral surgery under general anesthesia. This is best done in consultation with an endocrinologist, especially if treatment is necessary.

B. Thyroid hormone is one of the most indiscriminately prescribed medicines. It is frequently given in the treatment of obesity presumed due to hypothyroidism, even without laboratory assessment of thyroid function.

C. In the absence of physical symptoms, a patient generally is unlikely to be suffering from significant thyrotoxicosis. However, hypothyroidism is a more elusive diagnosis.

D. Infection, trauma, and surgery under general anesthesia may be poorly tolerated by patients at either end of the spectrum of thyroid dysfunction. A patient should be made euthyroid before any major elective procedure is undertaken.

E. Minor oral surgical procedures under local anesthesia should be well tolerated by the patient who does not have overt symptoms.

F. Hyperthyroid patients exhibit exaggerated responses to vasoactive drugs and catecholamines and may be prone to cardiac arrhythmias.

G. Hypothyroid patients may respond in an exaggerated manner to sedative and narcotic medications, necessitating, in extreme instances, respiratory support until such drugs are metabolized or eliminated.

Adrenal dysfunction and patients taking steroids

I. Each adrenal gland actually consists of two separate endocrine glands: the medulla and the cortex.

A. The adrenal medulla, part of the sympathetic nervous system, secretes epinephrine and norepinephrine and participates in the marshaling of physiological resources in "fight or flight" emergencies.

B. The adrenal cortex secretes numerous steroid hormones including sex hormones, mineralocorticoids, and glucocorticoids.

1. Adrenal sex hormones are important in sexual maturation and development but play a relatively minor role in adult reproductive function.

Table 4-1 ADRENAL DYSFUNCTION

Hormone	Hyposecretion	Hypersecretion
Epinephrine-norepinephrine	Very rare (hypoglycemia)	Pheochromocytoma, hypertension
Mineralocorticoids	Rare (salt wasting)	Conn's syndrome (primary aldosteronism)
Glucocorticoids	Addison's disease	Cushing's syndrome
Adrenal androgens	Rare	Adrenogenital syndrome

2. Mineralocorticoid activity is essential to the maintenance of sodium balance and the regulation of extracellular fluid volume.

3. Glucocorticoid activity is essential to carbohydrate and protein metabolism and resistance to stress.

4. In the absence of mineralocorticoids and glucocorticoids, cardiovascular collapse and death occur.

II. Hypo- and hypersecretion of each of the adrenal hormones are associated with a classically described clinical condition. Although these disease entities are, for the most part, rare (Table 4-1), the oral and maxillofacial surgeon should nevertheless be acquainted with them. A discussion of their diagnosis and treatment is beyond the scope of this chapter.

III. Glucocorticoid therapy

A. Glucocorticoid hormones in normal physiological quantities have numerous biological effects. These include

1. Increased protein catabolism in the liver and periphery as part of gluconeogenesis. Via this mechanism, glucocorticoid hormones elevate serum glucose and produce a glucose tolerance curve suggestive of diabetes mellitus. (Conversely, when glucocorticoid hormones are deficient, normal blood glucose levels are maintained only when food intake occurs at regular intervals. Fasting in the face of glucocorticoid deficiency leads to hypoglycemia and collapse.)

2. Glucocorticoids have a permissive action in a variety of physiological mechanisms. The hormones do not produce these effects but allow them to occur. Thus small amounts of glucocorticoid are required for both glucagon and catecholamines to produce an increase in serum glucose. Glucocorticoids are also necessary for vascular smooth muscle to contract in response to norepinephrine and epinephrine. This mechanism is important in the cardiovascular compensation for hypovolemia.

3. Whereas mineralocorticoids regulate Na metabolism, glucocorticoid deficiency leads to an inability to excrete excess body water.

B. In high doses a different spectrum of activities is observed, including the classical stigmata of Cushing's syndrome:

1. Somatic changes

Moon face
Red cheeks
Cervical fat deposition (buffalo hump)
Muscle wasting
Easy bruisability, capillary fragility with ecchymoses
Pendulous abdomen, purple abdominal striae
Inhibition of hair growth
Poor wound healing

2. Osteoporosis
   a. This occurs because excessive protein catabolism inhibits new bone formation while at the same time glucocorticoids inhibit the activity of vitamin D and increase glomerular filtration.
   b. These activities lead to a loss of calcium and demineralization of bone. Clinically there may be collapse of vertebrae, pathological hip fracture, and skeletal deformities.
3. Inhibition of the inflammatory response to tissue injury and infection
4. Inhibition of the manifestations of allergic and autoimmune disease
5. Exacerbation of hypertension, diabetes mellitus, and peptic ulcer disease
6. Production of characteristic psychological disturbances and mood changes
7. Reduction of host defences against a variety of infections, including tuberculosis and viral illnesses

C. It is important to recognize that the desirable antiinflammatory and antiallergic effects of glucocorticoids are seen only at dosage levels that also produce undesirable stigmata of Cushing's disease, especially if treatment is continued for a protracted period. Some undesirable effects are reduced by alternate-day drug therapy. Short courses of glucocorticoids with rapid tapering of dose produce minimal side effects.

D. Conditions for which glucocorticoid therapy may be useful include severe rheumatoid arthritis, systemic lupus erythematosus, severe asthma, and other allergic or autoimmune entities. Such therapy is also used to suppress the rejection of transplanted organs. The subject of steroids for reduction of postoperative swelling in oral and maxillofacial surgery is controversial, since they have been implicated in cases of Bell's palsy.

IV. Management of the patient receiving steroid therapy includes the following:

A. The principal source of concern is that high-dose glucocorticoid therapy, if extended for more than a short period, suppresses both the secretion of ACTH by the pituitary gland and the ability of the adrenal glands to secrete hormones in response to stress. In chronic glucocorticoid therapy profound suppression occurs and the adrenal glands atrophy. The time that it takes for the adrenal glands to return to a normal level of activity is a function of the duration of suppression. In a patient chronically supressed for a long time, there are grounds for concern about his ability to respond to stress a year after cessation of therapy, and perhaps even longer.

B. The concern over adrenal suppression is moot when the patient is receiving glucocorticoids in excess of the daily physiological requirement. It is only when steroids have been discontinued or the dosage has been tapered to a low level that the risk of an addisonian crisis in the face of stress becomes real.

C. It is possible to assay adrenal function, but much easier simply to provide a patient with supplemental glucocorticoid in the perioperative period if a stressful surgical procedure is to be undertaken. The steroids can be rapidly tapered to the previous maintenance dose or to zero.

D. The definition of *stress* is important. From the standpoint of adrenal physiology the term refers to noxious stimuli of sufficient impact to lead to an increase in ACTH secretion and, in turn, an increase in the release of glucocorticoids into the circulation. In point of fact, the term stress is wrongfully applied to most dental or outpatient oral surgical procedures. These procedures may be "stressful" in the colloquial sense that they evoke nervousness; but when a decision about steroid dosage in the perioperative period has to be made, stress probably should be considered to be an attribute of more protracted invasive procedures under general anesthesia. However, given the innocuous nature of a short course of steroid therapy, it is advisable to overtreat rather than undertreat when in doubt.

Dysfunction of the immune system

I. General considerations

A. The oral and maxillofacial surgeon is privileged to work in an area of the body where host defenses are strongly marshaled against infection and allow the healing of wounds that frequently prove troublesome elsewhere in the body. On the other hand, the oral cavity is often the first area to become symptomatic when the immune system is malfunctioning. Thus, for example, the presenting symptoms in acute leukemia may be painful hemorrhagic swelling of inflamed gingival tissues. Biopsy will typically show a leukemic infiltrate, which is the response of a compromised immune system to the presence of oral flora. Such organisms, usually benign, become pathogenic when host defenses are inadequate.

B. The science of immunology is one of the most rapidly evolving areas in medicine. It is an active front in the battle to understand and rationally treat cancer, and a growing number of diseases are now identified as being caused by autoimmune phenomena. Progress in the realm of organ transplantation is based upon evolution of surgical technique, but even more so on our growing ability to manipulate some of the immunological factors underlying histocompatibility.

C. The oral and maxillofacial surgeon is likely to encounter patients with dysfunction of the immune system in the following contexts:

1. Malignancy—marrow replacement by tumor cells, leukemic or metastatic, leads to neutropenia and immunological compromise.

2. Chemotherapy for tumor—in addition to killing or suppressing the growth of rapidly dividing tumor cells, chemotherapy also kills or suppresses rapidly dividing normal cells (e.g., marrow cells). Thus, along with other forms of toxicity, immunosuppression sets a limit to the use of such drugs.

3. Immunosuppressive therapy—such therapy is used in organ transplantation to prevent rejection. It is also employed in the management of a broad spectrum of autoimmune disorders including severe rheumatoid arthritis, systemic lupus erythematosus, and pemphigus vulgaris.

4. Marrow suppression and immunological compromise—these result from whole body radiation, as may be employed therapeutically prior to marrow transplantation or as might occur in the event of a thermonuclear war or an accident at a nuclear facility.

5. Aplastic anemia or pancytopenia—these occur idiopathically, as a consequence of an overdosage of marrow suppressive agents, as a result of exposure to industrial chemicals, or as an idiosyncratic reaction to medications such as chloramphenicol, antihistamines, and phenylbutazone.

D. Within the last several years a new disease entity known as the acquired immunodeficiency syndrome (AIDS) has appeared and caused great alarm. Primarily a disease of sexually active male homosexuals, it is transmissible hematogenously and may be on the rise in nonhomosexuals or both sexes as well.

1. As of mid-1984, there were fewer than 5000 cases reported in the U.S., but the number has been doubling roughly every 6 mo.

2. The causative agent for AIDS appears to be a retrovirus, and the incubation period is estimated to be about 2-3 yr. To date there are no documented instances of recovery from AIDS, although recent reports have suggested that some drugs (e.g., azidothymidine) may be useful.

3. The disease is characterized by lymphadenopathy, multiple opportunistic infections, and the multifocal Kaposi's sarcoma with lesions in the oral cavity. These, along with a variety of dental infections (e.g., oral candidiasis, herpes simplex, severe gingivitis, giant aphthous ulcer–like lesions), may necessitate oral surgical consultation.

II. Management considerations

A. When immunosuppressive treatment can be anticipated, patients should be screened in advance of therapy and any potential oral sources of sepsis treated preemptively. Thus, for example, in a renal patient with a history of recurrent episodes of pericoronitis, one would tend to remove the wisdom teeth to prevent such an episode from escalating into a major problem after the start of immunosuppression. Similarly, patients should be screened for dental disease prior to the start of chemotherapy for malignant disease.

B. During immunosuppression, oral care is likely to be supportive or palliative in the event of a dental emergency.

C. Immunosuppressed patients are prone to opportunistic oral infections such as candidiasis and are also subject to reactivation of viral illnesses such as herpes simplex. Oral candidiasis is well controlled by topical nystatin, but viral stomatitis is amenable mainly to palliative measures (e.g., institution of a bland diet, use of topical anesthetic mouth rinses, various oral coating agents, and in severe cases intravenous nutritional and fluid support).

D. The maintenance of hygiene is difficult in a patient with viral or other form of stomatitis. Half-strength peroxide rinses, or peroxide mixed with saline, can be useful when tooth brushing is too painful. The use of topical anesthetic agents (e.g., viscous lidocaine [Xylocaine] or dyclonine 0.25-0.5% solution) may be useful prior to hygiene activities or before meals.

E. The best time to undertake an elective or semielective oral surgical procedure in a patient receiving chemotherapy is midway between cycles of treatment, when blood counts are presumably on the rise.

F. Perioperative antibiotics are probably a good idea, but their use causes some risk of selecting out resistant organisms or opening various ecological niches for colonization by nosocomial organisms that may be both hard to eradicate and pathogenic in a compromised host.

G. Wound healing may be impeded in the patient receiving aggressive chemotherapy. Currently available chemotherapeutic drugs do not distinguish between one rapidly growing tissue and another; thus both tumor neoplasia and normal proliferation of tissues in a healing wound may be affected.

H. Since immunosuppressed patients are vulnerable to infection, they are frequently placed on precautions whose details are part of the standardized hospital protocol. It is appropriate to continue to observe these precautions for the protection of the patient when he is transferred to an outpatient facility for oral surgical treatment.

I. Special care is appropriate in the examination and treatment of patients with the acquired immunodeficiency syndrome (AIDS) for the protection of all directly and indirectly involved personnel. The precautions advised by the Centers for Disease Control are essentially the same as those applied to hepatitis:

   1. Accidental wounds from instruments contaminated with blood, saliva, or other secretions must be carefully avoided, as should exposure of open skin wounds or lesions to materials from AIDS patients.

   2. Gloves should be worn at all times when handling blood- or saliva-contaminated instruments or surgical specimens.

3. When the possibility of contaminating clothing with blood or secretions exists, gowns should be worn and disposed of properly.

4. All laboratory specimens should be labeled "AIDS precautions."

5. All blood spills should be promptly cleaned with a disinfectant (1:10 dilution of 5.25% sodium hypochlorite and water).

6. Masks and protective glasses should be worn if aerosolization of blood and saliva is anticipated.

7. Use of disposable instruments is encouraged, and they should be placed in a disposable container labeled "AIDS precautions."

8. Needles should *not* be bent or resheathed after use, for this is a common cause of needle injury. Instead, they should be placed in a puncture-resistant container.

9. Proper hand washing before and after treatment and after cleaning of instruments is mandatory.

10. Pregnant women should avoid direct contact with AIDS patients, since many of these patients excrete cytomegalovirus or other viruses.

GENERAL REFERENCES

Campbell, J.W., and Frisse, M., editors: Manual of medical therapeutics, Washington University, St. Louis, School of Medicine., Boston, 1983, Little, Brown & Co.

Condon, R.E., and Nyhus, L.M., editors: University of Illinois, Department of Surgery, manual of surgical therapeutics, Boston, 1985, Little, Brown & Co.

Ganong, W.F.: Review of medical physiology, ed. 12, Los ALtos, Calif., 1985, Lange Medical Publications.

Nora, P.F.: Operative surgery: principles and techniques, ed. 2, Philadelphia, 1980, Lea & Febiger.

Petersdorf, R.G., et al., editors: Harrison's principles of internal medicine, ed. 10, New York 1983, McGraw-Hill, Inc.

Sonis, S.T., et al.: Principles and practice of oral medicine, Philadelphia, 1984, W.B. Saunders Co.

Local Anesthesia and Sedation in Oral and Maxillofacial Surgery

LOCAL ANESTHESIA

I. Classification of anesthetic agents
   A. Amides, esters, and ketones constitute the major categories of local anesthetics. These designations refer to the molecular linkage between constituent hydrophilic and lipophilic groups. Because of their increased effectiveness and fewer hypersensitivity reactions, amides have largely supplanted esters; but ester-linked agents remain an appropriate alternative for patients with amide allergies. The ketone-linkage class of anesthetics has relatively little clinical importance and currently consists of a single topical agent.
   B. Metabolism of amide anesthetics occurs in the liver; ester-linked agents are hydrolyzed in the plasma by pseudocholinesterases. Water-soluble products are excreted by the kidneys.

II. Dissociation constants
   A. The pH of anesthetic solutions is low (typically 3.3-5.5). Such solutions contain hydrochloride salts of anesthetic bases and exist in the form of uncharged base (RN) and cation (RNH$^+$).
      1. An equilibrium between charged and uncharged forms is expressed by the equation

      $$RNH^+ \rightleftarrows RN + H^+$$

      The proportion of RN and RNH$^+$ at a given instant depends upon pH and the anesthetic molecule's dissociation constant (pKa).
      2. For a given molecule, pKa is characteristic and constant; it is defined as the pH at which half of the molecular species are ionized (RNH$^+$) and half are nonionized (RN) (see Table 5-2)
   B. After injection, anesthetic molecules are exposed to the pH of the injection site tissues. When tissue pH is below an anesthetic's pKa, excess H$^+$ is present and the reaction is driven to the left. The proportion of RN correspondingly declines. Since anesthetic diffuses into nerve membrane in the form of RN,

anesthetic effectiveness also decreases. The pH of infected tissues is low, so an anesthetic with a high pKa offers a smaller proportion of RN for diffusion through nerve sheaths and local anesthetic effect declines.

III. Composition of local anesthetic solutions
   A. Preservatives of various types may be incorporated into anesthetic solutions.
      1. Dental cartridges formerly contained the preservative methylparaben (1 mg/ml), but a significant incidence of paraben reactions confused whether the patient was allergic to the anesthetic or to the preservative. Since genuine allergies to amide anesthetics are extraordinarily rare, most hypersensitivity reactions have been attributed to methylparaben. This preservative is now omitted from most dental cartridges but may still be included in multidose vials.
      2. For anesthetic solutions containing a sympathomimetic vasoconstrictor, 0.5 mg/ml sodium metabisulfite may be present as an antioxidant.
   B. Anesthetic concentrations are expressed as percentages; vasoconstrictor concentrations are given as ratios. Knowing the volume of a standard U.S. dental cartridge to be 1.8 ml, it is possible to compute the anesthetic and vasoconstrictor content. (See bottom of p. 122.)

Drug doses are expressed either by stating the amount of each drug in milligrams (e.g., 36 mg lidocaine with 0.018 mg epinephrine) or by giving the concentration and volume (e.g., 1.8 ml of a solution containing 2% lidocaine and 1:100,000 epinephrine).

IV. Representative local anesthetic solutions
   A. Injectable agents are summarized in Table 5-1.
   B. Topical anesthetics decrease the pain and anxiety of anesthetic injections. Although they do not penetrate intact skin, they do provide superficial anesthesia for abraded skin and intact mucosa, deep tissues are not anesthetized. Topical agents are not completely innocuous, since application to intraoral mucosa permits rapid absorption and leads to significant blood levels. Representative topical anesthetic preparations include the following:
      1. Benzocaine—this ester-linked, water-insoluble agent is poorly absorbed. Overdose reactions are virtually nonexistent.
      2. Lidocaine—this agent is the only amide-linked anesthetic with clinically important topical properties. It can be employed in *base* or *salt* form. The base form (lidocaine 5%) is poorly soluble in water and is used for abraded, lacerated, or ulcerated tissues. The salt form (lidocaine HCl) is used as a 2% preparation and, being water soluble, is potentially more toxic.
      3. Dyclonine—this agent represents the only ketone-linked

local anesthetic. It does not cross-react with the other anesthetic classes. Its low water solubility accounts for a low systemic toxicity. It is available as 0.5% solution; the maximum recommended dose is 200 mg (40 ml).

4. Butacaine sulfate—this ester is more potent and toxic than cocaine. It is available as a 4% ointment; the maximum recommended dose is 200 mg (5 ml).

5. Tetracaine—this highly water-soluble ester is more than 5× as potent as cocaine and has a relatively high potential for systemic toxicity. It is used as a 2% solution; the maximum recommended dose is 2 mg (1 ml).

6. Cocaine—the main use for this agent in oral and maxillofacial surgery is as a nasal mucosal vasoconstrictor prior to nasal endotracheal intubation. Highly water soluble, it is absorbed rapidly and eliminated slowly. It is available in 2-10% solutions; the recommended dose for oral topical application is 4%. Its lack of stability in solution and potential for psychic dependence and tolerance militate against its routine intraoral use as a topical anesthetic.

V. Vasoconstrictors

A. Vasoconstrictors in local anesthetic solutions are believed to enhance the depth of anesthesia, reduce the peak plasma concentrations of anesthetic, and control local hemorrhage. Today these assumptions have come into question, and potential benefits are known to be influenced by the specific local anesthetic used, the concentration, and the injection site. Sufficient dosages of all sympathomimetic vasoconstrictors can cause adverse reactions, particularly in the presence of predisposing conditions.

B. Catecholamines are sympathomimetic amines often used in combination with local anesthetics. Phenylephrine, a noncatecholamine, was formerly used with procaine; but neither procaine nor phenylephrine is widely employed in local anesthesia today.

C. Representatives of this class of drug are given in Table 5-2.

1. Epinephrine is the most widely used vasoconstrictor in oral and maxillofacial surgery. It stimulates both alpha and beta receptors, but its value in dentistry as a vasoconstrictor is based on the predominance of alpha receptors in the oral mucosa, submucosa, and periodontium. When it is used to enhance pain control, no distinction exists between 1:100,000 and 1:50,000 lidocaine-epinephrine. The more dilute solution (1:100,000) is therefore recommended.

a. Healthy adults may receive up to 0.2 mg epinephrine per appointment. This translates into 20 ml of a 1:100,000 solution (approximately 11 local anesthetic cartridges). The fact that anesthetic solutions contain multiple constituents must be recognized when determining the maximum permissible volume of an anesthetic to be

Table 5-1 INJECTABLE LOCAL ANESTHETICS

| | | | | Maximum dose* | | | Duration (hr) | |
| | | | | | Cartridges‡ | | | |
	pKa	Vasoconstrictor	mg†	Healthy	CV impaired	Pulpal	Soft tissue
Procaine HCl, 4%	9.1	Phenylephrine, 1:2500	418	5.5	2.0	0.5	1.5-2.0
Lidocaine HCl, 2%	7.9	None	300	8.0		0.1	1.0-2.0
Lidocaine HCl, 2%	7.9	Epinephrine, 1:50,000	300	5.5	1.0	1.0-1.5	3.0-4.0
Lidocaine HCl, 2%	7.9	Epinephrine, 1:100,000	300	11.0	2.0	1.0-1.5	3.0-4.0
Mepivacaine HCl, 3%	7.6	None	400	7.0		0.3-0.7	2.0-3.0
Mepivacaine HCl, 2%	7.6	Levonordefrin, 1:20,000	400	11.0	7.0	1.0-1.5	3.0-4.0
Prilocaine HCl, 4% §	7.9	None	400	5.5		0.2-1.0	2.0-4.0
Prilocaine HCl, 4% §	7.9	Epinephrine, 1:200,000	400	5.5	4.0	1.0-1.5	2.0-4.0
Propoxycaine HCl, 0.4%, and procaine HCl, 2%	7.9	Levonordefrin, 1:20,000	400 total amine	5.5	5.5	0.5-1.0	2.0-3.0

Propoxycaine HCl, 0.4%, and procaine HCl, 2%		Levarterenol, 1:30,000	400 total amine	5.5	2.0	0.5-1.0	2.0-3.0
Bupivacaine HCl, 0.5%	8.1	None	175	19.0			
Bupivacaine HCl, 0.5%	8.1	Epinephrine, 1:200,000	175	19.0	4.0	1.5-3.0	4.0-9.0
Bupivacaine HCl, 0.75%	8.1	None	175	13.0			
Bupivacaine HCl, 0.75%	8.1	Epinephrine, 1:200,000	175	13.0	4.0		
Etidocaine HCl, 0.5%	7.7	None	300	33.0			
Etidocaine HCl, 0.5%	7.7	Epinephrine, 1:200,000	200	22.0	4.0	1.5-3.0	4.0-9.0
Etidocaine HCl, 1.0%	7.7	None	300	17.0			
Etidocaine HCl, 1.0%	7.7	Epinephrine, 1:200,000	400	22.0	4.0	1.5-3.0	4.0-9.0

*Suggested doses are based upon maximum recommended doses of both anesthetic agent and vasoconstrictor for a healthy 70 kg adult per appointment. In computing them, it is necessary to use the amounts of vasoconstrictor shown in Table 5-2. Suggestions for local anesthetic doses from other sources may be based upon the amount of anesthetic rather than the amount of vasoconstrictor. As a result the recommendations from such sources may be more permissive than those presented here.

†Maximum doses of local anesthetic (in milligrams) are based upon the amount of anesthetic contained within the maximal permissible volume of anesthetic solution. Maximum volumes are established on the basis of the most toxic constituent (which may be either the anesthetic or the vasoconstrictor).

‡*Cartridges* refers to standard 1.8 ml dental cartridges (rounded to the nearest half-cartridge).

§Contraindicated in patients with methemoglobinemia and in those taking medications known to produce methemoglobinemia (e.g., acetaminophen, phenacetin).

⊃CONSTRICTORS

Maximum adult doses (mg)		
Healthy	CV impaired	Concentration*
0.20	0.04	1:50,000; 1:100,000; 1:200,000
0.34	0.14	1:30,000
1.00		1:20,000
4.00	1.60	1:2500

esent concentrations of vasoconstrictors commonly used in oral and maxillofacial

administered at a single sitting. Maximum doses for multicomponent solutions should be based upon the most toxic constituent. Though the maximum allowable dose of lidocaine is 500 mg (14 cartridges of a 2% solution), the maximum dose of epinephrine is only 0.2 mg; therefore the actual number of 1.8 ml cartridges permitted is only 11. The anesthetic and vasoconstrictor content of dental cartridges is shown below.

b. Cardiovascular impairment, when clinically significant, may render the patient "epinephrine sensitive." The maximum epinephrine dose for such a patient is contro-

Anesthetic concentration (%)*	Anesthetic content (mg)†
0.05	0.9
0.04	7.2
1.00	18.0
2.00	36.0
3.00	54.0
4.00	76.0

Vasoconstrictor concentration‡	Vasoconstrictor content (mg)†
1:2500	0.72
1:20,000	0.09
1:30,000	0.06
1:50,000	0.04
1:100,000	0.02
1:200,000	0.01

*In other words, a 1% solution = 1 g anesthetic/100 ml solution.
†These amounts are present in a standard 1.8 ml dental cartridge.
‡Expressed as ratios.

versial. Published recommendations have been d
gent and inconsistent. Based upon an extrapolation f
guidelines promulgated by the New York Heart Asso
tion in 1955, an epinephrine dose ⅕ that permitted fe
normal adult is suitable for use in a sensitive individu
This translates into 0.04 mg epinephrine per appoi
ment. In fact, such a low level of epinephrine (and oth
vasoconstrictors) can probably be used safely in ar
patient with mild to moderate cardiovascular diseas
However, the development of effective local anesthetic
that do not contain sympathomimetic amines (3% mepi
vacaine, 4% prilocaine) often makes this decision
unnecessary. When a vasoconstrictor is considered
desirable, solutions containing 1:200,000 epinephrine
can be used.

D. Vasoconstrictor use during general anesthesia may be complicated by the tendency of certain inhalational general anesthetics to sensitize the heart to the arrhythmogenic effects of the
vasoconstrictor. Halothane and cyclopropane are considered
sensitizing; fluroxene, methoxyflurane, and isoflurane are not.
Anesthetics (e.g., enflurane) may sensitize specific subsets of
patients, so limitation of sympathomimetic amine dosage is
advised.

VI. Techniques of regional anesthesia. Thorough knowledge of relevant anatomy is necessary for reliable success in regional anesthesia. Details of specific anesthetic techniques are available in standard textbooks and review papers; however, two recently
described alternative approaches for mandibular block anesthesia
have generated substantial clinical interest and will be considered
in detail:

A. Gow-Gates technique
1. Nerves anesthetized are the inferior·alveolar, mental, incisive, lingual, mylohyoid, auriculotemporal, and buccal.
2. Needle—25 gauge long (1⅝ in)
3. Site of penetration is the oral mucosa along the medial border of the mandibular ramus lateral to the pterygomandibu-
lar depression but medial to the temporalis muscle tendon.
The needle is inserted along a line extending from the cor-
ner of the mouth opposite the side of injection to the lower
border of the tragus on the same side as the injection. The
alignment of the needle should be parallel to the angulation
of the ear to the face on the side of injection.
4. Depth of penetration—the needle should be advanced until
bone is contacted and then withdrawn 1 mm. Anesthetic
solution is deposited after negative aspiration.

B. Tuberosity (Akinosi) approach
1. Nerves anesthetized are the inferior alveolar, lingual, long
buccal, and mylohyoid.
2. Needle—25 gauge long (1⅝ in)

penetration is the oral mucosa along the medial bor-
the mandibular ramus. The mouth is kept closed
in occlusion) with the cheek and muscles of masti-
n relaxed. The syringe is aligned parallel to the occlu-
plane, positioned at the mucogingival junction in the
ion of the maxillary third molar. The needle penetrates
e oral mucosa just medial to the ramus.
epth of penetration—the needle should be advanced 1½
n.

lications

cal

1. Needle breakage is rare and usually occurs because of unexpected movement by the patient or because of the (unjus-
tifiable) iatrogenic practice of intentionally bending the
needle. Broken needles seldom migrate within tissues. They
become encapsulated by fibrous connective tissue and
remain stationary until delayed recovery is feasible.
2. Persistent anesthesia and paresthesia are caused by direct
needle trauma to nerve trunks or by anesthetic solutions
contaminated with alcohol or cold sterilization media.
Abnormal sensation is usually temporary but may be permanent. Persistent sensory deficit may require surgical exploration, anastomosis of severed nerve ends, or anastomosis
after removal of a damaged nerve segment.
3. Trismus, spasm of the muscles of mastication, is common
after local anesthetic injections and results from trauma,
hemorrhage, and/or infection. Treatment includes heat
therapy, analgesics, muscle relaxants, and opening-closing
exercises.
4. Hematomas are caused by extravasation of blood after needle damage to a blood vessel. Resulting swelling may develop rapidly or slowly depending upon the consistency of the
surrounding tissue and whether an artery or a vein is
involved. Swelling and ecchymosis resolve over the ensuing
weeks, and no specific treatment is needed. In the case of
immediate swelling, application of pressure to the injection
site may minimize hematoma formation.
5. Infection after injections is uncommon. When it does occur,
management is the same as for any other intraoral infection
(i.e., systemic antibiotics and drainage of fluctuant
abscesses).
6. Sloughing because of tissue necrosis can result from ischemia associated with the use of vasoconstrictors or from
sensitivity to the anesthetic agent. Management of necrotic
areas is symptomatic and consists of supportive treatment
with analgesics, hygiene, and local protection with Orabase.
7. Lip chewing is most common in children and the mentally
handicapped. Prevention requires use of shorter-acting

agents, placement of protective gauze or cotton rolls between the lips, and careful instructions for parents or guardians.

8. Facial nerve paralysis may arise from introducing anesthetic solution into the substance of the parotid gland. This blocks the propagation of impulses along facial nerve branches that innervate the muscles of facial expression. Cessation of nerve transmission is temporary and no specific treatment is required, but closure of the eye on the involved side may not be complete. Retention of the corneal reflex is usually sufficient for normal eye lubrication until complete muscle function returns.

B. Systemic

1. Adverse drug reactions to anesthetic solutions (i.e., the local anesthetic agent, vasoconstrictor, preservatives, or other components) may result from direct extension of the agent's pharmacological effects, altered physiology, or allergy. Toxicity resulting from an extension of pharmacological properties includes side reactions, overdosage, and local toxic effects.

2. Intravascular injection is not a systemic reaction itself but greatly increases the possibility of an adverse occurrence. The probability of an intravascular injection is diminished (but not eliminated) by preinjection aspiration. Recent development of self-aspirating syringes may facilitate the aspiration procedure, but clinicians still need to recognize positive aspirates when they occur and to redirect the injection path accordingly.

3. An authentic allergic reaction to a local anesthetic may range from a minor skin reaction to life-threatening anaphylaxis.

   a. Prevention of allergic reactions requires a detailed medical history. Allergy to amide local anesthetics is uncommon; nonetheless assertions by patients of "Novocaine" reactions should be taken seriously. To many patients, "Novocaine" is synonymous with local anesthetics. This makes it difficult to know whether the patient experienced a reaction to an ester (e.g., Novocaine) or to an amide anesthetic. If the category of anesthetic can be definitively established, the alternate class can be used with confidence.

      (1) The possibility of previous overdosage or of reactions to vasoconstrictors or other agents must be considered. Inquiry should be made into whether the patient has been taking other medications, whether hyperventilation or syncope provides a more realistic description of the previous incident, how the reaction was managed, and whether the patient required hospitalization.

(2) An attempt should be made to contact the previous oral surgeon or dentist for an objective appraisal of the event and for positive identification of the anesthetic class. Elective therapy should be postponed until the nature of the occurrence is discerned.

b. Management can be difficult for patients in pain who require emergency treatment and who allege a history of local anesthetic allergy. Use of general anesthesia can be considered. Alternatively, the local anesthetic effect of injected antihistamines can be exploited. A 1% solution of Benadryl (diphenhydramine) with 1:100,000 epinephrine is relatively effective. Management of anaphylaxis and other allergic reactions is discussed elsewhere in this manual.

SEDATION

I. Definition

A. No completely satisfactory definition of sedation in oral and maxillofacial surgery has been devised, but generally sedation produces a minimally depressed level of consciousness that retains the patient's ability to maintain an airway independently and continuously and to respond appropriately to physical stimulation and verbal command. By contrast, general anesthesia produces a controlled state of depressed consciousness or unconsciousness, a partial or total loss of protective reflexes, and an inability to maintain an airway independently or respond purposefully to physical stimulation or verbal command.

B. Detailed consideration of the applications of sedation and ambulatory general anesthesia in oral and maxillofacial surgery cannot be adequately covered in this brief descriptive outline. The present section therefore will provide a general summary of commonly employed techniques. Application of such methods should be limited to individuals who have undergone appropriate hospital-based clinical training in general anesthesia.

II. Techniques of conscious sedation

A. Routes of administration for sedative agents may be inhalational, oral (p.o.), intravenous (IV), intramuscular (IM), or rectal (p.r.). Inhalational sedation utilizing nitrous oxide–oxygen (N_2O-O_2) and IV sedation has gained widest popularity.

B. N_2O-O_2 sedation requires O_2 (supplied as a compressed gas) and N_2O (provided in cylinders as a liquid that vaporizes during use). This distinction in physical state is clinically significant since the vapor pressure within N_2O cylinders is maintained at roughly 750 lb/in^2 until the cylinder is virtually empty. By contrast, as O_2 is depleted a proportionate decrease in O_2 pressure occurs.

	Tank color	Tank size	Volume (gal)	Pressure (lb/in²)
N_2O	Blue	E	420	750
	Blue	H	3665	750
O_2	Green	E	65	2100
	Green	G	1400	2100

1. Flow is measured as liters per minute (L/min) and expressed as a percentage; for instance, 2 L N_2O/min and 4 L O_2/min is expressed as

$$\frac{2\ L\ N_2O/min}{2\ L\ N_2O/min + 4\ L\ O_2/min}$$

or 33.3% N_2O; 66.7% O_2

2. Procedures are similar for all sedation machines. Each typically delivers an absolute minimum of 20-30% oxygen, has a "fail-safe" system that prevents N_2O delivery if O_2 administration is interrupted, and employs a "pin indexing safety system" or "diameter indexing safety system" to ensure correct cylinder attachment. The procedure for operating and testing N_2O-O_2 sedation machines is shown on p. 128.
3. Monitoring involves measuring and recording blood pressure and pulse (every 15 min) and respiratory rate (every 30 min) (Fig. 5-1).
C. Intravenous sedation may employ psychosedatives (major and minor tranquilizers), barbiturates, narcotics, and belladonna-like agents (Table 5-3). Previously popular "fixed dosage" methods have now been supplanted by individually titrated regimens of benzodiazepines, narcotics, or barbiturates used either alone or in various combinations.
   1. Diazepam (a benzodiazepine) remains the most important intravenous sedative agent in oral and maxillofacial surgery, despite continuing development of numerous related compounds (Table 5-4).
      a. Physical characteristics and composition are as follows: lipid soluble, water insoluble; available (as Valium) in a 0.5% solution compounded with 40% propylene glycol, 10% ethyl alcohol, 5% sodium benzoate, and 1.5% benzyl alcohol.
      b. Major routes of administration are oral and IV; IM absorption is poor and erratic. Low water solubility causes diazepam to precipitate when combined with water-based injectables. Injection into a running IV line should be made at the portal nearest the vein.

Operating and Testing N₂O-O₂ Sedation Machines

A. Turning machine on
   1. Turn on N_2O-O_2 tanks
   2. Turn machine's "on-off" switch to "on"
   3. Verify that N_2O flow valve is "off"
   4. Turn O_2 flow valve "on" to provide O_2 delivery rate of 5-8 L/min
   5. Place inhaler assembly (nasal mask) on patient
   6. Adjust total gas flow to patient's tidal volume by establishing that reservoir bag neither overinflates nor underinflates
   7. Allow patient to breathe 100% O_2 for 1 min
   8. Introduce N_2O at rate of 1 L/min by adjusting N_2O flow valve (be sure to decrease O_2 flow at an equivalent rate so total flow remains constant); pause 35-45 sec between increments; increase N_2O flow rate until baseline sedation is reached
B. Turning machine off
   1. Using N_2O flow valve, decrease N_2O flow to 0 L/min
   2. Increase O_2 flow rate so total flow remains constant (usually 5-8 L/min)
   3. After patient has breathed 100% O_2 for 2 min, remove inhaler assembly
   4. Turn off N_2O at tank
   5. Turn off O_2 at tank
   6. Turn sedation machine's "on-off" switch to "off"
   7. Turn O_2 flow valve to 0 L/min
C. Testing machine's "fail-safe" system
   1. Turn machine on as indicated in Steps A 1-4
   2. Turn off O_2 at tank
   3. "Fail-safe" mechanism is operational if N_2O flow drops to 0 L/min

c. Clinical effects of IV diazepam include disinhibition, drowsiness, muscle relaxation, and anticonvulsant activity. Specific circulatory, respiratory, and CNS effects have been described. Although metabolism is very slow ($t_{1/2}$ 20-40 hr), clinical effects terminate rapidly because of redistribution.

d. Potential hazards are CNS depression, respiratory depression, cardiovascular complications (cardiac arrest, hypotension, hypertension), allergic reactions, altered mental state (coma, hysteria, hallucinations), and visual abnormalities.

   (1) In the elderly patient a disproportionate sedative effect may be observed.

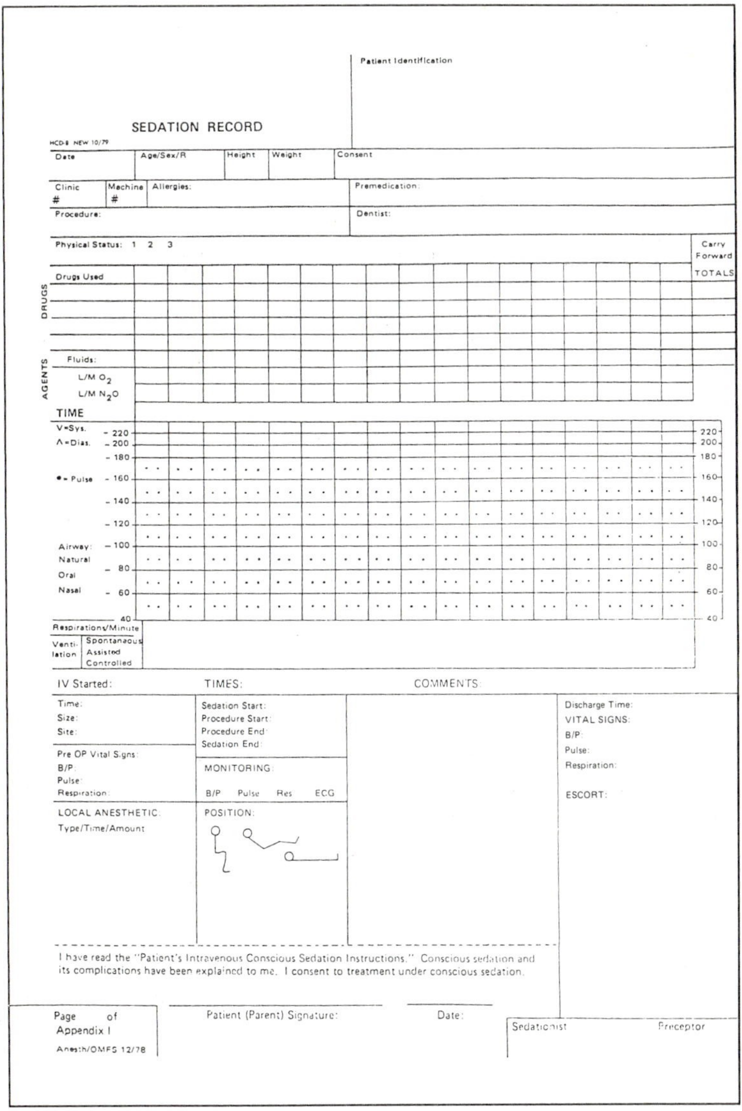

Patient Identification

SEDATION RECORD

HCD-8 NEW 10/79

Date | Age/Sex/R | Height | Weight | Consent

Clinic # | Machine # | Allergies: | Premedication:

Procedure: | Dentist:

Physical Status: 1 2 3 | Carry Forward

DRUGS: Drugs Used | TOTALS

AGENTS: Fluids: | L/M O_2 | L/M N_2O

TIME

V=Sys. Λ=Dias. • = Pulse

220, 200, 180, 160, 140, 120, 100, 80, 60, 40

Airway: Natural, Oral, Nasal

Respirations/Minute

Ventilation: Spontaneous, Assisted, Controlled

IV Started: Time: Size: Site:

Pre OP Vital Signs: B/P: Pulse: Respiration:

LOCAL ANESTHETIC: Type/Time/Amount

TIMES: Sedation Start: Procedure Start: Procedure End: Sedation End:

MONITORING: B/P Pulse Res ECG

POSITION:

COMMENTS:

Discharge Time: VITAL SIGNS: B/P: Pulse: Respiration:

ESCORT:

I have read the "Patient's Intravenous Conscious Sedation Instructions." Conscious sedation and its complications have been explained to me. I consent to treatment under conscious sedation.

Page of Appendix I

Anesth/OMFS 12/78

Patient (Parent) Signature: Date:

Sedationist Preceptor

Fig. 5-1 Sedation monitoring record.

(2) Thrombophlebitis is a common local complication. Its incidence increases when vascular access is through the small veins of the forearm and hand or when narcotics are injected through the same venipuncture site. No correlation has been established between thrombophlebitis and smoking, contraceptive use, or injection by needle versus plastic catheter.

Table 5-3 AGENTS COMMONLY USED IN INTRAVENOUS SEDATION*

	Multidose vial†	Disposable syringes†	Ampules	Usual adult dose‡	Duration§
Diazepam		5 (2)	5 (2)	10-20	30-45
Fentanyl			0.05 (2)	0.05-0.1	½-30
Meperidine	50 (30)	50 (2)	50 (2)	25-50	180
Methohexital	10 (50-500)			5-250	5-7
Nembutal	50	50 (2)		50-75	15-30
Naloxone			0.4 (1)	0.2-0.4	180-240

*Among manufacturers a wide variation exists in the concentrations, volumes, and forms of delivery of intravenous sedative agents. Values presented here are representative and considered to be particularly suitable for oral and maxillofacial surgery but should not be interpreted as a complete list of available products.

†Concentration in mg/ml. The number in parentheses indicates volume per vial, syringe, or ampule.

‡Expressed in mg. These are representative doses; all require individual titration and assessment of response.

§Duration of therapeutic effect must be assessed in patients individually. Wide variation exists. Values presented here are average effective durations of action for healthy adults expressed in *minutes*.

    (3) In general, diazepam enjoys a high therapeutic index. The very young and the elderly are most sensitive to its effects.

  e. Recommended dosage protocols recognize the wide variability in response to diazepam and mandate administration of small incremental doses that allow its effect to be assessed prior to giving more drug. In this manner dosage is titrated to the individual patient and overdosage is avoided.

    (1) The initial increment is usually 2.5 mg. Further increments of 2-3 mg are then given every 30 sec until an appropriate level of sedation is reached.

    (2) A dose range of 5-20 mg is common (average total dosage, 18 mg). The duration of an effective dose is generally about 45 min.

  f. Level of sedation is assessed on the basis of altered speech (most reliable index of sedation depth), ptosis (Verrill's sign), and blurred vision (least reliable index of sedation depth). Patients are carefully observed during the procedure, as described above; afterwards, they should be escorted home by a relative or friend.

  g. Combination techniques involving N_2O-O_2, narcotics, and barbiturates are common; but supplementing IV diazepam with either N_2O-O_2 or narcotics is generally unnecessary and carries the risk of unintended passage from a state of sedation into general anesthesia.

    (1) For mildly or moderately apprehensive patients diazepam alone is sufficient to allay anxiety. Complete control of pain is readily accomplished by regional anesthesia.

    (2) For more fearful patients local anesthesia and diazepam can be combined with low doses of the barbiturate methohexital. This method may approach or intentionally produce a controlled state of general anesthesia; however, with properly trained personnel and facilities, it makes diazepam's capacity for partial or total amnesia more predictable. Pain, anxiety, and recollection of the surgical procedure are thus minimized. Methods for combining diazepam and methohexital are described at the bottom of p. 134.

2. Narcotics (e.g., fentanyl and meperidine) are used because of their significant therapeutic value as sedatives and analgesics. They are employed alone or in combination with diazepam, N_2O-O_2, and/or barbiturates. As in all IV sedation techniques, primary pain control still relies upon effective local anesthesia.

Table 5-4 CHARACTERISTICS OF BENZODIAZEPINES

	Indications	Active substances in blood	Rate of elimination
Chlordiazepoxide	Anxiety Alcohol withdrawal Preoperative sedation	Chlordiazepoxide Demethylchlordiazepoxide Demoxepam Demethyldiazepam	Slow
Diazepam	Anxiety Alcohol withdrawal Muscle spasm Preoperative sedation Status epilepticus	Diazepam Demethyldiazepam	Slow
Oxazepam	Anxiety Anxiety-depression Alcohol withdrawal	Oxazepam	Intermediate to rapid
Flurazepam	Insomnia	Hydroxyethyl flurazepam Flurazepam aldehyde Dealkylflurazepam Demethyldiazepam	Slow Slow

Drug	Metabolite	Indication	Onset
Chlorazepate		Anxiety Seizure disorders Alcohol withdrawal	
Clonazepam	Clonazepam	Seizure disorders	Intermediate
Lorazepam	Lorazepam	Anxiety Anxiety-depression Preoperative sedation	Intermediate
Prazepam	Demethyldiazepam	Anxiety	Slow
Temazepam	Temazepam	Insomnia	Intermediate
Alprazolam	Alprazolam	Anxiety-depression	Intermediate
Halazepam	Halazepam Demethyldiazepam	Anxiety	Slow
Triazolam	Triazolam	Insomnia	Rapid

Modified from Greenblatt, D.J.: N. Engl. J. Med. **309**:354, 1983.

a. Fentanyl is 150-fold more potent than morphine (typical dose, 0.025-0.05 mg); onset is almost immediate, duration is short (30 min or less), and emetic activity is low. Like all narcotics, fentanyl is a respiratory depressant; resulting alterations in respiratory rate and alveolar ventilation may persist after sedative or analgesic effects have terminated. Reports of fentanyl-induced chest wall rigidity and potential need for treatment with narcotic antagonists and/or succinyl choline militate against fentanyl use by those untrained in general anesthesia or unprepared to ventilate and intubate the patient.

b. Meperidine is less potent than morphine and can be given p.o., IM, or IV in doses of 5-100 mg. In addition to the intended effect of analgesia (up to 3 hr), meperidine causes sedation, respiratory depression, euphoria, bronchoconstriction, constipation, nausea, postural hypotension, diaphoresis, and xerostomia.

3. Barbiturates designated "short acting" (secobarbital and pentobarbital) and "ultra–short acting" (methohexital and thiopental) are used in oral and maxillofacial surgery. Methohexital is the most widely employed barbiturate in both sedative and outpatient general anesthetic techniques.

a. Methohexital is administered as a 1% solution (10 mg/ml) given on an intermittent dosing schedule. In ambulatory general anesthesia an initial "test" dose of 20 mg (2 ml) is followed by an induction dose of 0.5-1.0 mg/kg and then by maintenance increments of 10 mg delivered at individually determined intervals. In outpatient anesthesia methohexital is used in conjunction with agents such as N_2O-O_2, fentanyl or meperidine, atropine or glycopyrrolate, naloxone, diazepam, and other substances.

b. Sedation and amnesia can be reliably obtained when methohexital is used to supplement IV diazepam sedation. An initial dose of diazepam (10-20 mg) is followed by small methohexital increments (5-10 mg). Local anesthesia is induced after the patient is adequately sedated. This technique offers the advantages of complete amnesia, intact reflexes (the patient remains conscious and can respond to commands), and the need for only a single operator.

c. Light general anesthesia with diazepam and methohexital is induced with a smaller initial dose of diazepam (5-10 mg) followed by a methohexital "test dose" and an induction dose (20-50 mg). Local anesthesia is recommended; N_2O-O_2 sedation is optional. This technique affords complete amnesia and is very effective for the intractable patient. However, reflexes are obtunded and two operators trained in general anesthetic techniques are required.

4. Narcotic antagonists of various types exist, but naloxone remains the most important. It is a synthetic agent whose configuration resembles that of oxymorphone. Naloxone reverses narcotic effects without exerting significant agonistic influences of its own.

   a. The initial IV dose for adults is 0.2-0.4 mg and may be repeated at intervals of 2-3 min until an effect is seen.

   b. Since the duration of narcotic-induced respiratory depression may exceed the length of time that naloxone is effective (3-4 hr), careful monitoring is needed to detect any recurrent respiratory depression.

III. Stress reduction protocol

  A. Several steps can be taken to help alleviate the anxiety that patients feel over the oral surgical experience.

  B. The "stress reduction protocol" printed below acknowledges a need for managing apprehension preoperatively, intraoperatively, and postoperatively. Note that it employs medications to help the patient relax prior to the procedure, obtain a restful sleep the night before the appointment, tolerate the procedure in comfort and feel less discomfort postoperatively.

Stress Reduction Protocol

A. Recognize medical risk and obtain necessary consultations
B. Recognize patient's anxiety about oral surgical treatment
C. Schedule patient appointment
  1. Usually in AM
  2. Minimize waiting
  3. Short treatment time
D. Control anxiety during therapy
  1. Suggestion
  2. Hypnosis
  3. Local anesthetics
  4. Oral sedation
  5. N_2O-O_2 sedation
  6. Intramuscular sedation
  7. Intravenous sedation
E. Control pain during therapy
  1. Local anesthetics
  2. Systemic analgesics
F. Control pain and anxiety postoperatively

GENERAL REFERENCES

Gustainis, J.F., and Peterson, L.J.: An alternative method of mandibular nerve block, J. Am. Dent. Assoc. **103**:33, 1981.

Malamed, S.F.: Handbook of local anesthesia. ed. 2, St. Louis, 1986, The C.V. Mosby Co.

Spiro, S.R.: Pain and anxiety control in dentistry, Englewood, N.J., 1981, Jack K. Burgess, Inc.

Trieger, N.: Pain control, Chicago, 1974, Quintessence Books.

Postoperative Care

6

BLOOD PRESSURE CONTROL

I. All blood pressure measurements should be interpreted relative to the patient's baseline values. If a preoperative value indicates an elevated (>140/90) or low (<90/60) blood pressure, several measurements should be performed.

II. It is important to realize that there are no absolute values. A wide spectrum of pressure readings exists—reflecting age, systemic conditions, medications, emotional status, and other factors. All readings should be interpreted along with other vital signs.

Hypertension

Hypertension, usually defined as blood pressure greater than 140/90, is a significant finding in a patient.

I. Etiology

A. In the older patient, previously uncontrolled borderline or frank hypertension is a leading cause of postoperative hypertension. A review of the patient's old hospital chart will be helpful, especially the anesthesia record and immediate postoperative vital signs.

1. If a patient is taking antihypertensive medication, one should carefully question him in regard to compliance.

2. A review of the medication chart will be helpful in assessing current medications for proper dosage and timing. (One must not assume that all orders are interpreted correctly.)

B. In the previously healthy younger patient, and for all persons, pain (with its catecholamine release) in the postoperative period is a significant factor in elevated blood pressure. Often, assessment of other vital signs may be helpful. The patient must be asked about his pain status and appropriate measures taken to ensure adequate dosage and timing of medications. The patient may appear quite sedated but actually be very uncomfortable.

C. Drugs may cause hypertension. Positive inotropes (e.g., ephedrine and phenylephrine) may have been administered intraoperatively. Pseudoephedrine is commonly used postoperatively for maxillary procedures. If the patient was paralyzed with pancuronium or gallamine and sedation not adequately reversed, hypertension may result.

D. Fluid gains and losses, including blood loss, transfusions, and urine output, may cause hypertension. The patient in significant positive fluid balance may appear uncomfortable and anxious and experience respiratory distress. One should assess pulmonary status, venous distension, and the extremities for edema.

E. Poor oxygenation and/or increased Pco_2 may result from postoperative atelectasis or preexisting pulmonary disease. Narcotics may have caused the patient to retain CO_2. Unreplaced significant blood loss may lead to poor tissue oxygenation. Arterial blood gas determinations are required for properly assessing any increase or decrease in Po_2 and Pco_2.

1. The Po_2, Pco_2, and pH comprise the arterial blood gas determination, which is a critical part of the preoperative workup and also the intraoperative and postoperative management of a case.

   a. Preoperatively it is needed for

   Evaluation of the respiratory status (e.g., in a patient with chronic lung disease, marginal oxygenation, or hypercapnia)

   Assessing the adequacy of ventilation (e.g., via endotracheal tube in a severe trauma patient with intracranial or thoracic injury)

   b. Intraoperatively it is used in

   Assessing the ventilatory status

   Measuring the acid-base balance

   c. Postoperatively it has multiple indications:

   Acute respiratory distress

   Cardiac emergencies

   Prolonged wakefulness or acute agitation

   Intubation or assisted ventilation

   Poorly controlled diabetes

2. Technique

   a. Equipment—5-6 ml glass syringe, 19-20 gauge needle, rubber stopper or cork (or metal cap), ice-filled container, alcohol swabs for preparing the skin, sponges for applying pressure after the puncture

   b. Method—1 ml of heparin (1000 units/ml) is aspirated into a syringe and is expelled with all the air after the barrel is coated; the syringe will then fill spontaneously by arterial pressure (plastic syringes do not offer this advantage)

3. Sites. The brachial, radial, and femoral arteries are available sites for arterial blood sampling. Each has advantages and disadvantages (see Table 6-1), but proficiency at each should be learned. A good pulse must be palable at the site.

Table 6-1 SITES FOR OBTAINING ABG SAMPLES

Site	Location	Comments
Brachial artery	Accessible as it crosses medial epicondyle of humerus proximal to antecubital space; median nerve is on medial side of vessel	Median nerve potential hazard
Radial artery	Crosses radial styloid; easily accessible with wrist and thumb extended	Allen test to confirm collateral circulation; use local infiltration to reduce spasm and provide patient comfort
Femoral artery	Largest; with patient in supine position and hip externally rotated, vessel is palpable distal to inguinal ligament; place one finger lateral to pulse, second medial to pulse; hold syringe perpendicular to pulse and puncture lateral to pulse	Puncture made lateral to pulse to avoid venous contamination

4. Interpretation
   a. Nomograms (Fig. 6-1) are available for bedside evaluation of results. The following axioms are also helpful:
      (1) The Po_2 is meaningless without knowledge of the inspired oxygen concentration at the time of sampling.
      (2) Assume a normal pH (7.40) and normal Pco_2 (40 mm Hg).
      (3) Each 10 mm Hg shift in the Pco_2 accounts for a pH shift of 0.08.
      (4) Changes in pH from metabolic causes or compensation occur slowly unless iatrogenically produced (e.g., bicarbonate infusion). Changes produced by respiratory function occur quickly.
   b. Oxygenation varies inversely with age. Thus the Po_2 is normally 80-100 mm Hg in room air containing 21% oxygen. A Po_2 of 80 may be "normal" for an elderly patient but not for a young one.
   c. Acidosis and alkalosis may have respiratory or metabolic causes. Multiple permutations are possible, since in most situations the observed pH is the end result of a primary derangement of either respiratory or metabolic function plus a secondary compensation. Bedside interpretation is possible using the axioms on p. 141. (See also Fig. 6-1.)

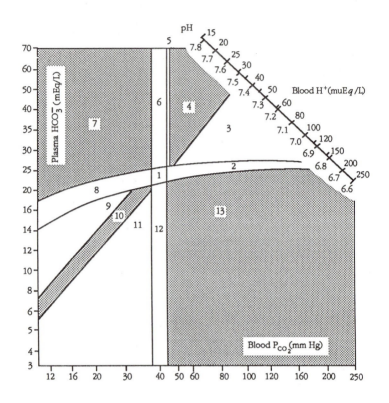

1. Normal
2. Respiratory acidosis
3. Respiratory acidosis (compensated)
4. Respiratory acidosis, metabolic alkalosis (mixed)
5. Metabolic alkalosis (compensated)
6. Metabolic alkalosis
7. Respiratory alkalosis, metabolic alkalosis (mixed)
8. Respiratory alkalosis
9. Respiratory alkalosis (compensated)
10. Metabolic acidosis, respiratory alkalosis (mixed)
11. Metabolic acidosis (compensated)
12. Metabolic acidosis
13. Metabolic acidosis, respiratory acidosis (mixed)

Fig. 6-1   Interpretation of arterial blood studies.

pH	Pco_2	Clinical status
<7.40	>40	Respiratory acidosis
<7.40	≤40	Metabolic acidosis
>7.40	<40	Respiratory alkalosis
>7.40	≥40	Metabolic alkalosis

(1) If the pH is less than 7.40, acidosis occurs; if greater than 7.40, alkalosis.

(2) If the Pco_2 is greater than 40 mm Hg, respiratory acidosis is occurring; if less than or equal to 40, the primary derangement is metabolic acidosis.

(3) For assessing the contribution of combined respiratory and metabolic factors to pH alteration: a Pco_2 of 60 mm Hg would be expected to lower the pH by 0.16 (0.08 for each 10 mm Hg difference from the normal of 40 mm Hg) to 7.24; if the actual pH is found to be 7.32, then partial metabolic compensation for the respiratory acidosis can be assumed (remember: metabolic compensation does not occur acùtely); similarly, if the Pco_2 is 60 mm Hg and the pH is 7.20, then a combined metabolic and respiratory acidosis exists, since the Pco_2 alone (respiratory component) would be insufficient to account for the observed acidosis.

(4) Above all, knowledge of and experience with the actual clinical setting are most important.

F. Urinary retention may cause hypertension. A noncatheterized patient with a full bladder who has not voided within a reasonable time (8-10 hr) after a surgical procedure will often display hypertension and tachycardia.

G. Rarer causes include renovascular hypertension, Cushing's disease, hyperaldosteronism, hyperthyroidism, coarctation of the aorta, pheochromocytoma, toxemia of pregnancy, and increased intracranial pressure.

II. Diagnosis

A. Blood pressure must be measured in both arms (or legs); several readings are necessary.

B. All other vital signs must be assessed and interpreted.

C. Additional indicators may be a visibly anxious patient, flushed skin, respiratory distress, epistaxis, retinal changes, proteinuria, and a full bladder (tender to palpation, dull to percussion).

D. Symptoms may include pain at the operative site, headache, nausea and vomiting, chest pain, and respiratory distress. Visual changes (e.g., scotomas) may appear. Disorientation secondary to stroke should be noted.

E. If chest pain or respiratory distress is present, cardiac enzymes, a chest radiograph, and an ECG must be obtained.

III. Treatment

A. Elevated pressure can be tolerated by a previously healthy patient over a short time. One whose cardiovascular status is compromised may be stepping in dangerous waters with higher than normal readings. It is important to treat the cause, not the numbers!

1. The previously poorly controlled patient needs to begin an antihypertensive regimen. A medical consultation is appropriate.

2. Control of postoperative pain is discussed on p. 145.

3. If the renal status is deemed adequate and the patient is urinating, pressure will often return to baseline within 12-24 hr.

4. Drugs are a possible cause. One must check for type, dosage, and adequate reversal.

5. Urinary retention is discussed on the facing page.

6. Rarer causes and those associated with cardiovascular-pulmonary complications should have an appropriate medical consultation as soon as possible.

B. Hypertensive emergencies (>180/115) or hypertension associated with cardiovascular-pulmonary findings may be treated with the following:

1. Diazoxide—300 mg IV push or 150 mg IV followed by 50 mg increments titrated to an end point

2. Hydralazine-propranolol—10 mg hydralazine in 10 ml normal saline with 1 mg propranolol (Inderal), given in 2 ml aliquots IV

3. Furosemide (Lasix)—initially 10 mg IV, if the patient is in positive fluid balance, or ½ the p.o. dose

4. Methyldopa (Aldomet)—250 mg IV, q.6h. in 125 ml D5W given over 30 min

5. Morphine if pain is the cause—begun with 5 mg IV and 2 mg increments added as needed; this will often lower blood pressure from its vasodilating effects

Hypotension

Hypotension represents a significant lowering of blood pressure below the patient's normal values.

I. Etiology

A. In a previously healthy patient, inadequate fluid replacement causing hypovolemia is a leading cause. The anesthesia record must be checked for all fluid losses and gains, including significant blood loss. Nasogastric suctioning, drains, and repetitive vomiting and diarrhea may be contributing elements. Polyuria associated with diabetes mellitus or insipidus may cause volume depletion. Occult blood loss, distant from the operative site, may be a causative factor; if it is suspected, stool guaiac tests are necessary. Fluid deficits are often associated with tachycardia.

  B. Reduction of cardiac output secondary to atrial or ventricular arrhythmias, congestive heart failure, myocardial infarction, or conduction deficits may cause hypotension.

  C. Drugs (e.g., narcotic analgesics, nitrates, droperidol, hydralazine, propranolol, or curare) may lower the blood pressure.

  D. Rarer causes include septic shock, adrenal insufficiency, large pneumothorax, and positive expiratory pressure treatment.

 II. Diagnosis

  A. Hypotension in the otherwise healthy patient is usually tolerated well.

  B. One must be very careful in the patient with existing coronary artery disease, since the heart receives its major blood supply during diastole, and in the compromised renal function patient, since significant or prolonged hypotension can lead to renal failure. Treatment of these patient groups is more aggressive.

  C. Diagnostic symptoms include

    1. Orthostatic vital signs supine, then sitting or standing, taken within 30 sec to 1 min of assuming each position—an increase in heart rate of 20 or a decrease in systolic pressure of 20 indicates significant volume depletion

    2. Syncope, tachycardia, arrhythmias, or other cardiovascular findings

    3. Laboratory values (hematocrit, osmolality, electrolytes, tests for occult bleeding)—can give clues as to the reason for an acute volume change

 III. Treatment

  A. In an emergency 300 ml of normal saline or Ringer's lactate is given IV over 10 min while observing response. Fluid deficits are best replaced by giving ½ volume over 12 hr and ½ over the remaining 24 hr (unless cardiopulmonary status is impaired).

  B. The patient is put in the Trendelenburg position.

  C. If drugs are the cause, ephedrine 10 mg IV or a phenylephrine drip (1 amp in 500 ml D5W with a "pedi" pump chamber) is given and titrated to response.

  D. Other causes demand prompt medical consultation and coordination treatment.

URINARY RETENTION

 I. A patient should normally void under voluntary effort within 8-12 hr postoperatively. Failure to do so is not an uncommon situation.

 II. Etiology

  A. The usual cause is retention secondary to anesthesia, drugs, and recumbency.

B. The causes can be categorized roughly as
1. Prerenal—secondary to decreased cardiac output (CHF, arrhythmias, etc.) or volume depletion
2. Renal (acute renal failure)—many underlying causes, but acute tubular necrosis the most common
3. Postrenal—obstructive uropathies, bladder atony secondary to medications (vagolytics, narcotics, etc.)
4. Urinary tract infection

III. Diagnosis
A. Physical examination is important. The patient should be asked if he desires to urinate. The bladder may be palpated and percussed for tenderness and dullness. Orthostatic vital signs can indicate hypovolemia.
B. Laboratory tests may be useful—serum hematocrit, osmolality, electrolytes, BUN, creatinine. If a urine sample can be obtained, specific gravity, occult blood, myoglobin (if transfusions were given), casts, and sodium are checked.

IV. Treatment
A. Treatment is directed toward the cause. The most common situation is a sleepy postanesthetic patient who has received one or two narcotic injections. If physical examination indicates a full bladder, suprapubic hot packs and assisted ambulation will usually suffice.
B. If after 10-12 hr no urine production is evident, a "straight cath" may be inserted, with care to remove no more than 500-700 ml since bladder spasm or syncope could result. After catheterizing a patient, it is wise to send a urine sample for analysis along with culture and sensitivity tests.
C. The box will serve as a guide for assessing urinary tests. Prolonged urinary retention demands medical evaluation to rule out renal failure.

RENAL CONSERVATION
Specific gravity high, 1.040
Osmolality high, 300 or greater
Na low (<10 mEq/L)
POSSIBLE RENAL FAILURE
Specific gravity isothenic or less, <1.010
Osmolality low, less than 275
Na high (>50 mEq/L)

D. For treatment of volume depletion, see the section on hypovolemia.
E. Cardiac or renal causes demand thorough and prompt evaluation and treatment coordinated with the proper medical specialty.

PAIN CONTROL

I. Patients may exhibit a wide variety of reactions to painful stimuli. After a major oral and maxillofacial surgery procedure, most patients will require narcotic analgesics for varying lengths of time.

II. Etiology. The source of pain is important. Besides the obvious surgical site, pain can arise from swelling, muscle spasm (secondary to intermaxillary fixation), and local factors (e.g., irritation of the gingivae from arch bars).

III. Diagnosis. A visibly anxious patient with guarding of the affected area usually tells the story. Associated tachycardia and hypertension can often result from pain.

IV. Treatment

    A. Systemic measures include

        1. Meperidine (Demerol)—50-100 mg IM q. 3-4 h.

        2. Morphine—5-10 mg IM q. 3-4 h.

        3. For less painful stimuli

            a. Codeine—30-60 mg and 650 mg acetaminophen q. 3-4 h.

            b. Diazepam (Valium) starting with 2 mg p.o. q.i.d. and increasing as needed for effect

        4. If these narcotic regimens do not sustain the patient, 50 mg hydroxyzine (Vistaril) IM along with the narcotic for increased efficacy

    B. Local measures are also important.

        1. Ice to the area for 24 hr followed by warm moist heat may decrease swelling and reduce muscle spasm.

        2. A rib graft donor site can be very painful. Local blockade of the afferent nerve fibers above, below, and proximal to the operative site is helpful. Bupivacaine (Marcaine) 5-10 ml of a 2% solution with epinephrine will often obviate the need for a heavier narcotic schedule.

        3. Wax (applied to arch bars) and lip creams are helpful.

        4. If the narcotic regimens do not sustain the patient, 50 mg hydroxyzine can be added IM with the narcotic for increased efficacy.

    C. The patient should begin taking oral pain medications at least 24 hr in advance of expected discharge so the efficacy of such a regimen can be ascertained. It may prevent an unexpected "emergency" call.

    D. The surgeon must always weigh the side effects and psychosocial implications of pain medications and try to weigh true patient need against possible drug abuse.

WOUND CARE

I. Wound care should be part of daily patient care. It includes direct observation, indirect observation (vital signs, laboratory values), and good surgical judgment.

A. All wounds should be observed for bleeding, discharge, suture breakdowns, erythema, and necrosis.

B. Experience is needed to distinguish between the expected amount of edema and tissue discoloration from surgical procedures versus that from wound breakdown.

II. Etiology

A. Wound dehiscence or infection may occur from poor surgical technique. Prevention is best achieved by proper debridement of all necrotic or compromised tissue, "sterile technique," irrigation, hemostasis, elimination of dead spaces, proper closure, and antibiotics.

B. Infection may result from intra- or extraoral sources. Cultures are absolutely necessary for determination of cause and selection of proper antibiotic.

C. Systemically compromised patients may be prone to infection by reduced host defenses.

III. Treatment

A. Routine care of intraoral wounds includes
   1. Daily observation
   2. A clear liquid diet for 24 hr; if the patient can be advanced to a full blenderized regimen, clear liquid rinses should follow
   3. Normal saline rinses starting 24 hr after the procedure; some clinicians claim that hydrogen peroxide dissolves existing clots, leading to fresh bleeding
   4. A Water-Pik started 5-7 da postprocedure, with light pressure
   5. Wax applied to arch bars to minimize gingival swelling
   6. Hydrocortisone cream 0.5% to lips pre- and postoperatively to reduce swelling and discomfort

B. Extraoral wounds require
   1. Daily observation
   2. Antibacterial ointment to sutures at each nursing shift
   3. Removal of sutures in 5-7 da, with Steri-Strips across the wound (perpendicularly) to reduce tension; collodion may be applied instead of Steri-Strips

C. Drains should be assessed daily and removed as soon as their purpose is finished. After 24-48 hr, entrance of microorganisms into the wound via the drain becomes more likely. Antibiotics are continued for at least 24 hr after removal of drains.

D. Compressive dressings may aid in reduction of postsurgical swelling. Gauze "fluffs" with Elastoplast and/or a neurosurgical head roll may effectively compress an extraoral surgical wound. Elastoplast placed across the chin for 3-4 da following anterior mandibular procedures is helpful for edema reduction.

E. External pin fixation devices should be observed for loosening and discharge around pin sites. Daily application of antibacterial ointment to pin sites should be routine. Indoform gauze between the skin and the acrylic bar of this device will help minimize irritation.

IV. Complications

A. Early wound breakdown generally results from excessive tension. If all other factors are healthy, the small wound will usually granulate in without complication. Wet dressings applied to the area help prevent dehydration.

B. Late wound breakdown (5 da) usually results from necrotic tissue or infection. More aggressive treatment is necessary—cultures, antibiotics, and thorough determination of cause.

POSTOPERATIVE FEVER

I. A fever may be defined as any body temperature that exceeds 1° above normal.

A. In assessing a patient's fever, it is important to remember the diurnal variation of 0.5-1° seen when AM and PM readings are compared. Also of importance in sequential temperature readings is to make certain that the mode of measurement (e.g., oral verses rectal verses axillary) is the same.

B. Temperature should be checked as part of every postoperative patient visit.

1. A low-grade fever (<100° F) is not an unexpected finding on the first 2-3 da postoperative. Fevers of this magnitude may be attributed to operative trauma or to tissue and protein absorption, and a cause need not be sought if no clinical suspicion of another source is evident.

2. If such a low-grade fever persists beyond 3 da postoperative, it is imperative that a fever work-up be carried out and a cause sought.

3. Fevers worthy of immediate work-up may be defined as

   a. Any that exceed 101.6° after a single dose of acetaminophen (Tylenol) (1.2 g p.o. or p.r.) on the first postoperative night

   b. Any above 101.6° thereafter (without antipyretic administration)

II. Etiology

A. In the search for a cause of postoperative fever, both the timing of its appearance and its magnitude (e.g., low grade verses hyperpyrexia) should be considered, as well as the pattern of temperature troughs and peaks and any associated systemic signs that give valuable clues as to etiology.

B. The timing of fever may be divided into three intervals:

1. Fevers that develop during surgery

   a. These are seen most often in patients who have had sepsis preoperatively. For example, in a patient with a non-reduced mobile mandibular fracture who has fever, swelling, and pain around the fracture site, manipulation of such a contaminated area will result in a bacteremia and temperatures spikes may well be noted intraoperatively.

b. Precipitous rise in body temperature after induction with general anesthesia (with temperature rise as high as 108° F) may herald malignant hyperthermia. This is an anesthetic emergency. The procedure should be terminated and anesthesia stopped immediately.

c. Intraoperative hyperthermia may occur in an anesthetized patient secondary to the thermal insulation provided by the drapes and by the loss of normal thermoregulatory mechanisms through the use of anticholingergic drugs and inhalation anesthetics.

2. Fevers that develop immediately postoperatively (0-6 hr)

a. Fevers within this time interval are commonly caused by either endocrine or metabolic abnormalities. Postoperative thyroid crises are now seen less frequently than in earlier days, before the use of medications that made it easier to attain a euthyroid condition preoperatively. The actual mechanism of thyroid crises remains obscure, but altered metabolism and sensitivity appear to play a role.

b. Blood transfusions may result in fever. This can be due to a full-blown transfusion reaction caused by administration of incompatible blood. Signs and symptoms are noted almost immediately after the transfusion is begun and may present as any of the following: hives, chills, palpitations, chest or flank pain, and shortness of breath, in addition to fever, headache, and flushing. When any of these signs are observed, the transfusion must be stopped immediately.

c. Dehydration secondary to inadequate fluid replacement intraoperatively and minimal oral intake postoperatively may result in fever. This is especially common in children and the elderly. Treating the underlying imbalance should normalize the temperature and help ensure adequate tissue perfusion.

3. Fevers that develop later

a. Postoperative atelectasis is produced by inadequate ventilation or by some obstruction of the tracheobronchial tree (e.g., a mucus plug). In addition to fever, the physical findings of tachypnea, tachycardia and moist rales upon auscultation (especially at the lung bases) are found. A fuller discussion of atelectasis and postoperative pulmonary complications is found on pp. 158-164. Fever secondary to pulmonary complications is most commonly found after the first 6 hr and any time thereafter and should always be high on the differential list of postoperative hyperpyrexia.

b. Another common source of fever spikes after the first 6 hr and as late as 4-5 da postoperative is urinary tract infection (UTI). This complication is more likely to be found in patients experiencing voiding difficulties (urinary stasis) or who have had an indwelling urethral catheter placed.

   (1) Upon questioning, the patient will complain of dysuria, frequency, and pain overlying the involved part of the GU tract (e.g., suprapubic, flank).

   (2) A clean voided specimen (midstream) should be examined microscopically for the presence of WBCs and bacteria.

   (3) Culture and sensitivity tests should also be ordered to ensure that antibiotic coverage is specific. The organisms most frequently isolated from patients with urinary tract infections are gram-negative enteric bacteria, enterococci, *Pseudomonas* species, and yeasts.

   (4) The most feared complication of UTIs is gram-negative sepsis. However, other worrisome sequelae of a chronic UTI are suppurative events (e.g., periurethral, prostatic, or perinephric abscess formation and acute suppurating epididymitis). Septicemia is accompanied by shaking chills and sudden temperature spikes along with the release of bacterial toxins, hypotension, and vascular collapse.

c. The postoperative examination of a patient should always include observation and palpation of the skin overlying the site and IV catheter placement. Nonsterile phlebitis is caused by the introduction of microorganisms into the venous system, with resultant pain, swelling, and edema surrounding the involved site. (The most common offender is thought to be a *Staphylococcus* species.) More often than not, however, phlebitis is a sterile process of vessel injury that is thought to be caused by the frequent infusion of irritating solutions (antibiotics, KCl, hypertonic fluids) into small venous channels.

d. Thrombophlebitis of the lower extremities is yet another later source of postoperative fever and may be suspected when a patient complains of pain and tenderness with palpation of the popliteal space, calves, or thighs. A positive Homan's sign (pain in the calf elicited by dorsiflexion of the foot) is also commonly found with this complication as well as an increase in calf diameter compared to the contralateral extremity. Factors that predispose to the development of thrombophlebitis include prolonged bed rest, long surgical procedures, unusual bed positions maintained postoperatively (e.g., with the pelvis the lowest point and the popliteal space being pushed upon by a flexure in the bed), a previous history of either thrombophlebitis or pulmonary embolus, heart disease (with venous stasis), obesity, polycythemia, and the use of birth control pills.

    e. Postoperative wound infections are generally a later (4-5 da postoperative) source of fever. Careful daily wound inspection will alert the surgeon to the possibility of infection. In addition to increased fever, there will often be tell-tale signs around the wound itself—increased tenderness, redness, drainage (often evidenced by dressing wetness), signs of necrosis and breakdown, reaction around sutures.

III. Formal fever work-up is a logical sequence of diagnostic tests and radiographic studies that address and focus on the common sources of postoperative fever. Results of the fever work-up, coupled with a thorough physical examination, should lead the surgeon not only to source identification but to prompt and appropriate treatment choices (e.g., the proper antimicrobial preparation).

  A. Fevers worthy of immediate work-up are

    1. Any greater than 101.6° F after a single dose of acetaminophen on the first postoperative night

    2. Any over 101.6° F thereafter (without antipyretic administration)

  B. Fever work-up should include

    1. Inspection—wound sites, drain and catheter sites, IV catheters or other lines, general cutaneous inspection for signs of urticarial drug rash or vasculitis

    2. Physical examination—pulmonary and cardiac, abdominal, palpation of extremities, measurement of calf diameter

    3. Cultures—blood from at least two sites, clean voided urine, any drainage from wound or IV sites (aerobic, anaerobic, and, if indicated, fungal); blood cultures must be obtained after careful preparation of the puncture site with antiseptic solutions (povidone-iodine and alcohol)

    4. Chest radiograph—may reveal atelectasis or pneumonitis; if the patient unable to travel, a portable flat chest film should be obtained

IV. Treatment

  A. General treatment of hyperpyrexia

    1. The primary treatment of postoperative fever is to identify its source and treat the underlying problem. In addition, measures should be taken to control hyperpyrexia, especially in patients at greater risk (children, the aged and infirm, the cardiovascularly impaired).

    2. Local measures include cooling mattresses and baths (which do little to affect temperature.)

    3. The salicylates act to reset the hypothalamic "thermostat"

for normal body temperature. Heat production is not affected, but dissipation is enhanced by the increased peripheral blood flow and sweating.

4. Acetaminophen (Tylenol), a para-aminophenol derivative, is an effective antipyretic mechanistically analogous to the salicylates and preferable for hospital use because of its decreased GI irritation. A typical (albeit somewhat arbitrary) postoperative Tylenol order for an adult may be written: 600 mg–1.2 g q. 4 h. when temp exceeds 101.6° F. It is imperative that nursing staff alert the doctor when fever of this magnitude develops in a postoperative patient.

B. Specific treatment when the cause of fever is known

1. For fever of malignant hyperthermia the patient's body is immersed in ice water. The stomach and body are lavaged with ice, and the body surface is cooled with ice packs. Pulmonary hyperventilation is instituted and sodium bicarbonate is given. Arterial blood gases and acid-base status are carefully monitored and abnormalities treated. A diuretic is given to avert development of acute tubular necrosis of the kidney.

   a. Cardiac arrhythmias may sometimes be the initial sign of malignant hyperthermia. Procainamide is usually the drug of choice in treating these. Hyperkalemia is treated with glucose and insulin infusion, and maintenance of fluid volume prevents circulatory collapse. Dantrolene, 1-10 mg/kg, is given as soon as possible.

   b. All of the above measures are continued postoperatively in an ICU since episodes may recur.

2. Treatment of a thyroid crisis as it develops consists of IV hydrocortisone, sedation, oxygen therapy, cooling of the febrile patient, and IV sodium iodide. Reserpine IM is given q.4-6 h. to reduce agitation and tachycardia (respiratory depression must be avoided). Guanethidine similarly is used to block the release of endogenous catecholamines, and IV propranolol is useful in the control of tachycardia. Hyperthermia is prevented by use of a cooling blanket.

3. Febrile reactions may occur to blood transfusions.

   a. Severe reactions secondary to bacterial contamination of blood (generally gram-negative anaerobes) (with temperature usually > 103° F) necessitate immediate cessation of the transfusion. The resultant septicemia is treated with IV fluid support, antibiotics, and steroids.

   b. Minor reactions to transfusions are occasionally seen and thought to be caused by leukoagglutinins or platelet agglutinins present in the recipient. They generally require more than ½ unit of infusion before symptoms (flushing, headaches, chills) are noted, and the fever is usually responsive to oral antipyretics.

4. Treatment of UTIs in a patient who is not acutely ill should

consist initially of hydration while the result of urine cultures is pending. If sepsis is likely, broad-spectrum antibiotics may be started after all cultures are obtained (both blood and urine).

5. In the case of noninfective phlebitis, treatment involves removal of the cannula, elevation of the extremities, and heat to the area. If septicemia is present, appropriate antibiotic treatment is begun (often requiring massive doses). If deep venous channels are involved, it is often necessary to remove the entire vein from the catheter entrance point to where it enters the next large venous tributary.

6. The risks and benefits of giving postoperative prophylactic anticoagulation therapy to those at high risk of thrombophlebitis must be weighed against the possibility of postoperative hemorrhage. If thrombophlebitis does develop, treatment includes bed rest, removal of all popliteal pressure, and anticoagulation as follows:

   a. Heparin is given by intermittent IV injection or by continuous infusion.
      (1) Intermittent: 10,000-15,000 units Na heparin initially and then 5000-10,000 units q.4h.
      (2) Continuous: 5000 units bolus and 1000 units/hr thereafter
      (3) Treatment should be monitored by the PTT, which is maintained at 1-1½ times normal (37-60 sec).
      (4) Heparin is usually continued 8-19 da or until symptoms have subsided and the patient is ambulatory.

   b. Warfarin (Coumadin) is not effective for 5-7 da, so it is not the agent of choice in treating an acute problem. Therapy is begun several days after heparin treatment is started and continued after the heparin is stopped
      (1) The efficacy of warfarin anticoagulation is monitored by serial PTs (obtained daily during the first week, twice weekly during week 2, and twice monthly while the patient is receiving the warfarin). The PT should be maintained at 1-1½ times normal.
      (2) The maintenance dose of warfarin varies between 2.5-12.5 mg/da, pending results of the PT.
      (3) If prompt reversal of anticoagulation is needed, vitamin K (5-25 mg IV) may be administered. (The complication of pulmonary embolism is discussed on pp. 161-164.)

POSTOPERATIVE NAUSEA AND VOMITING

I. The subjective complaint of nausea and the objective and measurable phenomenon of emesis are not infrequent problems in the immediate postoperative period (generally postintubation to 24 hr).

II. Vomiting may be an especially dangerous complication for a patient who has been placed in intermaxillary fixation. It is imperative that both a scissors (or wire cutter if IMF is via wiring rather than elastics) and a suction source be placed at the patient's bedside if extensive emesis that the patient cannot clear ensues and the jaws must be released. Generally, when the patient is fully awake and responding to verbal commands, the clearing of emesis will rarely require the release of IMF. Nasal suctioning and suctioning in the buccal vestibules will usually aid the patient in removal of emesis from the mouth. The patient should be placed on his side and the head of the bed lowered (Trendelenburg position) to enable gravity to abet clearing.

III. Aspiration of gastric contents secondary to vomiting may be a disastrous event and greatly increases the morbidity of a patient's postoperative course. The mortality from massive aspiration is reported as being as high as 90%. (A complete discussion of aspiration is found later in this chapter.)

IV. Etiology
   A. The cause may be one or a combination of the following:
      1. Use of morphine (or other opiates), which tend to increase gastric motor activity
      2. Inhalation general anesthesia (especially during induction and emergence), when the vomiting center is thought to be stimulated and protective reflexes have been lost
      3. Swallowing of blood and air intraoperatively and especially postoperatively (in which case nausea and vomiting are related to the site of surgery and it's extent); this is perhaps the most common cause of postoperative nausea in the oral surgical patient, especially when intraoral incisions continue to weep and blood-tinged saliva is repeatedly swallowed
   B. It must also be kept in mind that nausea and vomiting may be due to an acute problem not directly related to the surgery or the anesthetic (e.g., acute appendicitis, stress ulcer, small bowel obstruction).

V. Prophylaxis
   A. The use of nasogastric suction in oral and maxillofacial surgery has become an important part of prophylaxis for nausea, vomiting, and the potentially fatal complications of resultant airway obstruction or aspiration pneumonitis.
   B. The use of a Salem sump nasogastric tube is indicated if the patient is to be placed in IMF postoperatively, if the operation is expected to last over 3-4 hr, and if hemorrhage of greater than 100 ml from the operative sites or from the nose during or after surgery is expected. The nasogastric tube thus ensures that the stomach can be kept clear of any blood that leaks and (hopefully) removes this trigger for vomiting. The Salem sump is inserted after the patient is anesthetized. Auscultation while air is being forced through will help ensure proper placement in the stomach. The patency of the nasogastric tube should be checked each hour (irrigate with 30-50 ml H_2O). Thorough

suctioning before extubation is the rule, so the tube is left in place in the recovery room (and thereafter if it continues to drain when connected to wall suction). Before the tube is removed, the stomach should again be irrigated with normal saline and suctioned to remove any debris. The tube must be detached from the suction source before it is pulled.

C. Nasogastric suction, if prolonged, can remove large amounts of fluid from the upper GI tract and lead to resultant electrolyte imbalances (e.g., decreased K^+ or decreased H^+ [alkalosis]), which may require replacement therapy.

D. The tube must be securely taped in place so as not to apply excessive pressure to the skin, mucosa, or cartilage of the nose. A half-inch piece of tape is prepared with two tails by cutting the lower portion in half. The uncut portion is applied to the nose, and the tails are wrapped around the tube to secure it.

E. Complaints of nausea and vomiting after discontinuing naso-gastric suction are most frequently addressed by the use of antiemetic pharmacological agents (discussed next).

VI. Treatment

A. Following is a list of the more commonly used antiemetic prep-arations and recommended dosage schedules:

1. Promethazine (Phenergan)—this phenothiazine derivative is well tolerated by children. Usual dose: 12.5-25 mg q.4-6 h.

2. Trimethobenzamide (Tigan)—this drug depresses the "che-moreceptor trigger zone" in the medulla. Usual dose: 250 mg t.i.d. or q.i.d. It is not recommended for use in children since it is associated with Reye's syndrome. Extrapyramidal symptoms may be found.

3. Prochlorperazine maleate (Compazine)—use of this drug and other hepatotoxins is contraindicated in children and adolescents whose signs and symptoms suggest Reye's syn-drome. Usual dose: 5-10 mg p.o. q.6 h.; rectal dose: 25 mg b.i.d.; deep IM dose: 5-10 mg q.6h. There may be side effects of extrapyramidal tract involvement with severe opisthoton-os and risus sardonicus, which are dose related; in such cases less than 40 mg should be used per 24 hr.

4. Droperidol (Inapsine)—a neuroleptic, this drug experimen-tally antagonizes the emetic effect of apomorphine in dogs. Usual dose for prophylaxis: < 60 kg, 0.25 ml (0.7 mg); > 60 kg, 0.5 ml (1.4 mg). These are not sedating doses, and they have a good effect on nausea and vomiting.

5. Chlorpromazine (Thorazine)—this phenothiazine deriva-tive is contraindicated in children. Usual dose: 10-25 mg q.5-6 h. p.o. If no hypotension occurs, the dose may be increased to 25-50 mg q.3-4h. p.r.n. until vomiting is con-trolled.

B. Our institution has empirically found the following combination of medications particularly effective in the treatment of nausea caused by antineoplastic drugs:

> Droperidol (Inapsine)—5 mg, IM at 3 PM and 7 PM
> Diphenhydramine (Benadryl)—50 mg, IM or p.o.
>   at 2 PM and 8 PM
> Dexamethasone (Decadron)—12 mg, IM or p.o. in AM

C. All postoperative patient examinations should include both palpation and auscultation of the abdomen. If an acute process is responsible for the postoperative emesis, suspicion will be raised by rebound or pointing tenderness, loss of bowel sounds, or abdominal distension.

POSTOPERATIVE CARDIAC PROBLEMS

I. A routine portion of the postoperative examination is careful cardiac auscultation for regularity, normal heart sounds, and no acute changes from the preoperative work-up (e.g., no onset of cardiac murmur or development of S_3 gallop).

II. Etiology
   A. The more common causes of cardiac arrhythmias in a postoperative patient include
      1. Ischemia—may be secondary to inadequate respiration with resultant hypoxia or to severe volume depletion and underperfusion
      2. Ectopy—may be due to excessive release of endogenous catecholamines secondary to pain
      3. Acid-base imbalance—especially acidosis and hypokalemia
      4. Drugs intraoperatively and postoperatively administered
      5. Preexisting cardiac problems—e.g., atherosclerosis, left ventricular hypertrophy
      6. Hypercapnia—often contributes to the development of arrhythmias
   B. Each of these should be considered individually whenever one thinks about etiology. Many cardiac arrhythmias are very serious and can lead to a precipitously downhill course.

III. Recognition and treatment
   A. This review is aimed at specific recognition of such problems so that prompt cardiac consultation can be sought. Treatment is aimed at identification and, if possible, reversal of the cause.
   B. Sinus bradycardia
      1. Normal sinus rhythm exists, rate less than 60 bpm.
      2. Causes include increased vagal tone, elevated intracranial pressure, and general anesthesia (cyclopropane, halothane). It is also found in trained athletes.
      3. Treatment uses vagolytics (atropine, 1 mg IV, repeated in 3-5 min) with or without inotropes (isoproterenol, IV infusion [1 mg/250 ml D5W], with a pediatric drip set at 10-20 mg/min).

    4. This relatively benign condition must be differentiated from complete heart block. An ECG is diagnostic, though IV atropine will also allow differentiation.

C. Sinus tachycardia
    1. Normal sinus rhythm exists, rate 100-180 bpm.
    2. Causes include stress (e.g., postoperative pain), fever, hypoxia, hypovolemia (with reflex tachycardia), congestive heart failure, anemia, and hyperthyroidism (thyroid storm).
    3. Treatment of the underlying cause usually is sufficient. Beta blockade with propranolol 1.5 mg IV (with increments up to 2 mg over 10-15 min) or propranolol 10-40 mg p.o. q.i.d. may be instituted.

D. Premature atrial contractions (PACs)
    1. Irregularity of the pulse is noted. The ECG will show a non-sinus tachycardia with occasional premature P waves of varying morphology that are conducted through to the ventricle, producing a normal QRS complex. There is an incomplete compensatory pause after the PAC complex. PACs are ordinarily benign but may anticipate other atrial arrhythmias that are more worrisome.
    2. If treatment is necessary, quinidine sulfate and procainamide (Pronestyl) are generally the drugs of choice. Dosage schedules and development of therapeutic levels are worked out with cardiac consultation.

E. Paroxysmal atrial tachycardia (PAT)
    1. In PAT there is atrial tachyarrhythmia with a 1:1 ventricular response. Heart rates may be between 140-240 bpm, and the QRS complexes may be distorted at these rapid rates.
    2. The cause is usually a reentry mechanism (part of the Wolff-Parkinson-White syndrome). It is often seen in patients with no cardiac history and may follow general anesthesia.
    3. Initial treatment is by vagal stimulation (e.g., carotid sinus massage). If this fails, pharmacological intervention may include edrophonium (Tensilon), a synthetic anticholinesterase, or use of digitalis, quinidine, or procainamide. Cardioversion may be necessary if these measures fail.

F. Atrial flutter and fibrillation
    1. The atrial rate with flutter is 250-350 bpm; with fibrillation it is 375-600. The pulse is often described as "irregularly irregular."
    2. Frequent causes are rheumatic or coronary heart disease, thoractomy, pericarditis, hyperthyroidism, and pulmonary embolization.
    3. Treatment (always done with cardiac consultation) includes
       a. For acute atrial fibrillation—rapid digitalization (1.5-2 mg q. 24 h.), to increase the AV block, and then propranolol in 0.5 mg IV increments. If no conversion occurs,

quinidine sulfate or procainamide may be employed.

    b. For chronic atrial fibrillation—digoxin for rate control. If cardioversion is contemplated, one must anticoagulate beforehand.

G. Nodal rhythm

    1. On the ECG this is characterized by a loss of P waves (no atrial depolarization) with a normal-appearing QRS. The rate may be slowed when impulses arise from the AV node. Hemodynamic consequences follow the loss of atrial systole and decreased filling of the left ventricle. This is of little consequence in healthy patients but is more worrisome in a person with already compromised function.

    2. Causes include SA node inhibition by vagal reflex, digitalis toxicity, and acute myocardial infarction (most often noted with the use of general inhalation anesthesia, especially halothane).

    3. Treatment is of the underlying cause.

H. Ventricular extrasystoles (PVCs)

    1. These consist of a premature QRS complex with widened abnormal morphology.

    2. They are most commonly associated with ischemia, digitalis toxicity, hypokalemia, acid-base imbalance, stress, and mitral valve prolapse.

    3. Treatment is indicated if there are more than 6 PVCs/min, if the complexes are multifocal, if they occur on or near T waves, or if there are bursts of 2-3 PVCs (or more) in a row.

    4. Lidocaine, 100 mg IV bolus, is given followed by an infusion (lidocaine drip) of 2 g/500 ml D5W at 4 mg/min or 1 ml/min. A second bolus of lidocaine may be given in 30-40 min. If not effective, 500 mg procainamide IV or p.o. q. 4 h. is administered. (Because of the risk of developing a lupus syndrome with long-term procainamide use, the patient may be maintained on quinidine 200-400 mg q. 6 h.)

I. Ventricular tachycardia

    1. On the ECG this is seen as abnormal QRS complexes at a rapid rate (150-250 bpm).

    2. Ventricular tachycardia is an ominous finding, often heralding the development of ventricular fibrillation.

    3. Treatment is lidocaine via bolus and infusion (as above) for immediate correction of hypoxia and the acid-base and electrolyte abnormalities. Pharmacological intervention may include procainamide, quinidine, disopyramide, or propranolol.

    4. Immediate countershock is needed if the hemodynamic state deteriorates.

J. Ventricular fibrillation

    1. On the ECG this is an unmistakable, chaotic, and rapid sine wave pattern.

2. Treatment is immediate cardioversion followed by lidocaine given as a bolus and infusion. Acidosis is corrected with bicarbonate (acidosis lowers the fibrillation threshold).

POSTOPERATIVE PULMONARY COMPLICATIONS

I. Despite many advances in the care of the postoperative patient, pulmonary complications continue to be frequent. To avoid dramatic increases in morbidity and even mortality of oral surgical patients, they must be addressed promptly and efficaciously.

II. Thorough postoperative examination will raise the strong suspicion of pulmonary distress, and early intervention is thus likely.

III. Many factors (both surgical and anesthetic) play a role in the development of the following entities:

Airway obstruction, acute or chronic
Atelectasis
Bacterial pneumonitis
Aspiration pneumonitis
Pulmonary emboli and pneumothorax
Preexisting asthmatic and obstructive pulmonary disease

Airway obstruction

I. Acute obstruction is heralded by the development of increasingly stridorous inspiratory sounds, dyspnea, tachypnea, cyanosis, and pronounced use of the accessory muscles of respiration (suprasternal skin retraction during inspiration). Additional discussion of airway management is found in Chapter 12.

II. The causes of postoperative obstruction are as follows:

A. Significant laryngeal edema secondary to traumatic intubation—this is not uncommon in oral surgery patients receiving blind nasotracheal intubation. It may have an insidious onset, with increased restlessness and irritability yet drowsiness due to the worsening hypoxia as early signs. It has been observed in patients with a history of recent respiratory tract infection or previous irradiation to the region of the cords.

B. Tracheal narrowing secondary to neck surgery with a significant amount of postoperative swelling or hematoma formation—this can occur with vallecula epiglottica and piriform sinus excisions, base of tongue resections, composite resections with flap procedures for head and neck cancer patients, and bilateral neck dissections. It may also result from a Ludwig-type infection or cellulitis secondary to a badly infected tooth. Other causes of tracheal narrowing are soft tissue masses (mediastinal, oropharyngeal, and nasopharyngeal tumors) of appreciable magnitude, accumulation of viscous secretions in enough quantity to block the tracheobronchial tree, and the restrictive action of dressings placed overzealously about the neck and chest.

C. Position of the head in the unconscious patient—this may

cause the tongue and epiglottis to be posteriorly displaced so they block the glottic opening and prevent exchange of air. It is noteworthy that children have significantly smaller laryngeal openings than adults and thus even small quantities of secretions or slight compression may be sufficient to cause complete obstruction. Children also lack the forceful clearing power (e.g., cough) of adults.

III. Treatment of airway obstruction includes the following:
   A. Early recognition of respiratory distress—this is the first step.
   B. Alteration of head position if the patient is supine and unconscious—pushing forward at the angles of the mandible may permit air exchange.
   C. Prompt application of a mechanical airway—if oropharyngeal and nasopharyngeal airways do not alleviate the distress, the patient must be reintubated without delay.
   D. Emergency tracheotomy—with significant laryngeal edema, extensive swelling, and hematoma formation postoperatively, prompt and effective intubation is often not possible; in this case, tracheotomy will be lifesaving and should proceed without delay under local anesthesia (in the operating room only if time permits).
   E. Frequent suctioning and removal of secretions, blood, and vomitus from the pharynx—use of nasogastric suction will decrease the likelihood of aspiration of gastric contents.
   F. Oxygen therapy—this should be initiated immediately after the airway is assured and modified pending the results of arterial blood gas analysis. There should be frequent postoperative inspection of dressings and bandages as well as routine catheter aspiration through the nose and mouth.
   G. In patients undergoing extensive resection of head and neck tumors, in which dramatic postoperative swelling is anticipated, elective tracheostomy may be performed to obviate the need for emergency tracheotomy (a procedure with increased risk to the patient). In these patients airway maintenance is often a critical problem for the first 48 hr and a serious one for the first 7-10 da after surgery.

Atelectasis

I. Atelectasis often presents as tachypnea, tachycardia, fever, and moist inspiratory rales (especially at the lung bases).
II. Several factors predispose to this problem:
   A. Narcotics, often given as postoperative analgesics, depress both the respiratory center and the cough reflex (deep breathing and periodic coughing tend to ameliorate atelectasis).
   B. Prolonged bed rest postoperatively hampers lung ventilation.
   C. Postoperative pain and splinting often make deep breathing difficult.
   D. Acute pulmonary obstruction will prevent large portions of the lung from being adequately aerated.

Bacterial pneumonitis

I. If atelectasis persists untreated, secondary bacterial colonization (bacterial pneumonitis) may result. This significantly complicates the patient's postoperative course, and requires the use of antibiotics.

II. As part of standard postoperative orders, the nursing staff is instructed to help the patient go through the exercises of deep breathing, coughing, and rolling from side to side every 2 hr while awake and before he is able to ambulate. These conservative measures significantly decrease the occurrence of extensive atelectasis.

III. In patients with a previous history of significant smoking or chronic obstructive pulmonary disease, a postoperative order for formal chest pulmonary therapy is indicated. If atelectasis does not respond to these conservative measures, tracheobronchial suctioning or transtracheal cough stimulation should be tried. If mucous plugging of a smaller airway is thought to be responsible for an atelectatic patch, removal by means of bronchoscopy is feasible.

Aspiration pneumonitis

I. Depending upon its extent, aspiration pneumonitis may be a disastrous postoperative complication with significant mortality secondary to respiratory failure. It is usually caused by gastric contents that enter the tracheobronchial tree either during anesthesia (e.g., passive aspiration with induction) or after extubation before the patient has regained protective reflexes.

II. There are factors in addition to general anesthesia that tend to obtund reflexes. These include trauma, alcohol intoxication, drug overdose with resultant CNS depression, seizure disorders, a previous history of CVAs, and tracheostomy. Similarly, esophageal motility disorders (e.g., achalasia, spasm, hiatal hernia with reflux) place the patient at increased risk of aspiration. Bowel obstruction, either paralytic or mechanical, may also predispose to aspiration secondary to emesis.

III. Aspiration of particulate matter may lead to occlusion of airways, hypoventilation of a lung segment, and subsequent collapse.

IV. The pH of the aspirate has also been implicated in the extent of damage. If the pH of gastric fluid is over 2.5, minimum lung damage ensues. However, with a pH less than 2.5 and the amount of aspirate over 50 ml, pulmonary parenchyma and blood vessels are severely damaged and significant bronchospasm (secondary to chemical irritation) ensues.

V. Several findings are diagnostic of aspiration pneumonitis.

　A. Physical evidence—dyspnea, cough, wheezing (rhonchi and rales), fever, tachycardia, hypotension, shock, and cyanosis

　B. Radiographic evidence—unilateral radiodense infiltrates, most commonly seen in the right upper lung if the patient is supine at aspiration, or possibly bilateral diffuse infiltrates

C. Laboratory evidence—leukocytosis (12,000-15,000 WBCs), ABGs with hypoxia, and normal or decreased Pco_2 (Some 30% of these patients will have negative bacterial cultures. When cultures are positive, the most common etiological flora is an oropharyngeal species, with anaerobes outnumbering aerobes 10:1.)

VI. As soon as aspiration pneumonitis is noted or suspected (with active vomiting or passive refluxing), the patient should be placed in the Trendelenburg position. Pharyngeal and endotracheal suction should be started immediately and, if necessary, bronchoscopy for the removal of particulate matter from the airway.

A. If the patient's level of consciousness is significantly deteriorating secondary to hypoxia (Pao_2 is a worrisome value) and he is laboring to breath, mechanical ventilation with positive pressure should be instituted (to maximize oxygenation).

B. If wheezing is present, bronchodilators (aminophylline) should be used. IV steroids are of value only if administered within 5 min of aspiration.

C. Antibiotic therapy should be started only in response to a strong suspicion of a bacterial component of the aspirant (e.g., organisms on Gram stain or, preferably, positive culture results) and should be specific for the major offending organisms isolated.

D. The most effective treatment of aspiration pneumonitis remains prevention. This includes identification and appreciation of patients who are at particular risk. They may be treated prophylactically with cimetidine or an antacid (e.g., Maalox) in an effort to decrease the acidity and amount of gastric secretions. Rapid-sequence intubation is recommended in these patients, and they should be extubated in an alert and fully awake condition. A suction source should be readily available at the bedside at all times.

Pulmonary emboli

I. The origin of PEs is most commonly thrombi in the venous circulation, especially the lower extremities, that affix themselves to the intima of the host vessel.

II. Factors predisposing to the development of PEs include

Prolonged postoperative bed rest
Bed positions favoring the stagnation of venous bleed
Previous history of thrombophlebitis or pulmonary emboli
Heart disease
Obesity
Polycythemia
Use of PCBs

III. Signs and symptoms of pulmonary emboli are as follows:

A. Positive leg signs (e.g., pain, tenderness) may occur in 10% of patients. However, frequently there will be no presenting symptoms.

B. The classical triad of acute onset of chest pain, dyspnea, and hemoptysis is seen in only a small percentage of cases.

C. The classical auscultatory sign of a friction rub may be present.

D. If emboli obstruct over 60% of the pulmonary artery tree, physical examination will show signs of acute cor pulmonale—loud P_2 sounds, distension of neck veins, hepatomegaly, tachypnea, tachycardia, cyanosis, and hypotension.

E. In such cases ECG signs will include definite evidence of right ventricular strain—right ventricular hypertrophy and right axis deviation, ST depression in II, III, aV_F, V_2, and V_3, and inversion of T waves in V_1-V_3. These findings usually precede the development of shock and vascular collapse.

F. The chest radiograph will show decreased lung markings (Westmark's sign) and evidence of right ventricular enlargement. The classical wedge-shaped density is frequently seen.

G. In less than ⅓ of the cases of PE, pulmonary infarction ensues. The patient may then have dyspnea, pleuritic pain, hemoptysis, cough, fever, tachycardia, and tachypnea.

H. Noteworthy laboratory results include an increased WBC count and increased lactate dehydrogenase level by chest radiograph.

I. Pulmonary emboli should be suspected in any postoperative patient who presents with the above symptoms and laboratory and radiological findings (especially one who is at greater risk). Small emboli are considerably more difficult to diagnose since they are often asymptomtic and show no characteristic ECG or chest radiograph signs.

J. The use of pulmonary scanigrams is often helpful in diagnosis, for they define the areas of perfusion.

K. The most reliable diagnostic technique is pulmonary angiography.

IV. Treatment is as follows:

A. Oxygen therapy is begun and, depending upon the patient's Pao_2, may be accompanied by intubation. Ventilatory assistance is begun if needed. Central venous pressure is routinely monitored.

B. If hypotension and heart failure develop, they must be promptly treated.

C. Either morphine or meperidine (Demerol) is given to decrease pain and anxiety.

D. Anticoagulation with heparin is begun right away. It may be given by either IV intermittent injection or continuous IV infusion after the diagnosis has been made or the index of suspicion significantly increased.

1. Intermittent injection—initial dose 10,000 units IV, then 7500-10,000 units q. 4 h. for 24 hr; thereafter, the dose is decreased and warfarin treatment is started concurrently

2. Continuous infusion—initial dose 5000 units IV, followed

by 100 units/kg thereafter; heparin therapy monitored by the PTT, which is maintained at 1-1½ times normal value (37-60 sec); this is usually continued for 8-10 da, by which time the venous thrombi have presumably become firmly adherent to the vessel wall

E. Warfarin therapy is begun 2-3 da after heparin and the drugs are given concurrently until the heparin is discontinued.

1. Usual dose of warfarin—10-15 mg/da (the PT is drawn daily during first week of therapy, twice weekly during second, and weekly or less thereafter); levels 2-3 times normal found to be therapeutic, and dosage may be adjusted to achieve this

2. Duration—anticoagulation maintained for a minimum of 6 mo after pulmonary emboli in an effort to prevent recurrence

F. The use of fibrinolytic agents (to speed dissolution of the clot) has been advocated, especially in the case of massive PEs. Two plasminogen activators, streptokinase and urokinase, have been extensively studied for this purpose.

1. Streptokinase—not suitable because of an increased incidence of allergic reactions

2. Urokinase (a natural fibrinolysin obtained from human urine)—more suitable although its use has been associated with a high incidence of bleeding and its prohibitive cost makes it a less than ideal agent; unequivocal demonstration of its efficacy in decreasing the mortality and morbidity of PEs remains to be shown

G. Surgical interruption of the inferior vena cava (IVC) is an effort to safeguard against recurrent and possibly fatal PEs. Surgery is indicated in patients who are unable to receive anticoagulation treatment (e.g., trauma patients with major visceral, brain, or cord injuries, patients with other bleeding lesions, patients with blood dyscrasias or clotting disorders secondary to liver disease) or those in whom anticoagulation has previously been unsuccessful. IVC interruption is also advocated in patients with a history of recurrent PEs and documented septic phlebitis. IVC ligation results in total impedance of blood flow through the vessel. Partial occlusion of the vessel may be obtained by use of a slotlike clip, grid, or IVC "umbrella." The principle of partial occlusion is that emboli will be trapped whereas some blood flow may continue. In actuality, it is likely that the small openings quickly become occluded with either newly formed thrombi or recurrent emboli. To date, no significant differences in results obtained from either technique have been demonstrated. Anticoagulation therapy should be reinstituted several days after IVC interruption.

H. Pulmonary embolectomy is mechanical removal of a clot from the pulmonary artery. This highly invasive and risky procedure is indicated only in patients with progressive circulatory collapse, chronic pulmonary hypertension, or documented occlusion of the right or left main pulmonary artery. At best, embolectomy under direct vision through pulmonary arteriotomy carries a 33% mortality risk.

Pneumothorax

I. Pneumothorax is defined as air entering the pleural cavity, which thereby reduces the normal negative intrapleural pressure and results in partial lung collapse.

   A. The index of suspicion of postoperative pneumothorax is raised when the surgical procedure itself involves an area close to the lungs (e.g., the harvesting of autogenous rib grafts for mandibular reconstruction). Supraclavicular approaches to the brachial plexus (for regional anesthesia) and the insertion of subclavian central venous lines likewise carry a finite risk (usually <1%) of producing a pneumothorax.

   B. Pneumothorax develops occasionally as a result of injury to the apex of the pleural reflection at the inferior limit of the neck during neck dissections. Care must be taken when approaching this area to avoid entering the pleura.

II. Signs of pneumothorax include tachypnea, tachycardia, and cyanosis.

   A. At physical examination there is hyperresonance over the involved area, absent breath sounds, and loss of normal diaphragmatic movement on the affected side (?).

   B. At chest radiography the margin of the collapsed lung is seen outlined by air.

   C. Decreased PaO_2 (secondary to a functional shunt) may be found.

III. Treatment consists of intermittent needle aspiration or prophylactic chest tube insertion. Treatment of all traumatic pneumothoraces is chest tube emplacement (with underwater seal) checked by sequential chest radiographs.

GENERAL REFERENCES

American College of Surgeons: Manual of preoperative and postoperative care, Philadelphia, 1983, W.B. Saunders Co.

Condon, R.E., and Nyhus, L.M.: Manual of surgical therapeutics, Boston, 1985, Little, Brown & Co.

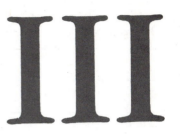

Dentoalveolar Surgery

7

Exodontia

GENERAL CONSIDERATIONS

I. A major goal of contemporary dental medicine is the preservation of the natural dentition. However, extraction of teeth is often indicated and remains an important part of oral and maxillofacial surgery.

II. The application of proper surgical technique and compassionate patient management will permit removal of teeth in a painless and atraumatic fashion. Managing a patient's fears and apprehensions is every bit as important as the execution of proper technique.

PREOPERATIVE MANAGEMENT

I. Patient treatment starts with the initial assessment. A concise history is obtained to determine whether preexisting medical or dental problems might affect the planned procedures.

II. A physical examination should precede any surgical intervention. The entire oral cavity is examined for other abnormal conditions that may exist in addition to that for which the patient was referred.

III. Radiographs are taken so the problem at hand can be evaluated as well as the teeth, alveolar bone, sinuses, etc. The relationship of the teeth to structures such as the inferior alveolar canal and maxillary sinuses should be ascertained.

IV. After a complete history, physical examination, and radiographic examination, a surgical plan is developed. This plan includes a determination of the patient's general management, surgical management, and anesthetic needs.

V. Several surgical principles must be considered.
   A. The surgeon must have good access to the surgical field. The patient is positioned to allow maximum exposure. Good lighting is essential. The assistant should also be able to suction the field as necessary.

1. Bleeding in the field must be controlled and attention given to maintaining good surgical anesthesia.
2. Whenever necessary, a flap should be developed to afford maximum access to the field. A flap will heal much better and faster than a torn, traumatized area of tissue.

B. The forces used to remove teeth must be under control at all times. The force used with rotary drills must also be carefully controlled. The surgeon has to develop a feel for the amount of bone removed by the drill with light pressure and must be careful to protect the adjacent tissues.

C. The path for removal of a tooth must be unimpeded. An adjacent tooth may block the extraction path of a malpositioned tooth, in which case the tooth to be removed may need to be sectioned before removal.
1. A multirooted tooth may need to be sectioned because the curves in the roots may be blocked by bone or the distance between the roots may be too wide for removal through the tooth socket.
2. Sectioning of teeth when indicated reduces trauma and prevents complications related to the use of excessive force as in extensive bone removal, maxillary tuberosity fracture, or sinus exposure.

D. When access to the surgical field is compromised by soft tissue or when bone removal is necessary, a soft tissue flap should be raised to provide access to the field. The flap should be large enough for access to the entire field of surgery.
1. To ensure adequate blood supply, the base of the flap should be wider than the crestal margin.
2. The flap should be designed so that, when repositioned, the marginal incision rests on bone.

VI. Following are some of the common indications for removing teeth:

A. Carious destruction that cannot be restored

B. Extensive and advanced periodontal disease that cannot be treated

C. Malpositioning that jeopardizes adjacent structures or teeth

D. Orthodontic therapy

E. Caries and/or periodontal disease along with impacted teeth in a patient undergoing radiation therapy (These teeth should be removed a minimum of 7-10 da before therapy.)

F. Tooth infection that is considered to be a potential source of systemic bacteremia in a patient with cardiac valvular and septal disease or with prosthetic valves (Teeth with extensive caries and periapical or periodontal disease are the potential problem. Coronary artery bypass surgery is not an indication for extraction. [A complete discussion of this important topic is found in Chapter 4.])

G. When they interfere with the placement of protheses

TREATMENT PROCEDURE
Elevator and forceps extraction

I. Elevators are very useful in the removal of teeth. They should, how-ever, be used with care because serious complications can occur when they are used improperly. Most problems with elevators stem from misjudgment of the amount of force delivered or from improper positioning.

   A. Trauma can result in fracture of the mandible, tuberosity, or alveolar bone and tooth segments or in loosening of teeth.

   B. Bone, not an adjacent tooth, should be used as a fulcrum when positioning the elevator.

II. Elevators are used in the following ways:

   A. Straight elevator (no. 40 or 301). This is the most versatile type.

      1. It is used to luxate an erupted tooth. Placed perpendicular to the long axis of the alveolar ridge on the mesial of the tooth with the rounded side of its tip resting on bone, it is rotated away from the tooth, creating a "scooping" action to elevate the tooth. The elevator may also be rotated toward the tooth to luxate and move it posteriorly. Once the tooth has some mobility, the elevator can be worked in an apical direction on the labial side. The labial bone plate is used as a fulcrum for further elevation.

      2. The straight elevator is also useful for sectioning a tooth. After a slot is made with a rotary drill at the point where the tooth is to be split, the elevator is placed in the slot and rotated to separate the halves.

   B. Bayonette elevator. This offset-shaped instrument is designed for removing maxillary and mandibular third molars.

   C. Potts and Miller elevators. These are useful for removing deeply impacted maxillary third molars. Their curved shape allows them to be seated at the cervical area to prevent the tooth from being inadvertently pushed superiorly into the maxillary sinus.

   D. Cryers or east-west elevator. This type is useful for removing fractured roots of molars.

III. Extraction forceps are designed to fit the anatomical shape of the crown and root of specific teeth and for the application of specific forces on individual teeth in different anatomical positions. Gener-ally speaking, straight-handled forceps are used for anterior teeth and curved- or bayonette-handled forceps are used for posterior teeth.

IV. Proper use of forceps and elevators promotes the efficient removal of teeth with a minimum of discomfort and tissue damage. There are many types of forceps available, all variations of a few basic designs. It is important to select the proper forceps for the specific tooth to be removed.

V. The basic techniques for removing teeth are as follows:

A. Maxillary incisors and canines. The upper straight forceps (no. 99-C) is used to remove maxillary central and lateral incisors and canines. It is placed on the crown, and apical force is applied to seat the beaks at the neck of the tooth. The tooth is removed with alternating labial and palatal pressure, followed by mesial rotation.

B. Maxillary premolars. The upper universal forceps (no. 159) is used to remove these teeth. The first premolar frequently has two roots and is removed by buccopalatal pendulum movements until loose. Slight rotation may be used to deliver the tooth, preserving the buccal plate. The second premolar has a more conical root and is removed in a similar fashion except that more rotation may be employed.

C. Maxillary molars. The upper universal (no. 150) forceps is used for most maxillary molars. More difficult or extensively decayed molars may be removed with the upper molar cowhorn forceps (no. 88-R or 88-L). Great care is needed with the latter, since the risk of bone fracture is increased by the large forces that these forceps can deliver. Buccal movement is used to remove the maxillary first and second molars. A firmly anchored molar may occasionally need to be sectioned with a rotary drill so it can be removed without damage to surrounding structures. The two buccal roots are sectioned from the crown, and the forceps is used to remove the crown and palatal root. The buccal roots are then removed individually.

D. Mandibular incisors. Mandibular incisors are most efficiently removed with the Ashe forceps, but the lower universal forceps (no. 151) may also be used. The roots of the incisor teeth are delicate and relatively flat on their mesial and distal surfaces, with thin labial and lingual plates. To prevent labial bone destruction, short buccolingual movements are best for removing these teeth.

E. Mandibular canines and premolars. The Ashe forceps is the most efficient for removal of mandibular canines and premolars. The lower universal (no. 151) forceps may also be used. Short buccolingual forces followed by a rotary motion are used to remove the canines, preserving the buccal plate.

F. Mandibular molars. The lower universal forceps (no. 151) is used for most mandibular molars. The lower molar cowhorn forceps (no. 23) is useful for difficult molars with divergent roots. The cowhorn forceps has sharp buccal and lingual beaks that seat between the mesial and distal roots. As the forceps is firmly seated between the roots, a vertical force is placed on the tooth and the tooth is delivered with buccal movement. If the crown fractures in the process of removal, the roots will usually be separated and this makes their removal relatively simple. It is occasionally necessary to section a molar between the roots with a rotary drill and remove the roots individually.

Postoperative complications

I. Most of the complications of exodontia can be avoided with proper presurgical planning. These problems are usually the result of poor access and visualization, poor surgical technique (most often the use of excessive force), or incorrect use of instruments.

II. Surgical complications should be approached with a specific plan and not as a haphazard addition to the procedure. Poorly handled complications often lead to more extensive problems. It is important that the patient be informed when problems occur.

 A. Fractured roots (mandible). When a portion of a root is fractured, the operator should stop and take a few moments to analyze the situation and plan an approach to the problem.

  1. The following should be reevaluated before proceeding:
   a. Patient position—should promote optimum visualization
   b. Light—should be adequate and positioned to give maximum visibility
   c. Suction—along with adequate irrigation, essential for keeping a clear field
   d. Assistants—positioned to retract the soft tissues effectively and suction without obstructing the surgeon's field of vision
   e. Surgical access—the field well suctioned and flaps retracted if necessary for optimum visualization (A radiograph may occasionally be useful in locating the root fragment.)

  2. The root segment should be gently manipulated with the appropriate elevators to luxate it superiorly. Excessive force in the posterior region can cause displacement of a tip mesially through the thin lingual bone plate into the submandibular space or inferiorly into the inferior alveolar canal.

  3. When a root is displaced mesially, it can be palpated with a finger in an attempt to manipulate the tip back through the lingual plate defect into the extraction site, permitting removal through the socket. If this is unsuccessful, a mucoperiosteal flap is elevated and the tip visualized and removed. It is important that the lingual tissues be well protected with retractors.

  4. If a root tip is displaced into the inferior alveolar canal, it is almost impossible to remove bone through the socket to retrieve the root. Excessive bleeding from the socket may make visualization difficult, increasing the risk of damage to the neurovascular bundle. These root tips may sometimes be left if there are no symptoms. If removal becomes necessary, it is best done in the operating room by an experienced surgeon.

 B. Fractured roots (maxilla). The same principles of access discussed for recovery of mandibular root tips are true for the maxillary teeth. Every attempt is made to remove the root with minimum damage to adjacent structures and minimum resection of bone.

1. Fractured premolar roots are easily removed by elevating a conservative mucoperiosteal flap for access and removing a portion of the buccal plate. The root tip can then be elevated or extracted with a root tip elevator or forceps.

2. Molar root tips may be removed in a fashion similar to that used for premolars. It is important that force applied with the elevator not push the tip apically. If this happens, the tip may be displaced into the maxillary sinus. Such a root may then be

   a. Displaced apically but still within the bony socket

   b. Displaced through the buccal bone plate and into the lateral soft tissues

   c. Lodged between the socket apex and the bony sinus floor

   d. Lodged against the sinus membrane at the socket apex, within the sinus, having penetrated the sinus membrane

3. A minimally displaced root may be removed using a small suction tip placed in the socket. If the root penetrates the membrane, it can usually be removed with small instruments through the socket. If the root has penetrated the membrane, it is often best to close the socket and recover the root tip via a Caldwell-Luc operation.

C. Postoperative bleeding. In patients without a defective coagulation mechanism this is usually avoidable with good surgical technique and appropriate postoperative care by the surgeon and patient.

1. Attention to the following points will significantly reduce the incidence of postoperative bleeding problems:

   a. History. A patient with a history of postoperative bleeding, easy bruising, etc. should be evaluated in the appropriate manner to rule out a bleeding disorder before surgery.

   b. Patient instructions. These should be clearly explained to the patient or to the person responsible for the patient as well as given to the patient in written form. The patient should be instructed to bite on a compact gauze sponge placed directly over the socket for at least 30 min after surgery without checking to see whether the bleeding has stopped. He should be instructed in the proper placement of the sponge in case it becomes dislodged.

   c. Foreign bodies. Fragments of tooth, bone, calculus, etc. should be removed from the socket, since these may become a focus for bleeding or infection. If the buccal or lingual bone plates have been expanded, they should be compressed before suturing the socket.

   d. Active bleeders. Any active bleeding sites in soft tissue or bone must be controlled. Soft tissue bleeding can usually be stopped with pressure; however, it may be necessary to ligate a large vessel or compress the bone around a nutrient vessel.

e. Sutures. Adequate sutures should be placed to close the soft tissues and approximate the papillae to bone since most postoperative bleeding is from unsutured papillae.

2. If bleeding occurs after the patient has left the office, he should be instructed to replace the gauze sponge directly over the socket and bite firmly for 20-30 min. A tea bag over the socket may also prove helpful. If bleeding persists, the patient must be seen so the problem can be evaluated. The following steps should be used in managing these cases:

a. Anesthesia. The surgical area should be obtunded with a local anesthetic agent containing a vasoconstrictor. This will allow the patient to be thoroughly examined without pain and will help reduce bleeding.

b. Access. A patient with postoperative bleeding will usually be apprehensive and need reassurance. It may occasionally be necessary to administer a sedative to comfort him. A calm patient as well as good light and suction is essential for a thorough examination and treatment.

c. Surgical site. The old clot should be cleared from the socket so the operator can examine the socket and surrounding tissues. A large clot protruding from the socket is easily disturbed by the tongue and teeth, causing continuous and prolonged bleeding.

d. Pressure. A gauze pack is placed over the site and firm pressure maintained until bleeding is controlled. The socket should be coapted with sutures through the papillae to put pressure on the soft tissues.

e. Direct hemostasis. Any soft tissue bleeding sites not controlled by pressure over the socket may be clamped and sutured or cauterized. Bone bleeders may be compressed around the site. If bleeding is over a large area or persistent, it may occasionally be necessary to place bone wax or a hemostatic agent (e.g., Gelfoam, Surgicel, Avitene, or topical thrombin).

f. Assurance. The patient should not be discharged until it is clear that the bleeding has been controlled. He should then be reassured that the problem is under control and will remain so if instructions are followed precisely.

D. Tuberosity fracture. This is usually the result of excessive force during removal of maxillary second and third molars.

1. When removing teeth, the surgeon should keep the tooth and surrounding soft tissues visible at all times and should palpate as pressure is applied. Particular attention should be given to teeth that stand alone in the arch and to those that

have a low extension of the maxillary sinus viewed radiographically.

2. When a fracture occurs, the segment should be retained if possible. If the segment is relatively large and well attached to periosteum, it should be replaced and the mucosa closed. If the segment is excessively mobile, it may be necessary to splint until it heals. If it is small or detached from periosteum, it should be removed and a flap rotated to close the defect.

3. It is important to recognize the fracture immediately, while it is occurring, so the soft tissue over the defect can be retained. If a tooth is being removed blindly, bone and attached mucosa may be removed with it, leaving a large sinus communication that may be difficult to close.

E. Postoperative pain. Pain following exodontia is usually well controlled with mild or moderate analgesics.

1. When it persists, it is usually a sign of an underlying problem. The patient should be examined clinically and radiographically.

2. Following are some of the common causes of persistent pain after tooth extraction:

   a. Postoperative infection. This should be treated as soon as possible with antibiotics (and drainage when indicated). Localized osteitis ("dry socket") can occur in teeth other than third molars and is caused when the blood clot in the socket is lost prematurely, exposing the bare walls of the socket. The patient has delayed increasing pain not controlled by mild analgesics. Appropriate antibiotics, analgesics, and a topical analgesic dressing are used. The dressing is placed in the socket and changed daily until the symptoms have resolved:

   b. Retained root, bone, or foreign body. The extraction site should be examined clinically and radiographically for any extraneous fragments. They may appear within the socket or between the alveolar plate and the mucosa.

   c. Alveolar plate fracture. The socket should be examined for evidence of alveolar plate fracture. Small fragments of bone may need to be removed, but larger ones with periosteal attachment can be left and supportive care given until the symptoms resolve.

   d. Maxillary sinus problems. Persistent pain in maxillary teeth after surgery may be the result of odontogenic infection or a coincidental sinusitis (nonodontogenic pain). The sinus should be evaluated clinically and radiographically and treated with appropriate antibiotics and surgical intervention when necessary.

   e. Adjacent teeth. The teeth adjacent to an extraction site should be examined to determine whether the pain is arising from another tooth or associated tissues.

f. Muscle spasm. Postoperative pain may be caused by prolonged mouth opening during a procedure, aggravation of a chronic or subclinical problem, or trismus from an anesthetic injection.

g. Nondental origin. Facial pain may persist after an extraction and have no obvious dental source. Various problems should be considered when a patient reports this. The oral surgeon must always look carefully before performing further extractions. It is not at all uncommon to see a patient with a history of multiple extractions done prior to the diagnosis of trigeminal neuralgia.

h. Prevarication. Finally, one must be mindful that there will be the occasional patient who complains of pain falsely in an attempt to secure narcotic medications.

Preparation of the Mouth for Dentures

GENERAL CONSIDERATIONS

I. The removal of teeth and preparation of the mouth for dentures require attention to numerous details so the alveolar bases will be suitable for long-term function and comfort.

A. To prevent root fracture and destruction of the labial plates, teeth are removed as atraumatically as possible.

B. Flaps should be kept to a minimum since excessive flap elevation may compromise the labial vestibule. This can be particularly damaging in the anterior mandible area, where the vestibule may be lost when the flap is sutured.

C. Alveoloplasty is kept to a minimum. If the width of the ridge is to be reduced, the buccal plate should not be removed if possible. To reduce the amount of resorption, the interradicular bone is removed and the plates compressed (or osteotomized and then compressed) to narrow the ridge over time.

II. Providing a patient with an immediate "surgical" denture is a very satisfying experience for the surgeon and a service for which patients are extremely grateful.

A. It has several advantages over the conventional:

1. The patient is never without teeth.

2. The immediate denture acts as a surgical bandage to reduce postoperative bleeding.

3. Postoperative edema and discomfort are reduced.

4. The patient is able to eat with relative comfort, thus assuring adequate nutrition. This may be of particular importance for patients such as diabetics in whom the nutritional status is critical.

5. Speech is not significantly impaired.

6. The denture acts as a stent to preserve the vestibules.

B. Although the immediate denture is only a "temporary" prosthesis and often has to be replaced by a "permanent" denture 6-12 mo after surgery, this is not always the case. The immediate denture patient is followed closely by the prosthodontist and the denture is adjusted or relined as indicated.

C. The disadvantages of immediate dentures include
1. Possible unsatisfactory healing
2. Need for a second regular prosthesis
3. Discomfort if not done optimally

SURGICAL TECHNIQUE

I. There are two techniques for placement of immediate dentures—a two-step and a one-step.
A. The two-step technique is used when the patient has a full complement or a significant number of posterior teeth. This method requires two surgical procedures. The posterior teeth are removed at the first procedure, and the ridge is allowed to heal. The anterior teeth are removed at a second procedure, and the denture is placed.
B. With the one-step technique, all remaining teeth are removed and the immediate denture is placed at the same time. To preserve alveolar bone and the vestibule, the teeth are removed as atraumatically as possible.
II. A clear acrylic tray and a duplicate of the trimmed cast are used at surgery to reveal where the prosthodontist has anticipated bone removal when making the denture. The tray may be used to fine-tune any necessary alveoloplasty. Small high spots that prevent the denture from seating may sometimes be corrected by selective trimming or thinning of hyperplastic gingival mucosa and fibrous papilla rather than removal of bone. Minimizing surgery is the best rule in immediate denture patients.
III. The immediate denture placed at surgery should be checked by the dentist within 2-3 da. If the patient is relatively comfortable the denture should not be removed prematurely, since it will quite likely not be possible to replace it until all the swelling has resolved.

Impacted Teeth

GENERAL CONSIDERATIONS

I. Third molars are the largest group of impacted teeth and the most frequently removed.
II. The indications for removal are as follows:
A. Infection. Pericoronitis is a common infection associated with impacted third molar teeth. It occurs when food and debris collect under the mucosal covering or operculum of the impacted tooth. The infection should be controlled before the tooth is removed. Treatment consists of appropriate antibiotic therapy, irrigation to remove debris, and incision and drainage if necessary. Any source of irritation (e.g., an opposing erupted maxil-

lary tooth) should be removed. Uncontrolled pericoronal infection can lead to more serious infections.

B. Pathological conditions. Clinical or radiographic evidence of disease associated with a third molar is indication for removal.

C. Pain. Caries, inflammation, and infection may all cause pain, which is an indication for removal.

D. Effect on adjacent teeth. Third molars that contribute to infection of adjacent teeth (e.g., caries and periodontal disease) should be removed.

E. Orthodontic considerations. Third molars may need to be removed to facilitate orthodontic therapy.

PREOPERATIVE PREPARATION

I. Patient preparation

A. Explanation of the radiographic and clinical findings and of the surgical procedure removes the mystery from the experience and also helps correct any false preconceptions that a patient may have regarding the surgery. The anesthesia to be used should also be discussed prior to surgery.

B. Potential complications should be explained and discussed without unduly frightening the patient. These should include, when applicable

1. Possible lingual and labial paresthesias
2. The possibility of mandibular fracture with deep mandibular impactions
3. Anesthetic complications
4. Damage to adjacent teeth
5. Possible sinus involvement with high maxillary impactions

C. Finally, the postoperative course should be discussed. The patient should know what to expect after emerging from anesthesia. He should have some general idea of how long he may need to recuperate, how much pain to expect, and how long he can expect to be swollen.

II. Radiographs

A. Appropriate radiographs are important in planning for third molar surgery. Classification of the teeth according to their anatomical position (mesioangular, distoangular, horizontal, vertical) aids in determining the surgical approach.

B. The relationship of impacted teeth to important structures (e.g., the mandibular canal, adjacent teeth, the maxillary sinus, the infratemporal space) should be assessed.

III. Clinical examination

A. It is essential in every case that a thorough examination be done before surgery. One needs to be sure that any pericoronal or other infection is resolved.

B. Restorations in adjacent teeth are noted and their effect on the surgical plan considered.

SURGICAL TECHNIQUE

I. General considerations

    A. Use of the surgical drill rather than the hammer and chisel is suggested for the following reasons:

        1. Modern technology has produced high-speed turbine drills that allow fast, efficient, low-temperature bone removal.

        2. The drill is much more comfortable for the awake patient.

        3. It is technically easier to use and safer.

        4. Bone can be removed in a more controlled fashion, reducing the amount of osteotomy.

    B. The importance of good access can hardly be overemphasized. Before bone surgery is begun, a flap should be raised for clear and unobstructed access to the surgical area. It must be retracted to prevent damage to it by the rotary drill. An envelope flap raised to the first molar area is adequate for removal of most impactions.

II. Mesioangular impactions

    A. The rotary drill with a fissure bur is used to remove labial bone from around the crown. It then makes a slot in the buccal groove following the long axis of the tooth into the pulp chamber.

    B. A thin straight elevator is used to section the tooth and remove the distal root and crown. The mesial section is then elevated and removed. To avoid rotating the tip of the root onto the roof of the mandibular canal, the surgeon should be careful to elevate the mesial section in the direction of its long axis rather than vertically.

    C. The socket is generously irrigated to remove bone and tooth fragments, and any remnants of the dental sac are removed.

III. Vertical and distoangular impactions

    A. The drill removes labial bone and bone covering the crown. This creates a groove extending to the cemento-enamel junction. A horizontal slot is made in the tooth at the CEJ extending into the pulp chamber.

    B. A straight elevator placed in the slot is rotated to separate the crown from the tooth. The labial groove is deepened with the drill, and a purchase point made just below the horizontal cut.

    C. A Crane pick is used to elevate the tooth.

    D. If the roots are curved or widely separated, they may have to be separated and removed in sections.

IV. Horizontal impactions

    A. The crowns of horizontally impacted teeth are frequently covered with bone. The drill removes the bone, exposing the crown to a point below the CEJ. Then a vertical slot is made at the CEJ and the crown is separated.

    B. The crown often cannot be delivered intact and must be divided horizontally and removed in sections.

    C. Superior and labial bone is removed from the roots, and a labial purchase made.

    D. The Crane pick is used to elevate the roots anteriorly. The roots may have to be separated and removed in sections.

Surgical Endodontics

  I. Conventional endodontic therapy should always be the treatment of choice in treating irreversible pulpal and periapical disease. There are, however, indications for surgical management of endodontic problems.

    A. A periapical lesion that does not resolve following conventional endodontic therapy should be surgically treated.

    B. Periapical lesions other than granulomas should be treated surgically, and the lesions examined histologically.

    C. Endodontically treated teeth in which the canal has not been completely filled can be treated surgically.

    D. Teeth in which endodontic instruments have been broken can be treated surgically.

    E. Teeth with a wide or "blunderbuss" apex that cannot be filled by conventional therapy may be treated surgically.

    F. Overfilled canals that are symptomatic can be treated surgically.

    G. Teeth that continue to be symptomatic after conventional therapy often respond to surgical management.

    H. Teeth with fractures in the apical third to half can often be treated successfully by surgical means.

    I. Teeth into which access is impossible because of the presence of crowns or posts can be treated surgically.

  II. Apicoectomy

    A. Two types of incisions may be used to approach the apical region for apical surgery.

      1. A mucoperiosteal flap elevated from the necks of the teeth with a relaxing incision is used in most cases.

      2. If the involved tooth is crowned, it may be advisable in some cases to use a semilunar incision placed over the apical area, although healing is often associated with a scar into the bone defect.

      Regardless of the design, it is important that the incision provide good access to the surgical field.

    B. If the periapical lesion has not perforated the labial plate, a hand chisel or air drill is used to remove bone for access to the apex of the tooth. It is important that adequate bone be removed to allow complete extirpation of the lesion and resection of the apex.

    C. The apex of a resected root must be completely sealed. If the tooth has been filled with gutta-percha, its apex may be sealed by heating the gutta-percha. If the root filling is inadequate, if the apex is wide or blunderbuss, or if the canal cannot be filled, the

apex should be sealed with a retrograde amalgam filling.
- D. The amputation cut is beveled so the apex can be visualized. The apical defect is thoroughly irrigated and the flap carefully closed with 3-0 or 4-0 gut sutures.

Replantation and Transplantation of Teeth

REPLANTATION

I. The oral surgeon is frequently called upon to replace teeth that have been partially or completely avulsed. The success of these procedures depends in large part upon the timing of treatment.

II. Partially avulsed teeth should be returned to the proper position and stabilized. To avoid unnecessary tissue damage, surgical intervention is kept to a minimum. Gingival lacerations are sutured, and the alveolar bone is remodeled around the tooth with digital pressure. Intruded teeth are brought back to their proper position, as are teeth that have been extruded. If partially avulsed teeth are stable, they may not require any splinting. When stabilization is required, rigid fixation should be avoided; periodontal packing or acid-etched resin splinting is recommended.

III. The prognosis for avulsed teeth is indirectly proportional to the time that the tooth is out of the socket. Teeth replaced within 30 min have the best prognosis for long-term success without root resorption.

IV. Avulsed teeth are managed as follows:
- A. Storage. The best recommendation is for the lost tooth to be immediately replaced in its socket. When this is not possible, the tooth should be retained in the buccal sulcus while the patient is transported to the office. Since it may not be a good idea for a young child to hold an avulsed tooth in his mouth, in these cases the tooth should be transported in milk or tap water.
- B. Root cleaning. The tooth should be handled by the crown, not the root. The root should not be touched before replantation unless there is dirt or debris on it, in which case it may be gently rinsed with saline and the debris removed with cotton pliers. The root should not be scraped, brushed, or cleaned with medicines or chemicals of any kind.
- C. The socket. The socket should be left alone unless it contains dirt, debris, or a blood clot, in which case it should be gently irrigated and suctioned. The tooth is replanted in the socket, and the socket manually compressed.
- D. Splinting. The tooth is splinted with acid-etched resin with or without an arch wire. In some cases it can be stabilized with sutures over the occlusal surface. It should remain splinted for at least 7-10 da, with the patient ingesting a soft diet.
- E. Endodontic therapy. A tooth with an open apex will usually reestablish its blood flow and remain vital. A replanted tooth should be followed closely and, if signs of pulpal disease devel-

op, the pulp extirpated and the canals filled with calcium hydroxide. A tooth whose apex is closed will usually not remain vital, and its pulp should be extirpated within the first 2 wk after replantation. The canals are filled with calcium hydroxide, which should be removed and replaced every 3-4 mo; after 1-2 yr a permanent root filling (e.g., gutta-percha) can be inserted. However, such therapy should never be started while the tooth is out of the mouth and socket, for this wastes time during which the tooth could be returned to the mouth.

   F. Antibiotics. A patient should be given antibiotics for 1 wk after treatment and tetanus toxoid as necessary by the history.

TRANSPLANTATION

 I. The third molar is the most commonly transplanted tooth. The usual situation is for an unerupted or partially erupted third molar to be transplanted in the site of a first or second molar that has been lost prematurely.

   A. The prognosis is best when cases are selected in which the roots of the tooth to be transplanted are approximately one third to one half formed, with wide-open apices, and the labial plates of the recipient site are intact. The space available at the recipient site must be assessed for adequacy. When the crown of a first molar is decayed, the second molar may drift forward, reducing the mesiodistal space.

   B. The surgical technique is as follows:

   1. The first or second molar to be replaced is removed as atraumatically as possible, to preserve the labial plate of bone. It may be necessary to section the tooth to prevent damage to the plate. The interseptal bone is removed to make room for the transplant, and the socket is curetted to remove any periapical disease, bone fragments, or soft tissue. The socket is then irrigated.

   2. An envelope flap is reflected to expose the impacted third molar, which is removed atraumatically to prevent damage to its root structure.

   3. The tooth is placed in the recipient socket and positioned slightly out of occlusion. It should not be wedged into the socket. If it does not fit, bone should be removed from the socket to allow the tooth to fit without being wedged.

   4. A transplanted mandibular tooth can frequently be secured with a suture or small-gauge wire placed over its occlusal surface. It may also be stabilized by placing acid-etched resin at the contact points.

   5. The patient is given appropriate antibiotic coverage for 7-10 da postoperatively and advised to maintain a soft diet and avoid masticating on the transplanted side for 2 wk.

 II. Canines are the next most frequently transplanted tooth. Transplantation is not a substitute for orthodontic positioning and should be performed only when the tooth cannot be positioned by conventional means.

A. The surgical technique is similar to that for third molar transplantation except that the socket usually must be better developed. The socket should be large enough that the transplant does not require wedging into position and is slightly out of occlusion. Splinting can be accomplished with periodontal packing, cold-cure acrylic, or acid-etched acrylic placed at the contacts.

B. As is true with a transplanted molar, it is important that a canine not be in a functional position during the healing period.

Alveolar Ridge Retention

I. Once the teeth are removed, the alveolar ridges undergo progressive bone resorption. As resorption progresses, denture function is increasingly compromised. Many of the factors that cause resorption are difficult to control. It has been observed, however, that as long as a tooth is present the alveolar bone is preserved.

II. The following procedures are designed to preserve bone by retaining or replacing the tooth roots.

A. Supramucosal root retention

1. Teeth are amputated above the mucosa and copings are placed on the root stumps. A complete denture prosthesis, referred to as an *overdenture,* is constructed to fit over and be partially supported by the prepared root stumps.

2. The patient must be observed closely so that any periodontal or periapical problems can be intercepted early.

B. Submucosal root retention

1. Teeth that have sound root structure may be amputated at the level of the alveolar bone and covered primarily with alveolar mucosa. The roots may be vital or may have undergone root canal therapy before being buried.

2. The success of this procedure depends upon keeping the roots covered with mucosa. The mucosa is permitted to heal before denture construction so the risk of dehiscence over the roots will be minimized.

C. Hydroxyapatite root cones

1. Hydroxyapatite cones have been used to prevent ridge resorption in patients for whom retention of natural tooth roots is not possible because of extensive periodontal and/or periapical problems. The cones, which are supplied in an assortment of sizes and shapes, are placed in the tooth sockets after the teeth are removed.

2. After removal of the remaining teeth, the sockets are sized with stainless steel socket gauges. The corresponding hydroxyapatite cone is placed in the socket so it is approximately 2 mm below the crest of the ridge.

3. Labial and lingual mucoperiosteal flaps are mobilized for primary closure over the ridge.
4. The incision is closed primarily with absorbable sutures, and a denture can be placed immediately or the incisions can be allowed to heal and a denture placed later. If a dehiscence occurs, it is best treated by cutting the cone down below the crest of the ridge and closing the mucosa again primarily.

Canine Exposure to Assist Orthodontics

I. Impacted canines can often be moved into position orthodontically. To do this, the canine tooth must be exposed so that an orthodontic appliance can be placed on its crown.
II. Soft tissue and bone are removed to the cervical area of the tooth.
   A. Electrocautery is used to remove the mucosa directly over the crown of the tooth and also to remove the dental sac and other soft tissue around the crown.
   B. Bone is removed to the cementoenamel junction to allow unobstructed eruption of the tooth. The rotary air drill carefully removes bone in conjunction with a hand chisel. The surgeon must be able to pass an instrument such as a small curette completely around the crown.
III. At this point, some orthodontists will instruct the surgeon to place a wire loop around the cervix of the tooth or place one of the various other appliances used to actively move the tooth. Our preference is to remove the obstruction to the eruption forces and allow the tooth to erupt naturally.
IV. When the bone and soft tissues are cleared from around the crown, an aluminum or other crown form is cemented over the crown with zinc oxide—eugenol cement. This prevents granulation and other soft tissue from healing directly around the crown and allows the tooth to erupt over the following 6-8 wk.
V. After the crown has erupted, an appropriate orthodontic appliance can be placed to allow the desired forces to be applied to position the tooth properly.
VI. The same technique can be used in managing other impacted teeth for orthodontic exposure (e.g., incisors and premolars).

GENERAL REFERENCES

Guernsey, L.H.: Preprosthetic surgery. In Kruger G., editor: Textbook of oral and maxillofacial surgery, ed. 6, St. Louis, 1984, The C.V. Mosby Co.

Kruger, G.O.: Impacted teeth. In Kruger, G.O., editor: Textbook of oral and maxillofacial surgery, ed. 6, St. Louis, 1984, The C.V. Mosby Co.

Obwegeser, H.L.: Surgical preparation of the maxilla for prosthesis, J. Oral Surg. **22:**127, 1964.

Starshak, T.J.: Preprosthetic oral and maxillofacial surgery, St. Louis, 1980, The C.V. Mosby Co.

Preprosthetic Oral and Maxillofacial Surgery

8

GENERAL CONSIDERATIONS

I. Preprosthetic surgery is that part of oral and maxillofacial surgery designed to establish the best hard and soft tissue bases for prosthetic appliances. Its scope spans the spectrum from simple extraction technique and preparation of the mouth for dentures to bone grafts and alloplastic implants.

II. The development of new biomaterials and improved prosthetic techniques, along with a better understanding of oral physiology, has contributed to great strides in the success of prosthetic appliances for edentulous patients.

PREOPERATIVE MANAGEMENT

I. A thorough evaluation of the patient is most important in determining whether he is a candidate for surgery and which procedure would be appropriate to treat his problem.

II. The patient's physical and psychological ability to tolerate a conventional prosthesis must be determined early in the evaluation process. Some patients will not be able to adapt to a conventional denture regardless of how well made and well fitting it is. A clue in this regard may be the patient's intolerance of multiple apparently well-made dentures. Such a person may be a candidate not so much for a ridge extension procedure as for an implant (e.g., a mandibular bone staple or an osteointegrated device).

III. Consultation with the prosthodontist is most important in determining the appropriate procedure to address each individual patient's prosthetic requirements.

IV. Other considerations—the patient's age, physical and mental health status, and financial constraints as well as the condition of the hard and soft tissues of the alveolar ridges—must be taken into account.

SIMPLE TREATMENT PROCEDURES

I. A poorly fitting denture can be a major contributor to alveolar ridge resorption.

II. Minor osseous and soft tissue defects can prevent proper denture fit and contribute to the need for later major reconstructive pre-prosthetic surgery. A number of limited surgical procedures can be performed under local anesthesia to improve denture fit.

Alveoloplasty and mylohyoid ridge reduction
Alveoloplasty

I. Conservation of alveolar bone is of paramount importance; therefore, any hard tissue corrective procedures should be conservative. Minimum flap deflection is recommended for preservation of the vestibulum.

II. When isolated prominences of the alveolar ridge must be removed, an incision is made directly over the prominence and a minimum flap is elevated for exposure. Rongeurs and bone files are used to reduce and smooth the area, and the incision is closed with absorbable sutures.

III. A knife-edged ridge is reduced by making an incision along its crest. A mucoperiosteal flap is elevated, exposing the ridge, and the sharp portion of the ridge is appropriately recontoured and smoothed with a bone file. A rotating bur or rongeur and file may be used as indicated.

Mylohyoid ridge reduction

I. A prominent mylohyoid ridge may prevent proper lingual flange extension and cause pain from impingement by the denture.

II. To remove this prominence, an incision is made along the crest of the ridge adjacent to the area. A mucoperiosteal flap is elevated over the mylohyoid ridge and a wide periosteal elevator is placed to retract and protect the lingual tissues. The ridge is removed or reduced with a chisel that is approximately 1 cm in width. A bone bur is used to smooth the area further. The operative site is irrigated and closed with absorbable sutures.

Tuberosity reduction

I. Enlargement of the maxillary tuberosity may result from excessive fibrous tissue or bony enlargement.

II. Fibrous tissue reduction is accomplished via a wedge resection over the crest of the ridge followed by submucosal resection of fibrous tissue under the buccal and palatal flaps. If bony enlargement is present, it may be reduced with rongeurs and smoothed with a bone file. The operative site is irrigated and closed with interrupted or continuous absorbable sutures.

Removal of maxillary and mandibular tori and exostoses
Maxillary tori

I. These may interfere with denture placement and cause discomfort by irritation of the thin overlying mucosa.

II. A maxillary occlusal radiograph is taken before removal to disclose whether the torus is pneumatized, since removal of such a torus could create an oronasal communication. An exploratory bur hole can be used to test for pneumatization.

III. A midpalatal incision is made over the torus, with a Y-shaped extension at one or both ends of the incision if necessary for access. A fissure bur is used to section the lesion, and each section is carefully removed with a curved chisel to prevent accidental creation of an oronasal communication. The site is smoothed with a bone file or bur, and the incision closed with interrupted sutures.

Mandibular tori

I. These usually occur on the lingual aspect of the mandible adjacent to the premolar area.

II. The incision for removal is made over the crest of the ridge and should extend beyond the immediate area of the lesion to allow for retraction of the mucoperiosteum without tension and to prevent lingual flap tears. A large periosteal elevator is used to retract and protect the lingual anatomy. Large broad-based tori are sectioned with a bone bur and removed with a chisel and mallet. Those with a narrow-pedicled base may often be removed with a mallet and chisel alone. After removal, the site is irrigated and the incision closed with interrupted sutures.

Exostoses

I. Lateral exostoses occur most frequently in the posterior maxillary areas. They should be removed when they interfere with proper extension of the buccal denture flange.

II. An incision is made over the crest of the ridge, and a mucoperiosteal flap is elevated to expose the lesion. A retractor is placed to protect the mucoperiosteum, and the exostosis is removed or recontoured to produce a smooth ridge. The incision is closed with interrupted sutures.

Submucosal vestibuloplasty

I. Submucosal vestibuloplasty may be used to restore maxillary vestibular depth when the bone height is adequate but the mucosa and muscles are attached on or near the crest of the ridge. Additionally, the overlying mucosa must be free of pathological changes.

II. A vertical incision is made through mucosa in the midline of the maxillary labial vestibule. Dissecting scissors are inserted into the incision, and a submucosal tunnel is extended from the midline to the tuberosities bilaterally. In wide broad arches additional vertical incisions may be required to gain access to the tuberosity regions. The vertical incision is then extended to periosteum and the scissors are again used to make a corresponding supraperiosteal dissection. Any abnormal muscle attachments are released from the crest of the ridge and displaced superiorly. If these tissues are redundant, they are simply excised. The incision is then closed with interrupted sutures, and a stent or denture is used to take a compound impression with the flanges extended to the depth of the newly created sulcus. The denture is secured with perialveolar wires for approximately 10 da. A palatal screw (in the middle of the hard palate) may also be used.

III. When redundant soft tissue is present, it is resected as necessary and the submucosal extension is performed through the open incision. In the open incision procedure, sutures may be placed to secure the mucosa in the depth of the sulcus to periosteum. The incision is then closed along the crest of the ridge. A stent is also used in this procedure and is placed as described previously.

Secondary epithelialization procedures

I. Over the years numerous secondary epithelialization procedures have been described to provide ridge extension in limited areas when adequate bone height is available. Such procedures are virtually limited to the mandible, however, since in the maxilla they have proved to be poor with respect to relapse.

II. Two of the more commonly used secondary epithelialization techniques are the Kazanjian and the lip-switch.

A. In the Kazanjian procedure a horizontal incision is made in the mucosa of the lip. A mucosal flap is reflected to the crest of the ridge, and a supraperiosteal dissection is extended to the depth of the labial sulcus. The success of this procedure depends upon maintaining a thin mucosal flap and a periosteal base free of muscle and submucosal fatty tissue. The mucosal flap is sutured to periosteum in the depth of the sulcus and the raw lip surface is left to granulate. A compound impression is taken with a stent or denture, and the denture left in place for 10 da.

B. The lip-switch procedure is similar to the Kazanjian except that the raw surface of the lip is covered with periosteum. After the mucosal flap has been developed, an incision is made through periosteum along the crest of the ridge and the periosteum is dissected from the labial side of the alveolar ridge and turned onto the raw surface of the lip. The periosteal flap is sutured to the lip mucosal incision. The remainder of the procedure is the same as described before.

COMPLEX TREATMENT PROCEDURES
Vestibuloplasty with grafts

I. The vestibuloplasty with split-thickness skin or mucosal grafts has been widely used in the U.S. since the 1960s for increasing the relative alveolar bone height and improving the soft tissue base for construction of a denture prosthesis. Suitable cases exhibit a relative loss of vestibular depth from a combination of alveolar bone loss and high soft tissue attachments; however, there should be adequate bone available if exposed.

II. The indications for vestibuloplasty with grafts include the following:

A. Severe atrophy of the alveolar ridge leading to poor retention. A minimum of 9-10 mm of residual bone is needed in most cases for an acceptable result. This is not the procedure of choice when severe resorption of basal bone has created a pencil-thin mandible requiring additional bulk for strength.

B. High soft tissue attachments that prevent adequate flange extension for denture stabilization. This includes high mucosal, muscle, and frenum attachments that cause displacement of the denture base.

C. High mylohyoid muscle attachments. A prominent mylohyoid ridge muscle attachment prevents adequate lingual flange extension and may also become painful from flange impingement.

D. Redundant soft tissue on the ridge and in the vestibulum. Soft tissue accumulations (e.g., epulis fissuratum) cause obliteration of the sulcus and also create a mobile soft tissue base that compromises denture stability.

III. Preoperative planning includes the following:

A. Thorough history and physical evaluation. The patient must be in generally good health and able to undergo general anesthesia lasting at least 3 hr. There should be no uncontrolled medical problems. Underlying disease of the mandible is eliminated prior to surgery.

B. Thorough oral examination. The alveolar ridge should be rounded rather than sharp or knife-edged. If it is sharp, this may require correction before surgery. The width of the ridge is equally as important as ridge height for denture retention and is therefore a presurgical consideration. The mylohyoid ridge also is examined so it can be determined whether revision will be necessary at the time of surgery.

C. Radiographic examination of the mandible. This should consist of at least a panoramic and a lateral cephalometric study, which are used in making determinations of the size and shape of the alveolar bases, the position of the mental nerves, and whether residual disease exists. The lateral cephalometric radiograph can be used to assess the angle at which the mandible flare as it extends toward the inferior border and will help in determining how much flare to give the extended flange of the denture or stent placed at the time of surgery.

D. Impression of the mandible. This is taken for stent preparation. A tray that is overextended with dental compound is used to fabricate a stone model. The labial vestibule of the model is further extended to the depth that is to be achieved surgically. The angle at which the vestibulum is to be extended inferolaterally is determined from the cephalometric radiograph. The flanges of the patient's denture or an acrylic tray is extended to the new vestibular depth and is used to maintain the graft during healing.

Mandibular split-thickness skin graft vestibuloplasty

I. Skin graft harvesting and donor site

    A. The donor site must be as free as possible of hair growth. The lateral thigh is a site commonly selected. The area is prepared and draped and the skin to be harvested is lubricated with mineral oil.

    B. The Brown or Padgett dermatome is set to take a graft approximately 0.012-0.015 in thick. A strip of skin 4-8 × 10-15 cm is usually required for vestibuloplasty. The harvested graft is stored on saline-moistened gauze until placed on the recipient site.

    C. The donor site is covered with a thrombin-soaked gauze pad and a temporary pressure dressing is placed until the intraoral procedure is completed. It is then covered with an Opsite dressing, which remains in place until spontaneously exfoliated. Compress gauze or scarlet red–impregnated gauze may also be used as a dressing.

II. Surgical technique

    A. The labial mucosa is infiltrated with 2% lidocaine–1:200,000 epinephrine.

    B. A no. 15 blade is used to make an incision just labial to the crest of the ridge, extending from the second molar region to the midline bilaterally. Posteriorly the incisions are extended distolabially ½-¾ in at a 45-degree angle to the ridge.

    C. Dissecting scissors and a periosteal elevator are used to perform a careful supraperiosteal dissection exposing the labial and anterior aspect of the alveolar ridge. The dissection should not extend below the external oblique ridge or a blind pocket may be created that will trap food.

    D. If the mentalis muscle is attached superiorly, only about half of it should be detached; otherwise, there may be prolapse of the soft tissue structure of the chin (the so-called "witch's chin").

    E. The mental nerves are protected during surgery.

    F. If the neurovascular bundle exits from the crest of the ridge or if there is a lateral bony prominence, it may be desirable to dissect the structure gently and create a new channel into which the bundle can be placed. However, even minimal manipulation of the mental nerve tissue will be attended by sensory disturbances at least temporarily and perhaps over a much longer time.

    G. Any fat or muscle remnants are removed from the periosteal base to allow firm healing of the skin graft to the periosteum.

    H. The small Obwegeser awls, designed for vestibuloplasty, are used to pass nine circummandibular (2-0 chromic) sutures around the inferior border of the mandible. These attach the lingual mucosa and muscle and the labial mucoperiosteal flap to the lower portion of the mandible. After all nine sutures are placed, they are tied into the labial sulcus to secure the repositioned lingual and buccolabial tissue. The inferior placement of the flaps creates a new deeper labial vestibule and a lower floor of the mouth. If the floor of the mouth does not require revision, these sutures may be placed through the floor adjacent to the lingual alveolus. The buccolabial flap can be further secured by suturing to the periosteum in the depth of the vestibule.

I. An impression of the newly exposed alveolar ridge is made with impression compound and the previously prepared stent. The compound should extend to the depth of the new vestibule. The inner aspect of the stent is painted with benzoin or other adhesive agent to secure the graft, which is then placed in the stent epithelial side down. When the adhesive has dried and the graft is securely attached to the stent, it is ready for placement. The graft and stent are carefully placed on the ridge and secured with two or three circummandibular wire or nylon sutures. The stent is held in place for 10 da and then removed for trimming of necrotic skin edges and removal of any debris from the sulcus. The stent is also trimmed slightly if necessary for comfort and is worn until a new denture is fabricated.

J. Antibiotics should be given prophylactically at the time of circummandibular suture removal. Penicillin-V or erythromycin in a dose of 2 g is given 2 hr before the procedure and 250 mg is given every 6 hr for 1 da after.

III. Factors contributing to success

A. When the basic principles of patient selection, technique, and skin grafting are followed, a consistently good to excellent result can be expected.

B. The principles essential to success of the vestibuloplasty procedure include

1. Selecting a donor site that is free of hair follicles. Harvesting from a hairless area as well as taking a very thin graft (0.012-0.015 in) reduces the possibility of having hair grow from the grafted site.

2. Preparing the alveolar recipient site by supraperiosteal dissection. This will create a clean periosteal bed. The periosteum should be free of fat and muscle tissue remnants so there can be firm attachment of the graft to periosteum.

3. Good hemostasis at the recipient site. Bleeding and subsequent hematoma will prevent complete attachment of the graft to periosteum.

4. Graft coverage of the entire recipient site. This will prevent granulation tissue formation and wound contracture and relapse.

5. Immobilization for 7-10 da. To ensure complete healing, a stent should hold the graft.

6. Leaving at least 9-10 mm of residual bone. The ridge should have a relatively broad and rounded shape, not a sharp crest.

7. Avoidance of extending the vestibular dissection into three critical regions:
   a. Posterior buccal area—the dissection should in most cases not extend beyound the external oblique ridge, since this will create a blind pocket that can trap food.
   b. Mentalis muscle—when the dissection must involve the mentalis, one third to one half of the muscle fibers should remain attached, to prevent the patient from having a "witch's chin."
   c. Genioglossus muscle—when the genial tubercles and attached muscle fibers are involved, approximately half of the genioglossus should remain attached to prevent postoperative tongue control problems.

Floor of mouth procedure

I. A floor of the mouth procedure is frequently necessary before the labial vestibuloplasty because, although infrequent, bleeding problems are more likely to occur in this location than in the labial vestibule.
II. The surgical technique is as follows:
   A. Lidocaine—1:200,000 epinephrine is injected along the lingual aspect of the mandible bilaterally for vasoconstriction.
   B. A no. 15 blade is used to make an incision just medial to the crest of the ridge extending anteriorly from the second molar area to the midline bilaterally.
   C. Using blunt dissection and finger pressure, the surgeon exposes the mylohyoid muscle and resects it at its attachment to the mylohyoid ridge. Extra care is taken to tie or coagulate any bleeding vessels immediately to prevent them from retracting and bleeding later.
   D. When the genial tubercles are superiorly positioned and would appear to interfere with future denture placement, they may be selectively reduced.
   E. The genioglossus muscles may also be resected at the bone attachment, but one third to one half of the muscle should remain attached to avoid postoperative tongue control problems that might result in airway obstruction or difficulties with swallowing or speech. Nine 2-0 chromic sutures are symmetrically spaced through the mucosa-muscle flap to be attached later to the labial flap.

Mandibular mucosal graft vestibuloplasty

I. Buccal mucosa and palatal mucosa have been used as an alternative to skin in the vestibuloplasty procedure. They have the advantage of eliminating an external donor site and may therefore be an excellent alternative when a skin graft is contraindicated, as in the patient with a history of keloid formation or other dermatological disorder.

II. Buccal mucosa may be used for full-thickness as well as split-thickness grafts. The full-thickness graft is taken freehand with a scalpel and dissecting scissors. After the graft is resected, it is carefully "defatted" before placement on the alveolar ridge. If fat is left on, the graft may not attach firmly to the periosteal base, leading to a mobile soft tissue base. The ridge extension procedure is performed as described for the split-thickness skin graft vestibuloplasty. The graft is secured with absorbable sutures, and a compound-lined stent or denture is placed.

III. Palatal mucosa may also be used as graft tissue for ridge extension procedures.

A. However, its use is limited by the amount that can be harvested. Removing the entire palatal mucosa leaves a wound that heals slowly and results in prolonged discomfort. Removing a horse-shoe-shaped graft and leaving a midpalatal strip of mucosa often will not provide sufficient mucosa for the procedure.

B. The palatal graft is taken freehand. Excess fat and salivary gland tissue are removed to prevent mobility of the graft after healing. The graft can be enlarged by means of a graft expander when necessary for complete coverage. The graft is sutured in place, and a stent is placed to secure it.

IV. A disadvantage of mucosal grafting is that the amount of mucosa available for harvesting may not be sufficient to cover the entire ridge. In such instances use of a graft expander will both increase the size of the graft and allow excellent adaptation to the ridge, thereby lessening the risk of hematoma under the graft because of the fenestrations present.

Alveolar ridge augmentation
Alloplastic augmentation

I. Hydroxyapatite implants

A. Hydroxyapatite (HA) is a biocompatible nonabsorbable calcium phosphate substance with physical and chemical characteristics similar to those of dental enamel and bone. Clinical and laboratory studies have produced no evidence of local or systemic inflammation or foreign body response to its use. It apparently can become strongly adherent to bone. It provides a nonabsorbable supporting matrix for deposition of bone by chemical bonding without an intervening fibrous capsule. Radiographic evaluation is easy because its high calcium content renders it radiopaque.

B. Hydroxyapatite implants alone can restore a variety of types of alveolar ridge defect. They may be used to restore the width of the ridge, ridge height, undercut areas, and mandibular height and width when moderate to severe loss exists as a result of resorption, prior surgery, or trauma. When extensive resorption has occurred with loss of basilar bone and the mandible is pencil-thin, it is suggested that HA be combined with autogenous bone.

C. The material is supplied in prepackaged 1-2 ml plastic syringes or in vials with syringes that are filled by the surgeon at the time of surgery. The HA-filled syringes use either saline or blood as a cohesive agent to aid in control of the particles during placement and to minimize postoperative migration. Approximately four syringes are required to augment the posterior ridge bilaterally or to augment the anterior ridge, and approximately eight syringes for a total ridge augmentation. The surgical procedure may be done under general anesthesia or in many cases under local anesthesia in the operatory.

II. Maxillary augmentation

A. The single vertical midline incision technique is sufficient for most maxillary augmentations.

B. The procedure may be done with or without a submucosal vestibuloplasty depending upon whether a ridge extension is necessary.

1. If the augmentation is done without a submucosal vestibuloplasty, the vertical incision is carried through periosteum immediately. A small periosteal elevator is used to develop a subperiosteal tunnel along the portion of the ridge to be augmented. It is sometimes necessary to elevate mucosa on the palatal side of the ridge to develop an adequate tunnel size.

2. When a submucosal vestibuloplasty is necessary, the initial vertical incision is carried through mucosa to periosteum. The submucosal dissection is then performed, with the vertical incision extended through periosteum and a subperiosteal tunnel formed. The periosteum is incised if a larger tunnel size is needed.

C. Traction sutures are placed on each side of the incision to aid in keeping the incisions open for insertion of the syringes that will be used to deliver the implant material.

1. The implant syringe is placed in the tunnel and the pockets are filled from the posterior aspect to the midline bilaterally.

2. To prevent the inclusion of implant particles in the incision during closure, the traction sutures may be used to lift the tissue edges away from the implant while the incision is being sutured.

D. The incision is closed with interrupted horizontal mattress sutures. Soft stents or dentures prepared on a preoperative model may help retain ridge form in maxillary cases but can cause tissue breakdown.

III. Mandibular augmentation

A. Bilateral vertical incisions approximately 1 in long placed over the lateral aspect of the alveolar ridge in the canine area are used for most mandibular procedures. Occasionally a single midline vertical incision is used for augmentation of the anterior mandible only.

B. The mental nerve is carefully visualized and protected during surgery.

C. A small periosteal elevator is used to develop a limited subperiosteal tunnel along the crest of the ridge from the vertical incision posteriorly to the third molar area bilaterally. If augmentation of the anterior ridge is necessary, the tunnels are extended anteriorly as necessary.

D. Care should be taken not to extend the dissection beyond the external oblique ridge, for this could allow excessive lateral migration of the implant particles.

E. Traction sutures are placed on each side of the incision to aid in keeping the incision open for insertion of the implant syringes.

F. In total mandibular augmentation the posterior pockets are filled with the implant first. The syringe is inserted to the posterior extent of the tunnel, and the pockets are filled from the posterior area to the canine area bilaterally. As the implant is injected, it is guided into position and molded to form with finger pressure as needed. The anterior pockets are then filled from the midline back to the canine incision.

G. When the implant is packed around the mental nerve, various alterations in nerve function have been noticed. Omitting the implant in this area does not compromise the prosthetic result.

H. Traction sutures are useful for lifting the tissue edges from the implant, and the incision is closed with interrupted horizontal mattress sutures.

I. Splints are not used as frequently in the mandible as in the maxilla but are helpful for undercut cases.

J. Antibiotics are started preoperatively and continued for 1 wk postoperatively.

K. Clinical judgment is the best indicator of when new dentures can be constructed. Most ridges are well healed and firm enough for denture construction approximately 6 wk after surgery.

L. When inadequate vestibular depth remains following augmentation, a secondary vestibuloplasty with a graft may be performed over the implant after sufficient healing has occurred. Some 3-4 mo healing time should be allowed before a vestibuloplasty is performed. The standard vestibuloplasty procedure is used.

M. Hydroxyapatite has several uses in mandibular augmentation:

    1. It can be applied in conjunction with the mandibular staple implant.

    2. It can also be mixed with cancellous bone. Augmentation of a very atrophic mandible is a suitable indication.

    3. In solid blocks it offers the clinician greater control over placement and reducing migration. The basic methods are

similar, although in the mandible more extensive lingual tissue dissection will permit tunnel development with less loss of buccal vestibular depth. Wound dehiscence is a common problem, and important.

Autogenous bone grafts

I. Autogenous bone grafts are the treatment of choice when maxillary or mandibular augmentation is deemed necessary. Despite graft resorption following the procedure, sufficient bulk for adequate function remains after the resorption has stabilized.

II. Bone graft augmentation is recommended in the followng circumstances:

A. When there is inadequate bone height and width for vestibuloplasty

B. When additional bulk is required to strengthen the mandible with extensive resorption

C. When the bulk of an implant substance (e.g., HA) would be too large to restore a functional denture base and strengthen the mandible

III. Superior border rib grafts

A. Superior augmentation of the mandible with a graft from the ribs placed via a transoral approach has been well described. Resorption is one half to two thirds within the first 18-24 mo, and vestibuloplasty procedures are often necessary following the graft. Thus the patient must be able to tolerate three procedures: harvest of the rib graft, placement of the graft, and vestibuloplasty.

1. Two rib segments 6-8 cm long are used. The first is contoured by vertical scoring on its internal surface to allow it to be bent and adapted to the curvature of the mandible. The second is cut into small pieces to be packed around the first after it is placed.

2. The buccal vestibule is infiltrated with lidocaine–1:200,000 epinephine.

3. An incision is made at the crest of the ridge from the retromolar region to the midline bilaterally.

4. The mucoperiosteal flap is elevated labially and lingually to expose the alveolar ridge, and a periosteal releasing incision is made to provide adequate tissue to cover the graft if necessary.

5. When the anterior mandible is higher than the posterior, a groove of sufficient width to accept the rib is made in the anterior region to compensate for the difference in bone height.

6. The rib strut is placed toward the lingual over the mylohoid ridge. Three wire sutures are used to secure it.

7. A continuous horizontal mattress (Dexon) suture is recommended for closure. Eversion of the tissue edges is stressed to encourage early closure and prevent wound

dehiscence. A periosteal releasing incision can be used to reduce flap tension. Closure is started posteriorly. As the closure proceeds anteriorly, a pocket develops between the graft and the mucoperiosteum; this is filled with the bone chips from the sectioned rib. Bone chips are placed primarily on the buccal aspect of the rib to form a well-contoured ridge.

8. After closure with the mattress suture is completed, a running spiral suture is recommended for added security of closure.
9. The patient is started on a regimen of antibiotics preoperatively and this continues for 1 wk postoperatively.
10. Some 4-6 wk is allowed for healing if a vestibuloplasty procedure is anticipated.

B. Augmentation of the maxilla
1. Ribs have also been used for maxillary ridge augmentation. Resorption is usually in the form of decreased ridge circumference, with more vertical bone loss anteriorly than posteriorly. The graft is therefore placed lateral to the atrophic ridge to compensate for the resorption and restore optimum alignment with the mandibular ridge.
2. The graft may be placed through an open incision extending from the tuberosity to the midline bilaterally. Lateral periosteal relaxing incisions are usually necessary to allow closure of the incisions with minimal tension. The graft is secured with four wire sutures. Anteriorly the strut is usually not in contact with the basal bone; posteriorly it is in direct contact. Two figure-8 wires are placed to secure the graft without basal contact. This area between the graft and basal bone is later filled in with bone chips. Two wires are placed posteriorly to further secure the graft.

IV. Inferior border rib grafts
A. Inferior border grafting for mandibular augmentation is designed to eliminate some of the problems associated with transoral graft procedures. Resorption is less with inferior border grafts because the graft does not bear the pressure of the denture and secondary vestibuloplasty is often not necessary. This is also an excellent procedure for the repair of fractures or malunions of the severely atrophic mandible. It does require an extensive extraoral approach, but with only slight added risk to the mandibular branch of the facial nerve.
B. Surgical technique
1. Two ribs are harvested, and each is scored on its inner surface with cuts approximately 1 in apart.
2. Rongeurs are used to remove every other notched section of bone to allow the ribs to bend easily. The bone sections removed are stored for use later.
3. The inferior border of the mandible is exposed from angle to angle through a submandibular incision.

4. One rib is adapted to the lingual aspect of the mandible, and the second is adapted to the buccal side. The bone segments previously removed are used to fill the space between the two rib struts.

5. Intraosseous or submandibular wires are placed as necessary to secure the grafts.

6. The surgical incision is closed in layers.

7. A temporary denture can be placed as soon as the patient is comfortable because it does not put pressure directly on the graft. If a vestibuloplasty is necessary, 2-6 mo of healing time should be allowed.

V. Superior border iliac block grafts

  A. Augmentation of the superior border of the mandible with iliac crest block grafts has been performed successfully for years.

    1. Treatment of atrophic mandibles with iliac crest bone placed transorally gives better results than treatment using cartilage. Iliac crest onlay grafts may be placed through an extraoral approach as well. The advantages of the extraoral approach are elimination of oral contamination, reduced risk of oral mucosal dehiscence, ease of closure of the surgical site, and reduced incidence of the need for secondary vestibuloplasty.

    2. The risks of an extraoral approach have already been discussed.

  B. Surgical technique

    1. The graft is placed through a submandibular incision adequate to expose the mandible from the second molar region to the midline bilaterally.

    2. The superior crest of the mandible may need to have any sharp areas reduced to allow good adaptation of the graft blocks.

    3. After the bone blocks are placed along the entire crest, the spaces between and around the blocks are filled with cancellous bone taken at the time the bone blocks are harvested. The bone blocks are secured by intraosseous wire sutures, and the incision is closed in layers.

    4. Three to six months' healing should be allowed before a functioning denture is placed or a vestibuloplasty is performed.

VI. Ridge augmentation with pedicled bone grafts

  A. Mandibular augmentation procedures using pedicled bone grafts are designed to take advantage of lingual muscle attachments, which provide a rich blood supply to the bone flap. Continuity of the blood supply may limit resorption associated with onlay graft procedures. Two types of osteotomy have been used for mandibular augmentation—the horizontal with an interpositional bone graft and the vertical or visor.

  B. Horizontal or interpositional osteotomy

    1. The horizontal osteotomy is generally indicated for

patients in whom resorption has been more extensive in the buccolingual dimension, producing a narrow mandible. This allows the osteotomy cut to be made above the mental nerve. A corticocancellous bone graft is taken before the procedure is started.

2. A mucoperiosteal incision placed just lateral to the crest is extended from the retromolar area to the midline bilaterally.

3. A buccolabial mucoperiosteal flap is reflected, and the mental nerves are exposed and dissected free of soft tissue so they can be protected.

4. A fissure bur is used to make vertical bone cuts through the posterior aspect of the alveolar ridge bilaterally. These cuts go through the buccal and lingual bone and extend from the crest of the ridge to just above the mandibular canal.

5. The lateral wall of the canal should be partially or completely uncovered so the level of the nerve will be revealed and the nerve protected against damage during surgery.

6. The horizontal bone cuts can be made with either a thin fissure bur or a reciprocal saw. The blade must be angled slightly inferiorly so it does not enter the canal.

7. Small osteotomes may be used to complete the lingual cortical cuts. The bone flap is reflected upward in preparation for placing the interpositional graft.

8. The corticocancellous graft is cut to the thickness corresponding to the desired increase in bone height.

9. The graft blocks are placed as necessary to fill the interpositional space and the remaining gaps are filled with cancellous bone and marrow.

10. Three wires or nylon sutures are usually adequate to secure the bone segment. The incision is closed with a continuous horizontal mattress suture followed by a continuous spiral suture.

C. Vertical or visor osteotomy

1. The visor osteotomy was first described by Hale in 1975. Other workers modified the procedure by raising the pedicled graft along the entire length of the arch, grafting the buccal aspect of the superior segment with cancellous bone, and performing a simultaneous vestibuloplasty.

2. Surgical technique

a. An incision is made just labial to the crest of the ridge and extended from the retromolar area to the midline bilaterally.

b. A vertical mucoperiosteal tunnel extending from the crest of the ridge to the inferior border is developed on the lingual side of the mandible in the third molar area.

    c. A fissure bur is used to make a vertical bone cut from the crest to the inferior border in this tunnel on each side. An air-driven reciprocating saw is used to make the sagittal cut between the buccal and lingual cortical bone.

    d. In the posterior mandible the saw blade must be angled laterally so the cut will extend through the inferior border.

    e. The mobilized segment is elevated to its new position and secured with wire or nylon sutures.

    f. Mucosal closure is started posteriorly with horizontal mattress sutures and the labial tunnel created lateral to the raised bone segment is filled with cancellous bone. A new denture is usually constructed 4-6 mo after surgery.

VII. Maxillary interpositional bone graft

    A. An interpositional bone graft for maxillary ridge augmentation has been suggested as an alternative to conventional onlay bone grafts. Less graft resorption is anticipated. Simultaneous interpositional bone graft with vestibuloplasty to restore the atrophic maxilla has also been described.

    B. A LeFort I osteotomy is performed in preparation for bone graft insertion. After the maxilla is inferiorly positioned, iliac crest bone struts are inserted to provide the preoperatively determined amount of augmentation, and the segments are stabilized with intraosseous wires or nylon sutures. The incision is then closed with absorbable sutures.

Dental implants

I. There has long been a search in the dental profession for a successful metal implant to stabilize or support artificial teeth. Endosseous implants, subperiosteal implants, and the mandibular bone staple implant have been the principal types available for clinical use.

    A. Endosseous implants are utilized primarily for fixed replacement in the partially dentulous patient and will therefore not be discussed here. More recently, osteointegrated implants have received considerable attention and early results are promising.

    B. Subperiosteal implants also will not be discussed except to say that a two-stage surgical procedure and a specially constructed denture are required. These procedures can be performed under local anesthesia.

    C. The mandibular bone plate can be placed in one surgical procedure and requires general anesthesia.

II. The mandibular bone staple implant is an orthopedic device designed to restore function to the edentulous atrophic mandible.

    A. Since 1968 the indications for its use have increased to include mandibles deformed by trauma and tumor surgery as well as by the usual bone loss due to years of denture wear and physiological resorption. Surgeons have reported using the device in patients with congenital ectodermal defects, cleidocranial dysostosis, and Parkinson's disease.

B. It can be placed through bone grafts and has been successfully used in patients with hydroxyapatite ridge augmentations. The implant has, in some special circumstances, been inserted into the body of the mandible rather than into the symphysis (for which it was originally designed). Hundreds of the implants are currently in place, with follow-up surveys reporting a success rate in excess of 90%.

C. The original three-pin model has been replaced by a five-pin and two seven-pin models.

   1. Each of the implants provides two transosteal (transoral) pins that penetrate the full thickness of the mandible and the intraoral soft tissues. These pins protrude into the mouth to provide abutments on which a stress-breaking attachment (e.g., a Dalbo or Ceka device) may be fabricated. Recently incorporation of a ball attachment on the transoral pins has simplified denture construction. The transoral pins are located at each end of the implant or in positions *2* and *6* in the modified seven-pin implant.

   2. The implants also provide three or five shorter intraossous pins approximately 8 mm high that are designed to increase the retention and stability of the implant.

   3. The implant itself is made of corrosion-resistant titanium, aluminum, and vanadium alloy.

D. It is important that the surgeon and the prosthodontist work together in rehabilitating the patient and that each understand the design and recognize the limitations of the implant. It is also vital that no occlusal forces be placed on the staple. The prosthesis must be entirely tissue borne with a balanced occlusion free of excessive interferences. The staple is designed as a stabilizing device, and the removable prosthesis must be constructed with this principle in mind.

E. Preoperative preparation of the patient includes a careful assessment of the mandibular hard and soft tissues. Requirements for use of the implant include at least 10 mm of bone height in the symphyseal region.

   1. If the patient does not have enough residual bone height, the area may be augmented with bone or hydroxyapatite.

   2. Any discontinuity or other osseous defects are best corrected before implant placement. Bone grafting procedures should be done at least 9 mo before the implant procedure is performed; augmentations may be done 6-8 wk before the implant.

   3. Other bone defects or problems (bone spurs, knife-edged ridges, etc.) are corrected, and retained roots and other foreign bodies are removed.

F. It is imperative that the patient be in overall good health and also be able to undergo general anesthesia of at least 2 hr duration.

G. The soft tissues are assessed so a determination can be made as to whether adequate attached mucosa exists in the area where the transoral pins will penetrate the mouth.

   1. If there is not adequate attached mucosa, a palatal mucosal or skin graft should be done before surgery to correct this critical problem.

   2. Redundant tissue problems or infection are also treated before surgery.

   3. Vestibuloplasty procedures, lowering of the floor of the mouth, or other revisions should be completed 6-8 wk before the implant. Recent reports of success with some of these accessory procedures (e.g., vestibuloplasty and hydroxyapatite augmentation simultaneously with staple implant placement) have appeared.

H. The operative technique used is that described by Small (1980) with some modifications.

   1. Under satisfactory nasotracheal general anesthesia, the submental region and oral cavity are prepared and draped in the standard fashion. Small believes that maintaining isolation of the surgical site from the oral cavity is extremely important to the success of the implant system; however, other authors have been less strict in this regard and have noted no adverse effects.

   2. Preoperative antiobiotics are given routinely and continued for 7 da postoperatively.

   3. After local anesthetic is administered with vasocontrictor, an incision approximately 4 cm long is made in a skin crease in the submental region following the curve of the mandibular symphysis.

   4. Dissection is carried down to the inferior border of the mandible. The periosteum is reflected, care being taken to clear all soft tissue from the exposed bone. Any irregularities in the bone surface may be smoothed with a bone bur for better adaptation of the staple base if necessary.

   5. The drilling chamber can now be tried in position along the inferior border.

   6. Attention is directed intraorally. An implant is chosen that, when inserted, places the transoral pins approximately 3 mm anterior to the mental foramina.

   7. The five-pin staple offers the easiest and most reliable fit. There are two methods of determining precise staple placement.

      a. The first utilizes a prefabricated clear acrylic splint to position the transoral pins. The splint is placed on the ridge, and the drilling chamber is placed and locked against the inferior border and the splint. The transosteal holes are drilled from the inferior border through the superior border and the oral mucosa.

    b. The second method does not use the acrylic splint. Bilateral ridge crest incisions are made in the attached mucosa anterior to the mental foramina, and the anchoring jaws of the drilling chamber are placed directly on the bony crest. Alternatively, the feet of the anchoring jaws may be placed directly on the mucosa.

  8. The drill guide must be placed so the lateralmost holes will be drilled directly over the center of the inferior border of the mandible. This can be checked by making a test mark with the drill tip.

  9. The distal ends of the drilling chamber should be no more than 2 mm off the inferior border of the mandible. If there is more space than this, the bone may be leveled. The chamber can be moved slightly posteriorly, or it may be necessary to use a five-pin staple. For this reason, it is advisable to have at least two staple sizes available at surgery.

10. A second surgeon now places the director rods on the crest of the ridge; or, if a splint is used, the rods are placed in two holes drilled into the splint before surgery. Tipping of the inferior border placement in a buccolingual direction permits proper ridge placement of the transoral holes.

11. The drilling chamber is now locked in place. A low-speed high-torque air drill is used with a tapered bit to place the holes. Initially, all the holes are placed to a depth 1 mm longer than the retentive pins.

    a. The lateral holes are placed first, and stabilizing pins are inserted into these two holes to maintain the position of the drilling chamber while the other holes are drilled.

    b. The surgeon should not run the drill in excess of 600 rpm, should maintain continuous irrigation while drilling, and should be careful to keep the holes parallel to each other.

12. If a modified seven-pin implant is to be employed, a twist drill without a drill stop is used to make the *2* and *6* position holes through the superior border of the mandible but not through mucosa. A small incision is later placed to allow the transoral pins to enter the mouth.

13. If the seven-pin implant is to be used, the stabilizing pins are moved to the *2* and *6* positions and the lateral holes are drilled into the mouth.

14. The outer edge of each hole is beveled slightly with the beveling instrument. The drilling chamber is removed, the holes are well irrigated, and the implant is gently and evenly tapped into place.

15. Locknuts or the new round balls are threaded over the transosteal pins until they are 1 mm above the gingiva. Fastener nuts are then placed over the locknuts.

16. The remaining portion of each transosteal pin above the fastener nuts is removed with the pin shortener.
17. The submental incision is copiously irrigated and closed in layers.
18. The patient may begin wearing his old dentures on the first or second postoperative day, provided the hard acrylic is completely removed from around the pins and the denture is lined with a soft tissue conditioner.
19. Postoperative treatment involves fabricating the metal suprastructure and the final removable prosthesis. Close routine follow-up and good oral hygiene are necessary to help ensure long-term treatment success.

I. Complications of this treatment are as follows:

1. Gingival hyperplasia—the most frequent sequela, this is usually due to chronic gingival infection or frictional irritation from the mobile mucosa adjacent to the transosteal pins. It can be treated with local excision if necessary, but electrocautery should not be used.
2. Acute infection—this may develop if attached mucosa is not maintained around the pins or if pocket depths greater than 3 mm develop around the pins.
3. Loosening or extrusion of the implant—this is the most significant complication and usually caused by occlusal loading. Once it occurs, the implant may never become completely firm again. Treatment consists of lining the denture to unload the implant. If the implant does not become firm in 3-6 mo, it may be used as the basis for an overlay denture.
4. Poor surgical placement, implant fracture, and dissimilar metal reactions—these are less frequent.

MAXILLOMANDIBULAR DISCREPANCIES

I. Severely compromised denture function may be experienced by a patient with sigificant maxillomandibular disharmonies. Compromised denture stability presents functional as well as esthetic problems and contributes to accelerated alveolar bone loss.

II. When severe discrepancies compromise denture function, an orthognathic surgical procedure should be considered. A complete clinical evaluation and diagnostic survey are as essential as they would be for the dentulous patient considering orthognathic surgery. A complete physical examination, radiographic examination and analysis, and analysis of mounted diagnostic casts are essential in developing a successful treatment plan. In addition, close collaboration with the prosthodontist treating the case is essential.

III. Developmental discrepancies may be accentuated by the normal resorption patterns of the alveolar ridges. A patient who did not have discrepancies with the natural dentition may exhibit relative discrepancies caused by the pattern of ridge resorption. The surgeon and prosthodontist should be aware of the differences in maxillary and mandibular resorptive tendencies.

 A. Maxillary resorption reduces the circumference of the maxilla because most of the bone loss is on the buccofacial aspect.

 B. The mandible loses bone primarily from the lingual aspect, with most of its vertical loss occurring in the posterior region.

 C. These patterns, together with overclosure from vertical bone loss, accentuate prognathic tendencies.

IV. When orthognathic surgical procedures are performed, stabilization of the osteotomized unit presents significant problems that must be considered in developing a treatment plan for the edentulous patient.

 A. Surgical splints secured to the mandible and maxilla are necessary for stability. The exact postsurgical positions must be established by use of mounted casts. When the new maxillomandibular position is determined, splints or dentures are constructed on the casts and interlocked in this position. The splints are secured to the mandible and maxilla and, when locked together, will secure the osteotomized units to the desired position.

 B. Lag screw and rigid internal fixation devices may also be useful.

GENERAL REFERENCES

Baker, R.D., and Connole, P.W.: Preprosthetic augmentation grafting—autogenous bone, J. Oral Surg. **35**:541, 1977.

Guernsey, L.H.: Preprosthetic surgery. In Kruger, G.O., editor: Textbook of oral and maxillofacial surgery, ed. 6, St. Louis, 1984, The C.V. Mosby Co.

Kent, J.N., et al.: Alveolar ridge augmentation using nonabsorbable hydroxylapatite with or without autogenous cancellous bone, J. Oral Maxillofac. Surg. **41**:629, 1983.

MacIntosh, R.B., and Obwegeser, H.L.: Preprosthetic surgery: a scheme for its effective employment, J. Oral Surg. **25**:397, 1967.

Schnitman, P.A., and Shulman, L.B.: Recommendations of the consensus development conference on dental implants, J. Am. Dent. Assoc. **98**:373, 1979.

Small, I.A.: The mandibular staple bone plate for the atrophic mandible, Dent. Clin. North Am. **24**:565, 1980.

Orofacial Pain and
Temporomandibular Joint
Problems

9

Orofacial Pain

GENERAL CONSIDERATIONS

I. Pain experienced in the orofacial structures is a common symptom. Although the cause in the vast majority of cases can be readily recognized, such is the complex anatomy of the area and the emotional significance of the pain to the patient that the diagnosis may be rendered extremely difficult.

II. Pain originating in the mouth and face is mediated mainly by the fifth cranial nerve (trigeminal), which has three branches: ophthalmic, maxillary, and mandibular. In addition, the facial (nervus intermedius root), glossopharyngeal, vagus, and cervical nerves innervate parts of this region. These nerves have a tortuous anatomical course and distribution. All pain fibers (except those from the cervical nerves) exiting this region travel to the spinal nucleus of the fifth nerve and are connected, by way of the bulbothalamic tract, to four sites:

  A. Inferior paracentral region of the cerebral cortex. The anatomical location and physical nature of the pain are perceived here (perceptual component).

  B. Orbital surfaces of the frontal lobes. Here the unpleasantness of pain (emotional component) is experienced.

  C. Cortex of the temporal lobe. Remembrance of past experiences in the oral cavity is a powerful motivating factor for many patients (memory component).

  D. Hypothalamic and reticular nuclei in the upper brain stem. Reflex responses in the endocrine and respiratory systems are mediated here (visceral reflex component).

III. In addition, the intensity of the painful experience can be modulated by the brain stem reticular system. Here the state of excitability of the cells is altered by humoral, metabolic, and pharmacological factors.

DIAGNOSIS AND TREATMENT

I. Pain history

    A. It is imperative that a thorough history be obtained before the patient is examined or special tests are ordered. In the majority of cases, the diagnosis may be made on this information alone.

    B. It is also important to obtain the patient's description of the pain, since primary neuralgias are frequently described as sharp and lancinating, vascular headaches as throbbing, and muscle pain as a continuous and dull ache. The patient may not be able to answer all these questions at the first interview. Collaborating information may need to be obtained from relatives and friends so that a general picture of the pain and its effect on and perception by the patient can be deduced. In the majority of instances this will readily lead to a diagnosis.

        1. The intensity of the pain needs to be measured against the patient's own experience of pain, need for medication, and effect on life-style (e.g., sleep, work, social activities).

        2. The origin of the pain should be ascertained by asking the patient to indicate this with one finger.

        3. Its distribution pattern should be accurately traced in terms of the local anatomy.

        4. The patient should be urged to remember the events surrounding the onset of the pain, even though this may have been several years ago. Any other incidents of similar pain should be ascertained even though the patient may not associate these with the present problem.

        5. The time relationships of the pain should be clarified in terms of duration and frequency of the attack as well as possible remissions.

        6. In many instances aggravating factors (e.g., lying down, chewing, the sight or smell of food, alcohol, stress) and in other instances relieving factors (heat and cold) are important clues.

        7. The effect of past treatment needs to be carefully elucidated (e.g., which medications helped, whether surgery altered the nature of the pain, whether endodontic treatment or extractions affected the pain).

        8. Finally, the presence or absence of associated factors (e.g., swelling, flushing, tearing, nasal congestion) needs to be ascertained.

    C. A complete physical examination and appropriate tests including blood and urine analyses, radiographs, and, when indicated, referral to other specialists and more sophisticated techniques (e.g., CT scan) will help confirm the clinical diagnosis and rule out other underlying conditions.

II. Classification of orofacial pain

    A. Pain due to local disease

        1. Teeth and jaws

   2. TMJ and muscles of mastication
   3. Salivary glands
   4. Nose and paranasal sinuses
   5. Blood vessels (arteritis)
   B. Pain from nerve trunks and central pathways
   1. No abnormal CNS signs (e.g., idiopathic paroxysmal trigeminal and glossopharyngeal neuralgia)
   2. Abnormal CNS signs (nerve involved by pressure, infiltration, or degenerative disease at an intra- or extracranial location)
   C. Pain from outside the face (eyes, ears, heart, cervical spine, esophagus)
   D. Psychogenic pain (atypical facial pain, atypical odontalgia, depression, psychoses, phantom tooth pain, conversion reaction, secondary gain, hysteria)
III. Characteristic features of orofacial pain
   A. Pain caused by local disease
   1. This category accounts for the greatest number of orofacial pains encountered in clinical practice. By means of a careful history and appropriate tests, the etiological abnormality can be detected.
      a. Pain arising from the teeth, supporting structures, and jaws is commonly diagnosed accurately by the patient.
         (1) Hypersensitivity of a tooth because of an exposed root surface or a recent deep restoration is described as a sharp, usually transient, well-localized pain aggravated by heat, cold, or sweet foods.
         (2) If the pulp of the tooth is involved in an inflammatory reaction because of dental caries, the pain will be spontaneous, severe, and less well localized. Heat will aggravate and cold relieve the pain, which may persist for minutes or hours. After a time the pain will suddenly stop, indicating complete necrosis of the pulpal tissue, which may progress to a periapical abscess with signs of infection and tenderness of the tooth to pressure and percussion. Endodontic treatment will save the tooth and eliminate the infection.
         (3) The infection may progress to cellulitis and abscess formation, in which case antibiotics and surgical drainage are indicated.
         (4) A particularly painful condition will occasionally arise after extraction of a tooth, most commonly a mandibular molar. This is termed localized osteitis (frequently called "dry socket"). The pain is severe and constant, starting 2-3 da after the extraction and lasting for 10-14 da. The socket should be irrigated and dressed on a regular basis until granulation occurs.

(5) Osteomyelitis of the jaws (usually the mandible) is rare but may present as an intense deep-seated pain with the appropriate physical and radiographic signs. The chronic sclerotic variety is much more insidious and less readily diagnosed. Treatment is surgical with vigorous antibiotic support.

(6) Osteoradionecrosis is a relentless extremely painful condition characterized by postirradiation bone necrosis, predominantly of the mandible, with exposure of bone in the mouth or externally. In most cases the condition can be controlled only by radical surgical excision of the affected bone.

b. Referred pain is occasionally encountered. The patient will complain of pain in the mandible, and a maxillary tooth will be found to be the cause. Even more common is the complaint of earache accompanying an unidentifiable toothache. Referred pain to the ear is a sure sign that a mandibular tooth is the offender. The mistaken perception occurs apparently within the branches of the trigeminal nerve.

c. The parotid and submandibular salivary glands are occasionally the site of infection or disease. In the more common condition of submandibular sialothiasis, Wharton's duct becomes blocked by a stone or nonopaque "sludge." Characteristically the gland swells and pain is experienced by the patient at the sight, smell, or thought of food. The swelling and pain may decline after the meal only to reappear at the next mealtime. If the stone is in the duct, a sialolithotomy will often bring relief. However, surgical excision of the submandibular gland is frequently necessary since the gland structure is considerably damaged by repeated infections.

d. Experimental stimulation of various areas in the nose and paranasal sinuses refers pain to well-defined regions of the mouth, face, and cranium. Therefore, in any diagnosis of pain, rhinological causes should be sought. The most common diagnostic dilemma is the confusion between maxillary toothache and maxillary sinusitis. On occasion, periapical infection from a maxillary premolar or molar may, in fact, cause sinusitis.

e. The plethora of names ascribed to facial migrainous neuralgias has served to confuse clinicians, as witness the considerable length of time elapsing between onset of symptoms and appropriate diagnosis and treatment of this condition.

2. The Subcommittee on Taxonomy of the International Association for the Study of Pain has provided interim conditional descriptions of pain of vascular origin (Merskey, 1983).

a. Cluster headache is most often unilateral in the ocular, frontal, and temporal areas but may also be situated in the infraorbital region. Such headaches predominantly afflict males and usually start when the patient is between 18 and 40 years of age. Bouts often last 4-8 wk, with one to three attacks every 24 hr to a maximum of eight attacks. The pain is excruciating and described as constant stabbing, burning, and throbbing. Pain-free intervals lasting several months occur between bouts. Associated features include ipsilateral ptosis-miosis, tearing, rhinorrhea, and nasal blockade. Treatment is with ergot preparations, prednisone, methysergide, etc.

b. Chronic cluster headaches are similar to cluster headaches but more rare. The diagnosis requires at least two or more attacks per week over a period of more than a year. Treatment is the same as for cluster headache, but lithium carbonate tends to work better for chronic cluster headache.

c. Chronic paroxysmal hemicrania involves the ocular, frontal, and temporal areas and occasionally the occipital, infraorbital, aural, mastoid, and nuchal areas, invariably on the same side. It occurs predominantly in females. Patients have attacks every day. Characteristically, the attacks fluctuate in frequency and severity; they may last 5-45 min and at their maximum are excruciating. Ipsilateral conjunctival injection, lacrimation, nasal stuffiness, and rhinorrhea are seen in most patients. Attacks occur at regular intervals through the day and night, and the patient may be awakened by a nocturnal attack. Indomethacin provides immediate and absolute relief.

d. Temporal giant cell arteritis afflicts patients over 60 yr of age. There is a dull persistent pain in the temple experienced after chewing. The temporal artery is nonpulsatile, tortuous, and tender. A biopsy will confirm the diagnosis. Referral to an ophthalmologist is essential to rule out ophthalmic artery involvement and the possibility of permanent blindness. Corticosteroids will ameliorate the condition.

B. Pain arising from nerve trunks and central pathways

1. No abnormal CNS signs present. These primary idiopathic neuralgias, which have been recognized for centuries, are among the most severe pains that afflict the human race.

a. The characteristics of trigeminal neuralgia are well defined and diagnostic. Characteristically, there is a "trigger zone" in the area of the nasolabial fold or upper or lower lip, which when stimulated by washing, shaving, talking, or any slight movement will cause the pain. There is no objective sensory loss. An untreated patient may therefore initially appear unkempt, drooling from the mouth, and unwilling to move or touch the trigger area. Injection of local anesthetic into the area will abolish the trigger for the duration of the anesthesia. Remission for months or years is to be anticipated.

(1) Although this description is classic and usually well recognized, patients who have had various treatments in the past may give vastly different descriptions that greatly confuse diagnosis. Furthermore, several less typical features may be reported—continuous or long-lasting aching or burning between paroxysms and spontaneous changes in sensation.

(2) No etiology has been found, but some patients describe a previous traumatic event. Pathology of resected nerve tissue shows evidence of hypomyelination or demyelination in the region of the trigeminal ganglion. Some neurosurgeons believe that impingement of blood vessels on the nerve, again in the region of the ganglion, is the cause. It is important to recognize that in some patients, especially those under 40 yr of age, symptoms of trigeminal neuralgia may indicate an underlying disease (e.g., multiple sclerosis or a space-occupying lesion at the cerebellopontine angle).

b. A similar condition, glossopharyngeal neuralgia, has the same characteristics except that the trigger zone is in the tonsil, lateral pharyngeal wall, or base of the tongue. This condition should not be confused with Eagle's syndrome, in which an elongated styloid process may impinge on the soft tissue of the throat during neck movement or swallowing, or with Trotter's syndrome, in which a tumor of the nasopharynx may give rise to pain in the lower jaw, tongue, and side of the head. In these cases, however, other signs—deafness (due to occlusion of the eustachian tube) and asymmetrical mobility of the soft palate (due to tumor invasion of the levator palati)—should be looked for.

c. Postherpetic neuralgia is occasionally encountered in the trigeminal (V) nerve distribution. The first division (ophthalmic) is especially affected and the possibility of corneal scarring should be borne in mind. Many patients are over 70 yr of age; the older the patient, the more severe the pain seems to be. Pain is described as a constant, burning type that may or may not be accompanied by a stabbing sensation and some hyper- or hypoesthesia. The diagnosis is readily made if a history of a painful rash in the area 1-2 wk previously is elicited, but this can be confused with trigeminal neuralgia or TMJ problems.

d. Treatment of the primary neuralgias is initially medical, carbamazepine (Tegretol) or phenytoin (Dilantin) being successful in many cases. However, some people are allergic to those medications or develop bone marrow depression. Surgical methods of treatment include the following:

(1) Traditionally, peripheral neurectomy of the maxillary or mandibular division of the fifth nerve or phenol or alcohol blocks have been used to denervate the area permanently.

(2) With the introduction of the radiofrequency lesion, the pain fibers specifically supplying the trigger zone may be selectively destroyed without necessarily impinging on sensory function. This is a relatively benign procedure with excellent long-term results.

(3) Other neurosurgeons prefer intracranial surgery to dissect vascular structures off the trigeminal ganglion. In their hands good results are obtained despite the greater risks of a major surgical intervention.

2. Pain arising from nerve trunks and central pathways in which abnormal CNS signs are present. The etiological agent may be extracranial (e.g., trauma, osteomyelitis, Paget's disease, tumors [either primary or metastatic]) or intracranial (including space-occupying lesions at the cerebellopontine angle or the middle cranial fossa). Other causes include disseminated sclerosis, cerebral vascular disease, syphilis, syringobulbia, and stilbamidine (antiprotozoal) therapy.

C. Pain arising from outside the face

1. Pain perceived in the face may be due to irritation of pain receptors in tissues that are embryologically related to the segmental innervation of the face. This pain originates in the eyes, ears, heart, or cervical spine. Common ocular causes of pain include

Refractive error
Convergence insufficiency
Extraocular muscle imbalance
Trauma (e.g., abrasion, contact lens damage, foreign body)
Iritis
Narrow angle glaucoma
"Dry eye" syndrome

2. Angina from coronary artery disease is classically described as substernal pain, referred to the left arm and side of the neck, brought on by physical exertion, emotional upset, or ingestion of food. It is rapidly relieved by rest or sublingual nitroglycerin. On occasion the pain sweeps up the neck and into the angle of the left jaw. If it occurs in the jaw without other related symptoms, the diagnosis may be missed.

3. Cervical disease may cause facial pain. The dorsal roots of cervical nerves 2 and 3 supply the skin overlying the angle of the mandible. A whiplash injury, cervical osteoarthritis, or

spondylitis may irritate these nerves and cause pain in that area.

D. Psychogenic facial pain

    1. It is unfortunate that psychogenic facial pain is frequently discussed last and is misused as a receptacle for all the hitherto undiagnosed pains. For the reasons alluded to earlier, many people with emotional and psychiatric problems focus their attention on the face and mouth. Some of these pains have, indeed, been characterized and a diagnosis can therefore be made. Other patients with overt or latent psychiatric problems are frequently less readily characterized and treated. Patients may exhibit a plethora of psychiatric symptoms and, on occasion, litigation or workmen's compensation may be pending after some traumatic event or dental or surgical intervention. Patients who malinger, abuse drugs, or exhibit Munchausen's syndrome may also be encountered.

        a. In a characteristic case of atypical facial pain the patient (usually female) complains of severe pain but rarely appears to be in pain at the time of the interview. The pain may or may not interfere with normal daily activities. The description of it is imprecise and variable with a nonanatomical distribution. Frequently the pain has been present for months or years, and remissions are rare. It is aggravated by fatigue, worry, tension, or emotional upset and is unrelieved by analgesics. The patient seldom has any insight into the origin of the problem and indeed may vigorously pursue an "organic diagnosis," going from practitioner to practitioner in a vain hope of finding the one "who can cure my pain."

        b. A variant of this is phantom tooth pain or atypical odontalgia, in which the patient complains of discomfort in a tooth or its supporting structures. Fillings, endodontics, extractions, and bone curettage may be performed, without relief, and the same sequence may be followed in the neighboring tooth until a whole region of the mouth is rendered edentulous.

    2. In all cases of atypical facial pain, a thorough physical and radiographic examination is necessary and a psychiatric work-up is indicated.

        a. Frequently, depression is associated with chronic pain, either as a preexisting condition or as a reaction to the pain.

            (1) The Washington University Research criteria for depression are

                Poor appetite or weight loss
                Sleep disturbance, including any type of insomnia or hypersomnia
                Fatigue, loss of energy, tiredness
                Agitation or retardation

Loss of interest in usually stimulating activities (job, hobbies, social interaction) or decreased sexual drive

Decreased ability to think or concentrate, slow or mixed-up thinking

Feelings of self-reproach or guilt

Recurrent thoughts of death or suicide, including the wish to be dead

(2) A patient with four of the eight criteria is probably depressed, and with five is definitely depressed. Whether the depression is endogenous or exogenous, the patient will greatly benefit from treatment.

(3) Antidepressant medications have a long history of effectiveness and safety and can be expected to reduce anxiety, reverse both mood and vegetative signs and symptoms of depression, and alter sleep dysfunction. The tricyclic antidepressants (amitriptyline and doxepin) are most widely used, and a bedtime-only schedule of 50-150 mg may achieve improvement in 1-2 wk. The treatment can be continued for several months and then tapered to a low maintenance dose. Monoamine oxidase inhibitors and lithium salts may on occasion also be prescribed.

b. Anxiety is a widespread experience and may or may not be associated with a specific major life change (e.g., illness, death, or acute stress).

(1) A careful history usually uncovers many symptoms—tachycardia, dizzy spells, headaches, unsteadiness, paresthesias, breathing difficulties, tremors, excessive perspiration, a choking sensation, hyperventilation.

(2) Relaxation techniques—meditation, hypnotherapy, behavior therapy, biofeedback—are useful, and the minor tranquilizers (chlordiazepoxide and diazepam) are widely prescribed.

c. Other psychiatric conditions may also be present with pain (e.g., hysteria, schizophrenia, hypochondriasis). Even when these diagnoses have been ruled out, there remain many patients suffering from a variety of emotional problems that may contribute to or cause pain.

d. Hackett has developed the MADISON scale to describe seven characteristics that correlate with psychogenicity of pain:

Multiplicity. This means that the pain is either in more than one place or of more than one variety. It also means that when one pain disappears through a therapeutic effort another will replace it.

Authenticity. Patients with pain having a high psychological titer often seem more interested in acceptance of their pain as genuine than in receiving a cure for it. They want to be believed. This has been found to be especially true for the pain that masks a depression.

Denial. Chronic pain patients often deny the presence of emotional problems. This denial can be highlighted when they give an exaggerated account of marital or family harmony. They paint a rosy picture of domestic bliss even in the face of impending divorce. Should they admit the occasional presence of anxiety or depression, it is with the proviso that these affects never influence the intensity of their pain. Pathological pain is a fluctuating state. It is highly sensitive to the influence of fear, anger, sadness, and tranquility. When a pain is reported to be unresponsive to these emotions, its nature should be questioned.

Interpersonal relationships. During the course of an interview, the patient may grimace or spontaneously complain of pain when a person's name is mentioned who has something to do directly, indirectly, or symbolically with the patient. Similarly, if that person should walk into the room during the interview, the patient will give evidence of being in immediate distress such as pressing the nurse call button. Yet, when the patient's attention is drawn to this relationship, the connection will be discounted.

Singularity. The following statement demonstrates singularity: "I'm sure you've never heard of a pain like this nor has any other physician who has treated me." It is a singular and unusual pain, one that puts the patient into a special category.

"Only you." This is perhaps the most pernicious factor in terms of the future of the physician-patient relationship. It reads, "Only you can help me, Doctor." One should immediately imagine the numerous other physicians who failed to meet this challenge.

Nothing helps, or no change. This means that the pain does not change from hour to hour, day to day, or year to year. If anything, it only gets worse. Nothing helps, including drugs. It defies all that is known about the nature of pathological pain. Distraction, suggestion, chemical interference, barometric pressure changes, circadian influences, and political upheaval fail to alter the patient's perception of the discomfort. Like the national debt, it remains forever present, and if a change should occur it invariably is toward the red. When asked "Why do you take so many medications?" the patient will respond with something like "What else is there to do? If I don't take them, I'll be worse off." When reminded of the statement that "nothing helps," he may respond with "Something is better than nothing" or some equally meaningless cliché.

e. All pathological pain changes for better or worse during a 24 hr period. Distraction plays a role, as does mood.

Appropriate pain medication invariably helps. In the absence of relief, either spontaneous or drug induced, the nature of the patient's pain is questionable.

Temporomandibular Joint Disorders and Diseases

DIAGNOSIS

I. Although it is a most common cause of facial pain (an estimated 20-40% of the population having experienced it), the TMJ syndrome nevertheless requires a thorough history and examination so that other potentially more serious diagnoses will not be missed.

   A. The previous history of pain and dysfunction should be detailed. In addition, the patient's previous family, social, and medical history should be ascertained.

   B. The clinical examination should include

      Palpation of the muscles of mastication (temporalis, masseter, pterygoidens medialis, pterygoideus lateralis)
      Observation of mandibular motion (opening, closing, lateral extension, protrusion)
      Palpation and/or auscultation of joint noises
      Examination of the dentition and occlusion

II. Masticatory system disorders have been classified in many ways. Because of the difficulty encountered in establishing a precise etiology, they are often defined on the basis of symptoms and signs. Following are some broad categories:

Masticatory muscle spasm
Internal derangement
Chronic hypomobility (ankylosis)
Trauma
Degenerative joint disease
Growth disturbances
Infections
Tumors

CLINICAL DISORDERS

I. Masticatory muscle spasm (TMJ or myofascial pain dysfunction syndrome)

   A. Epidemiological studies from many countries have clearly shown that the signs and symptoms of TMJ disorders are widespread and that 28-88% of people will have clinically detectable manifestations of dysfunction. Fewer individuals (12-59%) will be aware of the symptoms, and fewer still (5-25%) will require treatment.

      1. It is generally agreed that patients with TMJ dysfunction will exhibit one or more of the following signs:

        Decreased range of mandibular motion
        Impaired TMJ function (e.g., deviation, sounds, sticking)
        Pain on palpation of the masticatory muscles or TMJ or on movement of the joint

2. They may also have one or more of the following symptoms:

TMJ sounds
Fatigue or stiffness of the jaws
Pain in the face or jaws
Pain on opening the mouth wide
Locking

3. Radiographic studies of the TMJ will show no evidence of disease.

4. The etiology of this clinical complex is multifactorial—the factors most commonly cited being functional, psychological, and structural (i.e., occlusal). It is important to appreciate that for any individual patient one clear etiological component is rarely apparent. More often, several possible components will be identified. On the basis of this, the oral surgeon should formulate treatment goals bearing in mind the several likely etiological factors.

B. The vast majority of patients will respond to simple, noninvasive treatment plans. These should include, but need not necessarily be limited, to the following:

1. Reassurance. It is important that the patient realize he is not alone with his symptoms, that they are essentially self-limiting, and that no disorder exists. The role of muscle spasm and its benign nature should be carefully explained.

2. Rest. Although it is not prudent to immobilize the mandible entirely, the patient should be instructed to have a mechanically soft diet for 2 wk and to avoid yawning and laughing with his mouth open. Habits such as chewing gum and biting fingernails should be strenuously resisted.

3. Heat. The application of heat to the sides of the face by means of a heating pad, hot towel, or hot water bottle will be comforting and relieve muscle spasm. More vigorous treatment can be achieved with ultrasound or shortwave diathermy heat treatments, which are widely available in physical therapy departments.

4. Medications

    a. Nonsteroidal antiinflammatory analgesics are of value in the acute stage. Ibuprofen, naproxen, zomepirac acid, and indomethacin at a low dose for 2 wk are usually prescribed.

    b. Anxiolytic agents (e.g., the benzodiazepines) are by far the most widely used. Several regimens exist and dosages should be individualized; 2.5-10 mg b.i.d.-q.i.d. (with the nighttime dose increased as necessary to ensure restful sleep) is quite common. It is important that this treatment be limited to about 2 wk since there is drug tolerance and dependency beyond that time.

c. Narcotic analgesics should be rigorously avoided.

d. Antidepressants have a long history of effectiveness in the treatment of chronic pain; and in view of the strong association between TMJ dysfunction and psychological factors, their use is often justified, especially when the dysfunction is just a part of the complex of overall muscle pain with other signs and symptoms of depression. The tricyclic antidepressants are most widely used and a bedtime-only schedule of 25-150 mg amitriptyline or doxepin can be expected to relieve symptoms in 1-2 wk. Treatment is maintained for 2-4 mo and tapered to a low maintenance dose.

5. Occlusal therapy
   a. Appliances
      (1) A plethora of interocclusal appliances exist, and their multiplicity suggests that the optimum design has yet to be found. The devices are usually made of processed acrylic and do the following:

      Improve TMJ function
      Improve the function of the masticatory motor system while reducing abnormal muscle function
      Protect the teeth from attrition and adverse occlusal loading.

      (2) An excellent review of current splints and the theories on which they are designed is provided by Clark (Laskin et al., 1983). In essence, a full arch occlusal stabilizing appliance is the type that has proved most effective. Partial-coverage appliances tend to produce significant and irreversible changes in the dentition. It has been shown that an appropriate appliance can be effective in the majority (70-90%) of patients and will both reduce masticatory muscle pain and control attrition and adverse tooth loading.

   b. Occlusal adjustments. There have been numerous claims that occlusal interferences of various types are the chief cause of masticatory muscle pain and that their elimination will result in improvement. Since masticatory dysfunction is a multifactorial problem, this is not likely to be true. The negative influence of malocclusion, loss of teeth, and occlusal interferences on masticatory dysfunction is not well supported by the evidence. However, on general principle, occlusal disharmony (including premature contacts) should be eliminated and missing teeth replaced in an effort to achieve optimum occlusion for the patient.

   c. Repositioning. Perry (Laskin et al., 1983) summarizes repositioning by saying that its long-term evaluation in

       adult nongrowing jaws with occlusal splints or function-
       al appliances has not been satisfactorily proved.

   6. Behavioral modification. Since there is a psychological component of TMJ disorders, any attempt to lower the patient's
feelings of stress is important. Relaxation techniques, con-
ditioning, and biofeedback have all been shown to be advantageous. However, the most important technique undoubt-
edly is the therapeutic interaction of the dentist with the
patient.

II. Internal derangement of the temporomandibular joint.

   A. Despite the development of TMJ arthrography in the 1940s,
the dental profession has been reluctant to utilize it in recognizing internal derangement of the meniscus as part of the
spectrum of TMJ disorders. In recent years this lack of interest
has been replaced by an overabundance of interest. No doubt,
a balance will be found. It is quite clear that the meniscus can,
either temporarily or permanently, be displaced and give rise
to symptoms.

   B. The main categories of internal derangement are

     1. Anterior displacement with reduction. This occurs when
the meniscus is displaced in the closed-mouth position and
reduces (with a click) to the normal relationship some time
during opening. In these circumstances the patient complains of the click with a variable amount of pain. On opening, the jaw deviates toward the affected side until the click
occurs and then returns to the midline. Preventing the
mouth from fully closing with a splint, tongue blades, or
dental mirror handle eliminates the click. An arthrogram
will demonstrate the displaced meniscus, which reduces on
opening. This situation may worsen and include intermittent locking and then finally closed lock.

     2. Anterior displacement without reduction (closed lock).
The patient, again, has a variable amount of pain. If muscle
spasm has been adequately relieved, he may be pain free but
feel that something in the joint is stopping it from opening.
There is a history of clicking with intermittent locking.
Opening may be limited to 25-30 mm with restricted
motion to the contralateral side. An arthrogram will demonstrate a displacement without reduction (closed lock)
and may also demonstrate perforation and degenerative
changes. In such cases the signs and symptoms of degenerative joint disease may also be present.

   C. Initial treatment for internal derangement consists of the noninvasive therapies used for TMJ syndrome. In the patient who
has anterior displacement with reduction (intermittent locking) these strategies are often successful. In the patient with a
closed-lock, especially one of long standing, these treatments
may reduce muscle spasm and pain and restore some motion
but the underlying displacement will remain. When noninva-

sive treatment has been attempted for several months and the patient remains restricted, surgical repair should be considered.

1. Before beginning, the arthrographic technique is explained in full to the patient and consent is obtained. The patient is then placed on the fluoroscopic table in a lateral recumbent position with his head tilted so the joint projects over the skull above the facial bones. The side of the face to be examined is thus uppermost and is accessible for skin preparation and draping. Instructing the patient to open and close his mouth several times while under fluoroscopic observation allows rapid identification of the condylar head of the affected joint.

2. Under fluoroscopic guidance, the posterosuperior aspect (posterior upper quadrant) of the mandibular condyle is identified. Local anesthetic (1% lidocaine) is infiltrated locally into this region.

   a. A ¾ or 1¼ in scalp vein needle and attached tubing are filled with contrast material; care is taken to eliminate bubbles. In a direction perpendicular to the skin and x-ray beam, the 23-gauge needle is introduced into the predetermined region of the condyle with the jaw in the closed position. After advancement of the needle, fluoroscopic observation ensures proper positioning. When the condyle is encountered, the patient is instructed to open his jaw slightly and the needle is guided off the posterior slope of the bony margin. The needle will easily advance into the space behind the condyle without resistance. On fluoroscopic observation the needle will appear to be perfectly contiguous with the posterior condylar margin.

   b. Meglumine diatrizoate 3 ml (282 mg of iodine plus 0.03 ml of 1:1000 epinephrine) is drawn up into a 5 ml syringe. A test injection (0.2-0.3 ml of contrast material) will be observed to flow freely anterior to the condyle when the needle is properly placed in the lower joint compartment. Approximately 0.5 ml of contrast material completes the test injection. If there is simultaneous filling of the upper joint compartment with instillation of contrast into the lower compartment, another 0.5 ml of contrast material is usually needed for optimum visualization.

   c. The needle is immediately withdrawn and fluoroscopic-videotape images are recorded during opening and closing of the jaw.

3. During arthrotomography the patient lies prone on the radiographic tabletop with his face oriented in a lateral position or in such a way as to allow the flat surface of the mandibular ramus to be parallel to the tabletop. For images

of the TMJ in the closed and open positions, a tomographic unit with a circular motion is employed. The images are approximately 3 mm thick. Three tomograms at 3 mm intervals are obtained in each position of the jaw.

a. The objective of this series is to survey the joint space from medial to central to lateral compartments.

b. To minimize the dose of radiation to the patient, a rare earth film–screen combination is used throughout the entire radiographic protocol. This combination gives approximately one fourth the radiation dose that conventional film-screen combinations do.

c. In patients with clicking of the jaw, images are obtained in three positions: closed, just before the click, and maximum opening.

d. The radiographic protocol is tailored to the clinical presentation and fluoroscopic-arthrographic impression. Patients with painful clicking of the TMJ can be evaluated more thoroughly for jaw dynamics by means of videotape recording. Spot radiographs are obtained during fluoroscopy for a permanent record. The videotape record is available for review during subsequent and more detailed evaluations.

e. In patients whose meniscus is displaced without reduction or with perforation, arthrotomograms are obtained for a more detailed assessment of the anatomical derangement.

f. If the arthrogram appears normal or is indeterminate by fluoroscopy, then arthrotomograms are also necessary for further clarification or confirmation.

g. Spot radiographs under fluoroscopic guidance are obtained during the fluoroscopic procedure. If multidirectional tomograms are needed for a more complete evaluation, the patient is moved immediately to the unit for arthrotomography.

III. Chronic hypomobility (ankylosis)

A. Ankylosis is the persistent inability to open the jaws. It may be caused by pathological involvement of the joint structures (true ankylosis) or limitation produced by extraarticular causes (false ankylosis).

B. Infection and trauma are the primary causes of true ankylosis. The findings are severe limitation of opening, possibly with mandibular retrognathism if mandibular growth has been restricted. False ankylosis may be caused by a variety of disorders that can be categorized as

Myogenic, (e.g., contracture of the masticatory muscles)
Neurogenic (tetanus)
Psychogenic (conversion reaction)
Osteogenic (impingement of an enlarged coronoid process)

Histiogenic (following TMJ surgery, temporal flaps, trauma)
Neoplastic (nasopharyngeal carcinoma)

   C. Radiographs show destruction of the joint surfaces, loss of joint space, and in extreme cases ossificiation across the joint.

   D. The key to successful treatment is identifying as far as possible the cause of the ankylosis and addressing that as aggressively as possible. However, true ankylosis with fibrosis and calcification can be recalcitrant to treatment.

IV. Degenerative joint disease

   A. Degenerative joint disease (osteoarthritis, osteoarthrosis) of the TMJ may be the end point of several different insults to the joint structure exceeding its capacity to remodel and repair. These insults include trauma (acute or chronic), chemical injury, infections, and metabolic disturbances.

   B. The patient complains of pain on moving the jaw and of limited movement, with deviation to the affected side. There may be acute tenderness over the joint itself. Joint sounds are described as grating, grinding, or crunching but not clicking or popping.

   C. Initially radiographs may be essentially normal, but marked degenerative and remodeling changes will be noted later, possibly after symptoms have subsided.

   D. There is a strong predilection for females. A significant number of patients are in their third or fourth decade. A few will manifest generalized osteoarthritis.

   E. The natural course of the disease suggests that the pain and limitation may "burn themselves out" after several months in older individuals. The majority of patients can be kept comfortable until remission with the noninvasive techniques outlined above.

   F. Some patients require injections of corticosteroids into the joint. This treatment is generally reserved for older patients and is limited to two or three injections. (The technique is similar to that for arthrography.) In persons who prove refractory to these techniques, surgery may be indicated to remove loose fragments of bone ("joint mice") and reshape the condyle. Attention should also be directed toward the meniscus, since its displacement may be a primary reason for the degenerative changes.

   G. Rheumatoid arthritis can also affect the TMJ, and reports of its incidence are widespread. The disease may attack individuals of any age: in young persons an associated micrognathia may be noted; in advanced cases ankylosis may be the presenting complaint. Radiographic findings are of joint destruction possibly involving both the condyle and the articular eminence. Other stigmata of the disease will be evident. If medical management is ineffective, treatment of the degenerative joint disease or ankylosis as outlined may be necessary.

V. Growth abnormalities
  A. Studies of facial growth have demonstrated the major contribution made by the mandibular condyle to the adaptive growth of the mandible within the functional soft tissue matrix. Several conditions can reduce this growth—including hypothyroidism, hypopituitarism, and nutritional deficiency (e.g., vitamin D deficiency). In gigantism all the skeletal structures are enlarged, and in acromegaly a marked prognathism is produced.
  B. Several local conditions (trauma, infection, rheumatoid arthritis, radiation, scarring from burns or surgery) are causes of reduced postnatal growth.
  C. In congenital abnormalities the complex and coordinated growth of facial structures necessary for the achievement of normal form and function is altered and malformations occur. It is beyond the scope of this chapter to review all the possible anomalies that are encountered in clinical practice; suffice to say, most abnormalities of the TMJ occur in conjunction with recognized syndromes (e.g., lateral facial dysplasia, Treacher-Collins). A full clinical and radiologic work-up is necessary for full evaluation of the defect and to plan treatment with other specialists.

VI. Infections
  A. Infection of the TMJ can be due to an open wound or to direct extension from adjacent structures (e.g., osteomyelitis of the mandible, suppurative otitis media). More rarely it may be due to hematogenous spread from a distant site.
  B. With improved medical care, better nutrition, and the introduction of antibiotics, infections of the TMJ have diminished in frequency.
  C. Septic arthritis usually affects one joint, which becomes acutely painful, warm, and swollen. Characteristically the swelling in the joint prevents the posterior teeth from meeting. Diagnostic features are the systemic indications of an infection and bacteria in the joint fluid. As sequelae of acute infection, arthritis with ankylosis and growth retardations may develop. Treatment is directed at the underlying cause.

VII. Tumors
  A. Tumors of the TMJ are rare, but clinicians need to maintain a high index of suspicion since the signs and symptoms of neoplastic disease can mimic those of other, more common, TMJ disorders.
  B. Tumors may arise from the native cell population of the joint and invade the adjacent structures, or they may metastasize from distant primary sites.
  C. The benign connective tissue tumors (osteoma, chrondroma, osteochondroma) are most common. They may present with pain or limitation of opening and an open bite on the affected side.

1. In osteoma a globular expansion of the condyle (as opposed to an elongation or overall enlargement seen in condylar hyperplasia) is noted on radiographs, which should be taken in both the lateral and posteroanterior planes.
2. In synovial chondromatosis, foci of cartilage develop in the synovial membrane and occasionally radioopaque masses are seen within the joint.

D. Malignant tumors are rare and may be indicated by pain, swelling, and hearing loss (as the neoplasm expands into the external auditory meatus). Tumors may spread from surrounding structures or metastasize from distant sites. Radiographic changes are osteolytic or osteoblastic depending on tumor type.

GENERAL REFERENCES

Alling, C.C., and Mahan, P.E.: Facial pain, ed. 3, Philadelphia, 1985, Lea & Febiger.

Bell, W.E.: Orofacial pains, ed. 3, Chicago, 1985, Year Book Medical Publishers, Inc.

Feighner, J.P., et al.: Diagnostic criteria for use in psychiatric research, Arch. Gen. Psychiatr. **26:**57, 1972.

Hackett, T.P.: The pain patient: evaluation and treatment. In Hackett, T.P., and Cassem, N.M., editors: Handbook of general hospital psychiatry, St. Louis, 1978, The C.V. Mosby Co.

Helms, C.A., et al.: Internal derangements of the temporomandibular joint, Radiology Research and Education Foundation, San Francisco, 1983.

Laskin, D.M., et al., editors: The President's Conference on the Examination, Diagnosis, and Management of Temporomandibular Disorders, J. Am. Dent. Assoc. **106:**75, 1983.

Merskey, H.: Development of a universal language of pain syndrome, Adv. Pain Res. Ther. **5:**37, 1983.

Sarnat, B.G., and Laskin, D.M.: The temporomandibular joint. A biological basis for clinical practice, 3, ed. Springfield, Ill. 1980, Charles C Thomas, Publisher.

Zarb, G.A., and Carlsson, G.E.: Temporomandibular joint: function and dysfunction, St. Louis, 1979, The C.V. Mosby Co.

Orthognathic and Reconstructive Surgery

10

Orthognathic Surgery

Preparation of a patient for the surgical correction of a dentofacial deformity differs from that required for the evaluation and treatment of an acute problem. The patient who presents for orthognathic surgery is usually many months away from the actual surgery. However, to provide a successful outcome, the meticulous attention to detail in diagnosis and treatment planning required from the very beginning in caring for an acute surgery patient is also necessary from the very outset in caring for an orthognathic surgery patient.

INITIAL EVALUATION

  I. A thorough medical history is the essential first step. In this phase of evaluation, it is critical to determine

   A. Significant etiological factors of the deformity (acromegaly, birth injury, drug exposure, trauma, juvenile arthritis, etc.)

   B. Medical conditions that would contraindicate or require modifications in orthognathic treatment

 II. The patient's history must include recent growth experience, past dental history, and previous orthodontics or surgery.

III. The chief complaint must be recorded. The patient's major concern in seeking treatment may not coincide with the accurate diagnosis of or treatment plan for the deformity. When a discrepancy exists, there is need for careful patient education in the presentation of a treatment plan.

IV. Complete diagnostic records are obtained. These consist of

   Clinical examination
   Facial and intraoral photographs
   Radiographs
   Dental impressions and bite registration
   Facial moulage (in selected cases)

   A. The clinical examination is the most critical part of the diagnostic process.

      1. Components include the following:

         a. Frontal

Facial height
Facial symmetry
Eyes: interpupillary width and cant
Malar prominence
Nasal deviation, alar base width
Upper lip length and symmetry in function
Lower lip length and symmetry in function
Lower lip and chin length and symmetry
Maxillary incisor exposure at rest
Maxillary incisor exposure when smiling
Interlabial gap when relaxed

b. Profile

Eyes: enophthalmos, exophthalmos
Nose: convex, concave, tip deformity
Upper lip: procumbence, nasolabial angle
Lower lip and chin: depth of labiomental fold

c. Intraoral

Oral hygiene
Missing, decayed, or mobile teeth
Prostheses
Periodontal tissues
Tongue: function and posture
Dental midline asymmetries
Malocclusion (Angle's classification)
Maxillary occlusal plane to interpupillary plane
Mouth opening: maximum, deviation from midline
TMJ: pain, limitation, crepitus

2. Treatment planning will follow from the information obtained in the clinical examination, supported by the additional data provided through cephalometric analysis or study of the articulated dental casts.

B. Facial and intraoral photographs are then taken.
1. The following are needed:

Frontal—centric occlusion, lips relaxed
Frontal—centric occlusion, lips together
Frontal—centric occlusion, full smile
Profile—centric occlusion, lips relaxed
Profile—centric occlusion, lips together
Profile centric occlusion, full smile
Submentovertex or "horizon" view—facial asymmetries
Frontal—deficient mandible postured forward
Profile—deficient mandible postured forward
Frontal and both buccal views teeth in occlusion
Mirror view of maxillary arch
Mirror view of mandibular arch

2. Ideally photographs of the patient should be taken under conditions that are reproducible from one set of films to the next. This may be accomplished by permanently mounting

the camera so it can be used with the Cephalostat; alternatively, a single photographer or a well-defined list of camera lens settings may be sufficient. The photographs must include all poses needed in the treatment planning process. For example, if in the clinical examination the patient is asked to posture the mandible forward to demonstrate the effects of mandibular advancement, then photographs of this position should be taken so the "clinical examination" can be repeated even in the absence of the patient.

C. To have any value in the diagnostic and record-keeping process, cephalometric radiographs must be very carefully taken.

1. Following are the films usually needed:

> Lateral cephalometric with the teeth in centric occlusion and the lips in repose—provides good definition of soft tissue densities
> Panoramic of the jaws
> Periapical—when interdental osteotomies are planned
> Posteroanterior—when there is facial asymmetry
> Tomographic, CT, etc.—for evaluating precise anatomical abnormalities of the midface, orbits, skull base, or condyles
> Radionuclide bone scan—for evaluation of actively changing asymmetries
> Hand-wrist film—for evaluatng the completion of longitudinal growth

2. The head must be aligned in the natural head position, a relaxed balanced posture with eyes viewing the horizon, so the true vertical and horizontal axes will be normal. The teeth must be in centric occlusion. The soft tissues will be better visualized by using appropriate masking of the x-ray beam. The lips must be in repose, fully relaxed to show the position of the upper lip relative to the upper incisors and to demonstrate any incompetence that may be present.

3. The lateral cephalometric radiograph should be traced on standard acetate tracing paper with adequate landmarks to allow a standard cephalometric analysis.

   a. The Steiner analysis is the most commonly used (Fig. 10-1), although others may be chosen. The important consideration in choosing a method and implementing it is that the procedure be reproducible from one film to the next as well as from one observer to another.

   b. Newly available techniques using microcomputers and suitable software programs to trace cephalometric points with a digitizer and to perform analyses and storage of data electronically will become more widespread; and the information obtained thereby will be more easily obtained, manipulated, and stored.

4. The primary purpose of the standard cephalometric analysis is to confirm the clinical diagnosis; treatment is not determined by the numbers obtained from the analysis. An excep-

NAME _____ ORTHO NO. _____

CAUTION — Line SN must be 83° to true vertical!

		Ref. Norm										
SNA	(angle)	82°										
SNB	(angle)	80°										
ANB	(angle)	2										
SND	(angle)	76°										
1̱ to NA	(mm)	4°										
1̱ to NA	(angle)	22°										
1̅ to NB	(mm)	4										
1̅ to NB	(angle)	25°										
Po to NB	(angle)	Not established										
Po & 1̅ to NB	(difference)	Varies										
1̱ to 1̅	(angle)	131°										
Occl to SN	(angle)	14°										
GoGn to SN	(angle)	32°										
SL	(mm)	51										
SE	(mm)	22										
H-line to NB	(angle)	Varies with ANB										
3|3 width												
4|4 width												
6|6 width												
e|e present												
Tooth size relationship	(Bolton index)	6=77 12=91	6= 12=	6= 12=	6= 12=	6= 12=	6= 12=
Arch length discrepancy												

Fig. 10-1 Steiner cephalometric analysis form.

tion, however, may be considered if the mesh analysis of Moorrees et al. is used (Figs. 10-2 to 10-8). This method analyzes and compares facial proportions to population norms rather than to absolute measurements, as is customary with other methods. Once the patient's mesh is constructed, it is compared to an idealized mesh and treatment planning then determines which jaw movements will be necessary to approach the ideal. Nevertheless, even this method of cephalometric analysis, although superior to others for treatment-planning purposes, is still secondary to the clinical examination in determining the diagnoses and necessary treatment.

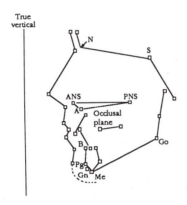

Fig. 10-2   Take a radiograph in the natural head position and draw a vertical (imagine a plumb line). Trace the radiograph and determine the indicated reference points (*ANS, PNS,* etc.)

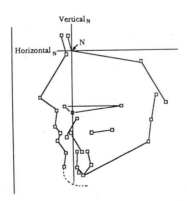

Fig. 10-3   Draw a horizontal and a vertical line through nasion *(N).*

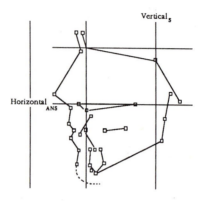

Fig. 10-4 Draw a vertical line through sella *(S)*. Draw a horizontal line through anterior nasal spine *(ANS)*.

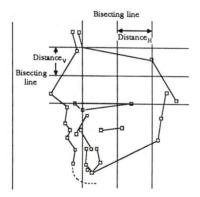

Fig. 10-5 Draw a vertical line bisecting the distance between the verticals through nasion and sella. Draw a horizontal line bisecting the distance between the horizontals through nasion and anterior nasal spine.

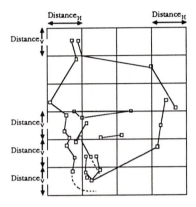

Fig. 10-6 Complete the basic mesh by drawing more vertical and horizontal lines, keeping distance *H* (half the distance between verticals *S* and *N*) and distance *V* (half the distance between horizontals *N* and *ANS*) at the original measurement.

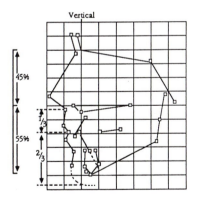

Fig. 10-7 For greater accuracy in locating points, it is often helpful to further subdivide each box of the mesh as shown. The points on this mesh were determined from radiographs of 18-year-old female subjects. The 18-year-old male is quite similar.

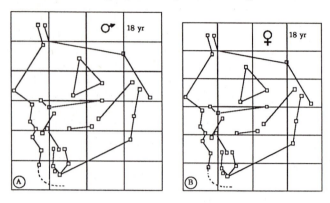

Fig. 10-8   Differences between the mesh norm for 18-year-old males **(A)** and females **(B)** are slight. In general, males have larger faces and a thicker soft tissue layer over the facial bones.

5. Other radiographic studies may be indicated in specific clinical situations:

Frontal cephalometric—to assist in the evaluation and treatment planning for patients with asymmetry

Hand-wrist—for assessment of the growth potential remaining in adolescent patients, in whom further growth may play an important role in the eventual size and position of the jaws and for whom appropriate timing of the surgery would be critical in maintaining a stable result

Tomographic—of particular value in assessing patients with condylar, orbital, and/or cranial base deformities

Radionuclide bone scanning—when the clinical history suggests the possibility of hyperplastic or neoplastic condylar growth

D. Accurate well-trimmed dental study casts are essential.
   1. Duplicate casts should be poured in dental stone. They must be indelibly marked with the patient's name and the date on which they were obtained.
   2. The bases must be of sufficient size to allow monoplane trimming of the posterior cast surfaces when the casts are held in the patient's present centric occlusion.
   3. One set of casts is retained for the patient's permanent record; the other may be used for further duplication or for any necessary model surgery.
   4. Not every patient's study models will require mounting on an articulator by means of a facebow transfer. An adjustable or semiadjustable articulator can be useful in certain cases of asymmetry or when precise three-dimensional registration of mandibular autorotation after maxillary movement is desired.

INITIAL DIAGNOSIS

I. The problem list is developed and enumerates the various diagnoses or conditions pertinent to the patient.

   A. Nonmedical problems must be included if they might influence the eventual treatment or outcome. (Socioeconomic conditions, type of employment, motivation for treatment, and the likelihood of cooperation with and completion of treatment are examples.)

   B. Only problems that are active or that contribute to the presently contemplated treatment should be listed. (A history of prior valve replacement or a family history of malignant hyperthermia would be a "contributory problem.")

   C. In the orthognathic portion of the problem list, each jaw must be considered as a three-dimensional structure with potential problems to be found in any of the three planes. (For example, the maxilla might be vertically excessive, horizontally [sagittally] excessive, and transversely normal.)

II. The initial diagnostic process is completed by listing all pertinent problems whose solutions can now be addressed:

   A. Nonmedical problems

      Employment
      Insurance
      Financial constraints

   B. Medical history problems

      Rheumatic fever
      Hepatitis
      Bleeding disorders
      Allergies
      Current medications

   C. Dental problems

      Restorative needs
      Periodontal needs

   D. Orthodontic problems

      Angle classification of malocclusion
      Crowding of dental arch
      Malposition of individual teeth

   E. Orthognathic problems

      Maxilla
         Vertical
         Horizontal
         Transverse
      Mandible
         Vertical
         Horizontal
         Transverse

Note: Wherever necessary to delineate the patient's problems more clearly, each jaw may be further subdivided into anterior and posterior or left and right.

TENTATIVE TREATMENT PLAN

I. The tentative orthognathic treatment plan begins with the incisal tip of the maxillary central incisor. The position of this tooth relative to the upper lip is the keystone of the architecture of the jaws. Therefore, one first looks to the problem list to determine whether any vertical or horizontal malposition of the maxilla exists. If so, a new position for the maxilla must be chosen (Fig. 10-9) (see also Algorithm 4).

    A. Using the tracing of the lateral cephalometric film, retrace the maxilla so the tip of the central incisor is positioned correctly in relation to the upper lip. This will usually place the incisal edge 2-3 mm below the drape of the upper lip at rest. The horizontal position is chosen from the desired nasolabial angle and midfacial prominence.

    B. Rotate the tracing of the mandible until the mandibular incisors are in 2-3 mm of overbite. Positive or negative overjet is temporarily ignored. The axis of rotation may be taken as the midpoint of the condyle.

    C. Without moving the tip of the maxillary central incisor, rotate the maxilla until the maxillary occlusal plane is aligned with the occlusal plane of the mandible as established in the preceding step.

    D. Determine whether the mandible requires advancement, retropositioning, or change to achieve a normal overjet.

    E. Make a new tracing of the lateral cephalometric film with the maxilla and mandible in the newly chosen positions; use a different color for this tracing. Now the two tracings can be superimposed to demonstrate clearly the amount and direction of movements that have been chosen. Construct a mesh diagram of the proposed new positions of the jaws.

    F. In case of asymmetry, similar tracings should be made of the AP cephalometric film.

II. The study models are evaluated as to whether the changes proposed by the cephalometric prediction will produce an adequate occlusion. Included in the concept of an adequate occlusion are such important considerations as

    A. The presence of dental compensations

    B. The significance of interarch problems (crowding, spacing, or rotation of teeth)

    C. The nature of interarch incompatibilities related to transverse width discrepancies, mismatch of the maxillary and mandibular occlusal curves, or discordance in the shapes and circumferences of the two arches

III. The need for presurgical orthodontic treatment is then determined.

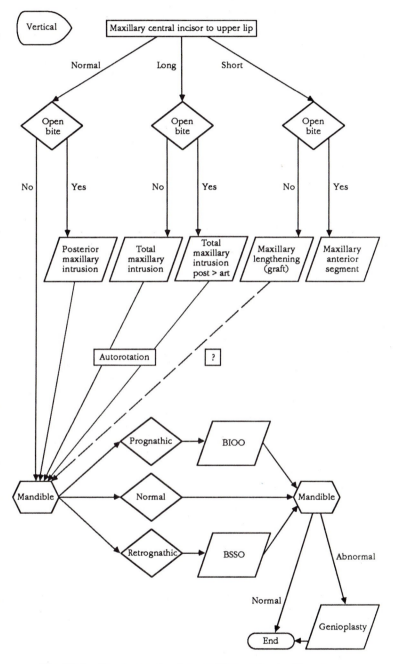

Fig. 10-9 Treatment plan for maxillary orthognathic surgery.

A. The surgeon must be aware of the goals of presurgical orthodontics: elimination of dental compensations and coordination of the two arches.

B. He must also know the feasibility of the orthodontic treatment; thus orthodontic consultation is critical at this time.

C. To aid in making the decision regarding the need for orthodontic treatment as well as to help in formulating the surgical plan, model surgery may be performed on duplicate sets of dental casts. Several "rules" must be followed:

1. Indelible reference marks should be placed on casts before the casts are cut.

2. All segmental cuts should be made completely through the bases of casts.

3. All cuts on casts should be realistic; root positions must be carefully estimated so the model surgery will reflect clinical reality.

4. The minimum amount of stone should be removed in areas of simulated osteotomies; this, too, will more accurately depict the clinical situation at the time of surgery.

5. Fewer is better: one large segment is surgically and biologically preferable to two or four smaller segments. Segmental surgery should not be thought of as a substitute for orthodontic treatment.

6. Repositioning of dentoalveolar segments should take into account the periodontal and dental stability of the new position. Large steps horizontally or vertically at the level of the crestal alveolar bone are unacceptable and would indicate the need for orthodontic rather than surgical movement of the teeth in question.

IV. After necessary orthodontic treatment is performed, the patient returns for assessment of his surgical "readiness." The steps of clinical evaluation, cephalometric prediction, tracings, and model surgery are repeated. The patient is evaluated as a new candidate, since changes in position of the teeth relative to the underlying bone and to the overlying soft tissues may necessitate significant revisions in the original treatment plan. A new or revised problem list is developed, and a final surgical treatment plan is formulated.

FINAL SURGICAL TREATMENT PLAN

I. Completion of the final surgical treatment plan requires a thorough familiarity with the various surgical procedures available as well as their indications, contraindications, and limitations. Full details of the surgical techniques are available elsewhere and will not be repeated here, but it is assumed that the user of this manual is knowledgeable in this area.

II. Maxillary problems

A. Vertical maxillary excess

1. When the excess is confined to the anterior region of the maxillary arch, implying a reversed curve of Spee with an acceptable posterior occlusion, an anterior segmental or dentoalveolar osteotomy is indicated. The method of Cupar (utilizing a labial incision and a palatal pedicle) may be chosen for this.

2. When the excess is confined to the posterior maxilla, producing an anterior open bite with a normal relationship of the upper lip and upper central incisors, either posterior segmental osteotomies or a LeFort I osteotomy is the preferred treatment (the latter in all but exceptional cases). The position of the mandible produced by its autorotation following the maxillary movement may require inclusion of a mandibular osteotomy in the final surgical plan.

3. Vertical maxillary excess involving both anterior and posterior areas, whether accompanied by an anterior open bite or not, necessitates a LeFort I osteotomy. Model surgery will demonstrate the need for segmental osteotomies in conjunction with the total maxillary procedure. Also the possibility must be considered that mandibular surgery will be necessary as a result of the maxillary change.

B. Vertical maxillary deficiency

1. When the deficiency is confined to the anterior maxilla (with an exaggerated curve of occlusion and acceptable posterior intercuspation), an anterior segmental osteotomy may be the surgical choice; either the Wassmund technique (vertical labial incisions, palatal tunneling) or the Wunderer (palatal incision, labial pedicle) may be used (the latter is preferred).

2. Vertical deficiency involving either the posterior or the entire maxilla may be corrected by a LeFort I osteotomy and interpositional bone graft, although long-term problems with stability of the procedure require careful consideration.

C. Horizontal (sagittal) maxillary excess

1. Premaxillary prominence with a satisfactory posterior occlusion is corrected with an anterior dentoalveolar segmental osteotomy; this procedure will usually require removal of the first premolars. The technique of Wunderer (palatal incision, labial soft tissue pedicle) is suggested. However, this solution is usually contraindicated when the premolars have been removed previously and all spaces have been closed; extraction of additional premolars and placement of the canines adjacent to the first molars by means of this osteotomy will generally result in unacceptable periodontal and esthetic configurations of the arch.

2. When anterior segmental osteotomy is contraindicated or when the entire maxillary arch requires posterior movement, a LeFort I osteotomy is chosen.

D. Horizontal (sagittal) maxillary deficiency
1. The LeFort I osteotomy is preferred for advancement of the entire maxillary arch. Bone grafting to maintain the stability of the advancement is usually not necessary.
2. Advancement of malar areas may be accomplished simultaneously by performing horizontal osteotomies high on the lateral maxillary walls or by implanting onlay bone grafts or alloplastic materials (Silastic or Proplast). True advancement of the infraorbital rims will require an osteotomy of the LeFort III type.

E. Transverse maxillary deficiency
1. The problem of a narrow maxilla will most often be addressed during the presurgical orthodontic phase of treatment. In adults, when conventional orthodontic appliance therapy for rapid palatal expansion is not successful, a minor surgical procedure may be necessary. A lateral maxillary osteotomy through the zygomatic buttress on each side will usually suffice, although separation of the midpalatal suture will be required in some patients for the palatal expansion appliance to be effective. Separation of the pterygomaxillary sutures or the interincisal bone is not necessary.
2. When expansion of all or portions of the maxilla is needed, either in the absence of orthodontic treatment or in cases of incomplete orthodontic expansion, segmental osteotomies can be planned in conjunction with a LeFort I osteotomy. Unilateral expansion of a posterior maxillary segment can be accomplished with a segmental osteotomy if there is no other concomitant need for a LeFort I osteotomy.

F. Transverse maxillary excess. When there is need to narrow the maxillary arch, palatal ostectomy can be performed at the time of a LeFort I osteotomy.

III. Mandibular problems (Fig. 10-10 and Algorithm 4)
A. Horizontal mandibular excess
1. If the entire mandible is prominent and the mandibular dental arch requires posterior movement, a mandibular ramus osteotomy is indicated. The vertical or oblique osteotomy, extending posterior to the inferior alveolar neurovascular bundle from the sigmoid notch to the angle of the mandible, is the procedure associated with least morbidity. An alternative would be the sagittal ramus osteotomy. Posterior body or ramus ostectomies are rarely used or indicated.
2. When the posterior occlusion is satisfactory and the prognathic relationship is confined to the anterior segment, a segmental osteotomy is the treatment of choice. Extraction of two premolars is required unless preexisting space within the dental arch can be used for retropositioning the anterior dentoalveolar segment. The position of the mental foramina must be considered in planning the procedure.

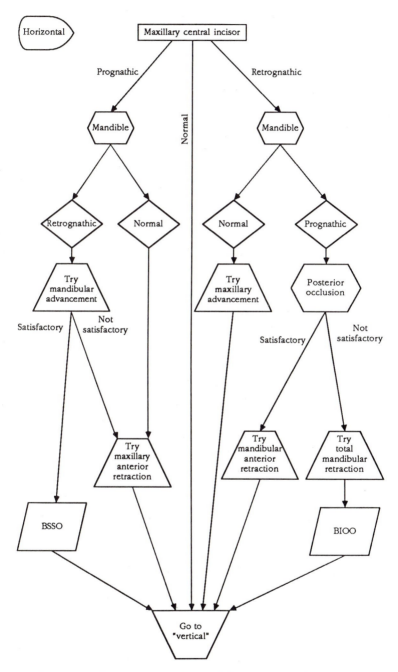

Fig. 10-10 Treatment plan for mandibular orthognathic surgery.

3. When the occlusion is satisfactory, the prognathic mandible requires contour reduction, either by reduction genioplasty or by ostectomy of the lower border of the mandibular body.

B. Horizontal mandibular deficiency
1. Autorotation will usually suffice for correction of relative mandibular deficiency—i.e., when the problem is in the maxilla and the surgical procedure can be confined to the upper jaw.
2. If the entire mandible and lower dental arch require advancement, the sagittal ramus osteotomy is the most reliable procedure; clinical stability can be anticipated as long as there is no elongation of the height of the ramus resulting from the procedure. This precludes any "closing" rotation of the distal mandible during the advancement. Advancement of the mandible *and* closure of an anterior open bite will require maxillary surgery in conjunction with the mandibular procedure. Alternatives to the sagittal ramus osteotomy include the inverted-L and the C osteotomies; the inverted-L requires a bone graft, and both the L and the C are usually performed from an extraoral approach (making them relatively less desirable than the sagittal osteotomy).
3. Advancement of the total mandibular alveolus without advancing the lower border and chin point has its advocates, but the growing consensus is that the total alveolar osteotomy is contraindicated by the relative avascularity of the dentoalveolar segment and by the unacceptable frequency of inferior alveolar nerve injury.
4. When the occlusal relationship of the mandibular arch with the maxilla is acceptable, advancement of the mandible is usually achieved by means of advancement genioplasty. Implantation of bone grafts or alloplastic materials is occasionally used, but the long-term results are not as satisfactory as those obtained with the sliding genioplasty.

C. Vertical mandibular deficiency
1. Advancement of the mandible will usually result in lengthening of the lower third of the face, the amount of vertical change being dependent upon the mandibular plane and the steepness of the occlusal plane.
2. Attempts to elongate the vertical dimension of the mandible by total alveolar osteotomy give unstable results, and this procedure is not recommended.
3. Horizontal genioplasty with interpositional bone grafts for lengthening the chin may be considered for correction of vertical mandibular deficiency.

D. Vertical mandibular excess
1. Elongation of the lower third of the face may be corrected by intrusion of the maxilla and thus require no mandibular surgery.

2. When no surgery is required in the maxilla or when the maxillary correction produces insufficient change in the lower third of the face, reduction genioplasty or contouring ostectomy of the lower border of the mandible may be included in the treatment plan.

E. Transverse mandibular deficiency

1. If the mandibular dental arch is too narrow for the maxillary arch, orthodontic treatment is the primary method for increasing the circumference of the arch. If the teeth are appropriately situated over basal bone and a transverse deficiency is still present, the discrepancy will usually require maxillary surgery to narrow the upper jaw. Surgical procedures to widen the lower dental arch are unsatisfactory.

2. If the occlusion is acceptable, transverse mandibular deficiency is generally managed by the use of onlay bone grafts to improve the contour of the jaw. This procedure is most often needed in cases of severe asymmetry.

F. Transverse mandibular excess

1. If the occlusion is satisfactory, excessive width of the mandible is corrected by reduction contouring of the jaw.

2. Relative excess of mandibular width may be corrected by altering the sagittal relationship of the jaws. If this relationship has been corrected and transverse discrepancy remains, one must consider either widening the maxilla (particularly if maxillary surgery is already planned for other reasons) or narrowing the mandible. Ostectomy in the symphyseal area, often in conjunction with an anterior dentoalveolar segmental osteotomy or together with extraction of an anterior tooth, will enable the mandible to be narrowed. Simultaneous "relaxing" osteotomies of the ramus may be needed, particularly if the posterior portion of the dental arch must also be narrowed either unilaterally or bilaterally.

PREADMISSION PREPARATION

I. The medical history obtained at the time of initial evaluation must be updated at the final preadmission visit so that any changes in the patient's health status can be determined. If indicated by this history, whatever medical consultation is necessary should be arranged in anticipation of the patient's being admitted to hospital. The physician must be apprised of the nature of the planned surgery, the anesthesia requirement, and the specific medical assistance being requested.

II. Communication with the patient's insurance carrier is often necessary at this time. A growing number of insurance companies stipulate a preadmission review of elective hospitalization; the insurer may expect the patient to obtain a second opinion before elective surgery or may have a program for predetermination of benefits that enjoins the surgeon to submit pertinent records before surgery can be performed. It is the patient's responsibility to comply with the demands of his insurance company, but the surgeon should remind the patient to ask about any preadmission requirements if this has not already been done.

III. If there is the potential need for transfusion of blood products during the planned surgery, arrangements with the hospital's blood bank should be made. Whenever possible, donation of the patient's own blood for autologous transfusion should be scheduled. One unit of blood may be obtained every 7-10 da, with the last unit collected at least 2 wk before the scheduled surgery. The patient must be given a prescription for ferrous sulfate, 300 mg t.i.d., from the time of the initial collection until admission. Two units of blood obtained in this manner will usually be adequate for use in uncomplicated orthognathic procedures.

IV. A final presurgical orthodontic consultation is necessary for any patient who has been undergoing orthodontic treatment in preparation for surgery. At this time the surgical treatment plan should be discussed with the orthodontist. After his concurrence on the proposed surgery, he will be able to construct surgical arch wires and make any necessary changes in appliances to facilitate the procedure. Final presurgical records, including photographs and radiographs, are also obtained at this time.

V. It should remain the surgeon's responsibility to construct any necessary templates or interocclusal splints that will be used during the procedure. Such devices are constructed on articulated casts after the final model surgery has been performed; cold-cure acrylic, preferably clear, is used. The appliances must be carefully trimmed and polished before they are taken to the operating room.

INPATIENT MANAGEMENT

I. At the time of admission a complete history is obtained and physical examination performed according to the prescribed format of the hospital.

II. Informed consent of the patient to the planned surgical procedure is obtained and documented in the hospital record.

III. Preoperative laboratory studies, as required by the hospital and the needs of the patient, are ordered. A complete blood count, urinalysis, and blood bank sample will usually be the minimum complement of tests. Evaluation of serum electrolytes, tests of renal and hepatic function, examination of chest radiographs, and the taking of an electrocardiogram will all be carried out according to the patient's history, as will evaluation of coagulopathies, endocrine disorders, and other pathological conditions relevant to the surgery and the anesthesia.

IV. The anesthesiologist will conduct a preoperative assessment of the patient. Close cooperation is essential between the surgeon and the anesthesiologist so the latter knows the nature, extent, and special needs of the planned procedure. Hypotensive anesthetic techniques are favored by some surgeons. The minimization of operative blood loss makes the surgical field cleaner and reduces the need for transfusion of blood products. However, the slightly head-up position of the patient, use of autologous transfusion, and ability to perform the surgery efficiently will, in most instances, render the advantages of hypotensive anesthesia negligible and thereby avoid the potential complications associated with the hypotensive technique.

V. Preoperative orders are written as usual.

    A. Most surgeons prescribe prophylactic antibiotics to be given as the patient is taken to the surgical suite. Penicillin, 6 million units per day in divided doses IV for 48 hr beginning at the time of surgery, is a widely used regimen. For patients allergic to penicillin, erythromycin or clindamycin may be used.

    B. Although there is little valid evidence to support their use, corticosteroids are commonly ordered at the time of surgery in the belief that they will lessen postoperative edema and thus reduce airway embarrassment for the patient whose jaws are immobilized. A common dosage schedule is 8 mg dexamethasone at the time of surgery and 4 mg t.i.d. for the next 48 hr. Some surgeons prescribe 100 mg of hydrocortisone or 40 mg of methylprednisolone instead of dexamethasone.

VI. A nasogastric tube may be placed at the conclusion of the procedure to empty the stomach of secretions and swallowed blood. This will usually aid in reducing postoperative nausea and vomiting. The tube is removed as soon as there is no active bleeding.

VII. Ice packs are used in the first 24-36 hr to help minimize postoperative edema.

IMMEDIATE POSTOPERATIVE MANAGEMENT

    I. Immediate postoperative orders are for the usual medications—analgesics, antiemetics, antipyretics, antibiotics. For patients who have undergone maxillary surgery, nasal decongestants and antihistamines may also be prescribed to aid in clearing the nasal airway and to promote drainage of the paranasal sinuses.

    II. Airway management is of paramount importance in the perioperative period. Close monitoring is necessary both in recovery and after the patient returns to his room.

        A. In settings where the nursing staff is unfamiliar with the needs of a patient in intermaxillary fixation, it may be necessary to utilize intensive care for the immediate postoperative recuperation before returning the patient to the regular hospital ward.

        B. The use of nasopharyngeal airways is not recommended except in the totally monitored environment of the recovery room or intensive care unit.

        C. When nasal, buccal, and labial edema makes air exchange difficult, the placement of plastic syringe barrels between the cheeks and the teeth may make the patient more comfortable.

D. Providing humidified air or oxygen via a loose or open face mask will often aid in loosening or preventing crusting of secretions in the airway.

III. In patients who have had ribs harvested for grafting, a postoperative chest radiograph should be obtained to rule out the possibility of pneumothorax.

IV. The hematocrit is usually checked in the recovery room. The test may be repeated as indicated if there is continued bleeding or if transfusions have been administered. Replacement of RBCs is not usually necessary if the hematocrit is greater than 30% and the patient shows no evidence of postural change in vital signs. When autologous blood is available, it is transfused even in the absence of postural signs if the hematocrit is less than 40%.

V. To minimize edema in the immediate postoperative period, the head is elevated above the level of the heart.

VI. Oral nutritional intake is encouraged as soon as possible, starting with clear liquids and progressing to a high-protein, high-calorie, fully blenderized diet. Consultation with the dietitian is recommended for patient and family to assist in nutritional management after discharge.

VII. Early ambulation is urged and should be started on the evening of surgery whenever possible.

VIII. Oral hygiene for the patient in intermaxillary fixation is achieved with the use of half-strength hydrogen peroxide rinses and the help of mechanical devices such as a Water-Pik. The latter must be used with caution in the early postoperative period, however, lest the intraoral incision lines be disrupted. Suction apparatus must be available at the bedside in the immediate postsurgical days but is not generally necessary after the patient has left the hospital.

IX. Scissors or wire cutters must be readily available for use in an emergency. The patient's family must be both reassured with regard to and instructed in the release of intermaxillary fixation before the patient is discharged from the hospital.

X. Appropriate postoperative radiographs, usually consisting of a lateral cephalometric film and a panoramic view, are obtained within 24-48 hr of the surgery. The mandibular condyles must be well visualized on these films, since any malpositioning would necessitate a return to the operating room at the earliest opportunity.

XI. Before discharge a final check on the adequacy and stability of the IMF is carried out. The patient must clearly understand the limitations on his physical activity, instructions regarding nutrition and hygiene, and how to reach the surgeon in case of emergency.

OUTPATIENT POSTOPERATIVE MANAGEMENT

I. Patients are usually seen weekly for postoperative care during the first 3-4 wk. Changing of elastics used for intermaxillary fixation is done at each visit.

II. The patient on whom only a segmental osteotomy was performed and who is not in IMF will need fewer postoperative visits—generally at the first, second, and sixth weeks following surgery. At the last visit the splinting appliances may be removed; the finishing phase of orthodontic treatment begins at this time.

III. The patient who has undergone only a total maxillary osteotomy will be held in IMF usually for 10 da to 2 wk (the minimum time). Then light guiding elastics are often used to aid in settling the occlusion and closing the path of the autorotated mandible. Six weeks after surgery any piriform, infraorbital, or circumzygomatic suspensory wires that may have been used are removed under local anesthesia infiltration.

IV. When mandibular ramus surgery has been performed, with or without simultaneous maxillary procedures, the IMF is maintained for 6 wk. The final orthodontic phase of treatment may be started after this time.

V. A lateral cephalometric radiograph and photographs should be obtained at the end of the 6 wk postoperative period. These will mark any subsequent tendencies toward relapse.

VI. The patient must be instructed in the gradual progression during the seventh and eighth weeks from a soft to a full diet. Mouth opening exercises may be instituted during this time for any patient who demonstrates trismus following the release of IMF.

VII. In the absence of any complications, routine follow-up visits with the patient are scheduled at 6 mo and 1 yr after surgery. Final records obtained at the last such visit will include a clinical examination, lateral cephalometric radiograph, and photographs. A review of these in comparison with the preoperative and immediate postoperative records will help assess the adequacy of the treatment plan in solving the problems that were so carefully delineated at the outset.

Reconstructive Surgery

I. Reconstructive surgery is viewed as the restoration of form and function that has been lost because of trauma, both surgical and accidental. Reconstruction may involve bone, soft tissue, or both.

II. The specifics of care for the patient who requires reconstructive surgery relate to the location of the defect, the type of tissues to be reconstructed, and the donor sites to be employed. These patients have many of the same preoperative and postoperative needs as do patients undergoing major oral and maxillofacial surgery. The principles of blood and fluid management, diet regulation, respiratory care, and wound management differ only to the degree that the reconstructive procedure is more complex than other surgery.

SOFT TISSUE RECONSTRUCTION

I. Replacement of missing soft tissue is indicated whenever there is insufficient local tissue to achieve adequate primary closure, when primary closure of the local tissue would compromise function, and when the quality of the local soft tissue would jeopardize the success of primary closure (e.g., tissues that have previously been irradiated). An additional indication for soft tissue reconstruction is the need to prevent or minimize wound contracture in areas that would otherwise be allowed to heal by secondary intention; such an indication is described in detail in the discussion of split-thickness skin and mucosal grafts for preprosthetic vestibuloplasty.

II. Choices for soft tissue reconstruction include the following:

Split-thickness skin or mucosal grafts
Full-thickness skin or mucosal free grafts
Local composite flaps (e.g., tongue, pharyngeal, Estlander, or Abbe)
Distant pedicled flaps of the axial type (e.g., deltopectoral, temporal, or trapezius)
Myocutaneous flaps (e.g., pectoralis, sternocleidomastoideus, latissimus dorsi, platysma)
Free composite flaps requiring microvascular anastomosis at the recipient site

III. The choice from among these alternatives will be made based upon the indications listed. The first two types are usually employed only when the objective is to minimize scarring and wound contracture. Local composite flaps are reserved for specific anatomical locations where relatively small amounts of soft tissue replacement are required. Both axial and myocutaneous flaps can replace large volumes of soft tissue; the latter is more often used today because of the greater certainty of its blood supply and, hence, the viability of the transferred tissue. Microvascular free grafts are employed when large volumes of tissue are needed in areas where muscle-based flaps have been already utilized or are not anatomically accessible.

IV. Preoperative care for the donor site is limited to thorough cleaning. To minimize bacterial colonization of the skin, shaving of hair from the donor sites is not recommended until immediately before or during the surgical procedure; microscopic shaving defects in the skin become heavily populated with bacteria if the shaving is done several hours before surgery.

V. Postoperative care for skin graft donor sites is discussed in Chapter 6.

   A. Flaps whose viability depends upon unimpeded circulation through a pedicle, whether the pedicle is composite tissue or a muscle body, must be protected from pressure. Both tension and compression are to be avoided, and the flaps should be inspected frequently in the immediate postoperative period.

   B. Some surgeons recommend the use of anticoagulants (either intravenous dextrans or low-dose heparin) to aid the circulation in myocutaneous or microvascular free flaps.

C. Suture lines at the recipient site should be kept meticulously clean; extraorally, they should be swabbed daily with hydrogen peroxide and are usually protected with an application of polymixin-B (Neosporin) or bacitracin ointment. Intraoral recipient sites are cared for with mouth rinses of half-strength hydrogen peroxide four times daily. Activities with the potential for disrupting the flap-recipient interface (e.g., positive-pressure inhalation therapy) are contraindicated.

OSSEOUS RECONSTRUCTION

I. Restoration of osseous continuity is almost always a procedure directed at defects of the mandible. In the maxilla the ability to restore both form and function with a prosthesis makes the need for bone grafting rare, even after extensive ablative surgery.

II. The indications for osseous reconstruction of the upper jaw are usually limited to situations in which there is nonunion or malunion following trauma or a discrete discontinuity defect of the alveolar process has resulted from trauma, severe atrophy, ablative surgery, or congenital deformity. Mandibular discontinuities require reconstructive surgery in almost all instances when there is a need to restore form and function; removable prostheses cannot be satisfactorily constructed.

III. The principles of osseous reconstruction require that there be

A. Sufficient numbers of viable osteocytes or cells capable of inducing osteogenesis at the host site

B. A form or shape to the bone graft consistent with that which is being replaced

C. The ability of the graft to function in a manner similar to that of the missing part

D. Stability at the graft-host interface during the period of healing

E. Adequate blood supply from surrounding soft tissues, even if this requires the insertion of vascularized soft tissue flaps as described above

F. Closure of soft tissues over the graft without tension or leakage

G. Meticulous attention to hemostasis at the host site to minimize or eliminate the formation of hemotoma

IV. Several substitutes for bone grafts have been popular for reconstruction of jaw defects. However, it must be recognized that the use of materials such as metal, acrylic, silicone, or hydroxyapatite alone does not fulfill the principles; similarly, cadaveric bone alone is inadequate as a bone graft material. Only autologous cancellous bone is capable of meeting the first requirement for successful bone grafting.

A. The autologous bone must be freshly obtained at the time of the reconstructive procedure. Two donor sites are commonly used, the ilium and the rib.

B. Cortical bone, which may be taken from the donor site with the cancellous bone, serves the purpose of providing form and stability to the graft, but it is not critical to the success of the graft. Alternative means of providing shape and a solid bed for the grafted marrow include metal plates, metal or Dacron-polyurethane trays, and freeze-dried cadaver bone; in each case, fresh autologous cancellous bone is densely packed into the chosen vehicle.

C. In certain instances (e.g., grafting alveolar defects) a soft tissue envelope may be sufficient to provide the appropriate shape to the bone graft material. Some surgeons have successfully mixed cancellous bone with hydroxyapatite, the latter material giving form and the former providing the osteogenic stimulus.

V. The requirement for stability at the graft-host interface during healing is met in ways not unlike those used for fixation of fractures.

A. Internal fixation by means of bone plates or rigid trays that span the grafted defect and that can be solidly attached to the adjacent host bone are frequently used.

B. Intermaxillary fixation is employed whenever there are adequate teeth or where intraoral prostheses can be used without the risk of pressure necrosis of the soft tissues overlying the bone graft.

C. Extraoral biphasic pin fixation is also a frequently used means of providing stability, having the advantage of making intermaxillary fixation unnecessary.

D. The care of reconstructed patients with these various fixation devices is no different from that employed for patients having fixation for fractures.

E. The duration of fixation differs from that of fracture patients and will depend upon the size of the graft, the blood supply of the recipient bed, and the radiographic appearance of the grafted site in the postoperative follow-up period; fixation for 8-12 wk is usually recommended, except when graft replacement of the TMJ has been done, with either a costochondral graft or an alloplastic prosthesis, in which case early mobilization of the mandible is desired (3-4 wk customarily used).

VI. Meticulous hemostasis of the graft recipient site must be obtained before careful closure of the overlying tissues in anatomical layers. To minimize the potential for hematoma or serous accumulation at the graft site, a low-pressure vacuum drainage system may be used in the first 48 hr; a small Jackson-Pratt drain will accomplish this task. The drain should be removed as early as possible lest it allow for the ingress of skin bacteria.

OSSEOUS DONOR SITES

I. Rib grafts
   A. Any patient in whom a rib is to be harvested for a graft should

have a preoperative radiographic series taken of the chest. This will allow the surgeon to assess the degree of osteoporosis that may be present, which might dictate another choice of donor site. In addition, the chest films will serve as a baseline study if respiratory problems develop postoperatively as a consequence of the rib harvesting.

B. Optimal pulmonary toilet should be attained preoperatively and the patient should receive instruction in the routine chest physiotherapy that will be expected postoperatively.

C. The location of the incision for the harvesting of the rib graft should be chosen so as to be as cosmetic as possible; the inframammary fold provides good access for the harvesting of as many as three ribs. No more than two consecutive ribs should be harvested if more than two ribs are needed, however, lest the chest wall mechanics be compromised; if after two ribs are taken the next rib is left intact before another is harvested, respiratory function of the thoracic cage will be preserved.

D. Intraoperative management of the rib donor site is the most critical factor in preventing postoperative problems.

  1. Careful attention to operative technique will allow the rib to be harvested in a completely subperiosteal fashion, thus avoiding any violation of the pleural space or disruption of the intercostal neurovascular bundle.

  2. Prior to closure of the wound, there should be thorough inspection for pleural leaks. If no obvious tears in the pleura are found, the wound should be flooded with normal saline and the anesthesiologist should then apply positive pressure via the endotracheal tube.

    a. If no bubbling is observed in the saline-filled wound, there can be reasonable certainty that no pneumothorax has been caused.

    b. If there are lacerations of the parietal pleura, they should be repaired with a 2-0 chromic suture on an atraumatic needle with a small-bore catheter brought out through one end of the tear. As the last suture is tied, suction is applied to the catheter and positive pressure ventilation is given; the suture is secured as the catheter is withdrawn. The saline bubbling test is then performed again as a check on the adequacy of the repair.

E. Postoperatively a chest film should be obtained to reveal the possibility of undetected pneumothorax. A small one (compromising 10-20% of lung volume) may be treated by observation; a larger one will necessitate placing a chest tube for evacuation of the air.

F. Pain and splinting in the area of the rib donor site may contribute to poor respiratory excursions, with increased potential for atelectasis or pneumonia. Rather than large doses of parenteral narcotics, which might decrease respiratory drive, an injection of a long-acting local anesthetic (e.g., bupivacaine [Marcaine]) should be given to block the intercostal nerves of the affected area. This will provide excellent comfort to the patient and promote good respiratory toilet.

II. Iliac crest grafts

A. The iliac crest is a favored donor site for large corticocancellous grafts and pure cancellous bone, since in most patients either type of graft can be readily obtained without any functional deformity.

B. Preoperative preparation of the patient may include a laxative or rectal suppository to aid in bowel emptying before the procedure. This measure will prove useful for patients who may experience ileus from peritoneal irritation as a result of the bone harvesting.

C. Intraoperative technique must adhere to the standard surgical principles of anatomical dissection, careful hemostasis, and protection of neighboring structures. Actual violation of the peritoneal cavity is rare even when both inner and outer cortical tables of the ilium are taken as part of the graft, but simple mechanical irritation of the peritoneum cannot always be avoided.

D. A drain, usually of the closed-system, low-vacuum type (e.g., Hemovac), is often employed because of the tendency of the exposed cancellous portion of the ilium to bleed into the dead space of the wound after the graft has been harvested. As with all drains, this should be removed as soon as it is no longer collecting significant amounts (less than 10-20 ml in a 24 hr period).

E. Postoperatively, the patient who has had iliac crest bone harvested must be examined for adequacy of bladder and bowel function.

1. It is not uncommon for the patient to experience bladder spasm or adynamic ileus as a result of local peritoneal irritation. Catheterization of the bladder is necessary if the bladder becomes distended and the patient is unable to void spontaneously.

2. The patient should not be given any oral food or drink until it has been determined that there is normal bowel function, as determined by the presence of normal bowel sounds and the passage of stool. If ileus is detected, nasogastric suction is instituted to aid in decompressing the adynamic bowel; the suction should be continued until bowel sounds have returned to normal. The fluid and electrolyte losses associated with the gastric suctioning must be taken into account during intravenous fluid management.

F. Physical therapy to aid in the early ambulation of the patient after harvesting of an iliac crest graft should be instituted. Use of a walker or a cane may be necessary.

GENERAL REFERENCES

Bell, W.H.: LeFort I osteotomy for correction of maxillary deformities, J. Oral Surg. **33**:412, 1975.

Bell, W.H.: Surgical correction of dentofacial deformities, vol. 3, New concepts, Philadelphia, 1985, W.B. Saunders Co.

Bell, W.H., Proffit, W.R., and White, R.P.: Surgical correction of dentofacial deformities, vols. 1 and 2. Philadelphia, 1980, W.B. Saunders Co.

Hinds, E.C., and Kent, J.N.: Surgical treatment of developmental jaw deformities, St. Louis, 1972, The C.V. Mosby Co.

Kawamoto, H.K., and Wolfe, S.A.: Treatment of the elongated face. In Symposium on maxillofacial surgery, Clin. Plast. Surg. **94**(9):479, 1982.

Moorrees, C.F.A., et al.: New norms for the mesh diagram analysis, Am. J. Orthod. **69**:57, 1976.

Shelton, D.W., and Irby, W.B., editors: Current advances in oral and maxillofacial surgery: orthognathic surgery, vol. 5, St. Louis, 1986, The C.V. Mosby Co.

Trauner, R., and Obwegeser, H.L.: The surgical correction of mandibular prognathism and retrognathia with consideration of genioplasty, Oral Surg. **10**:677, 787, 899, 1957.

Wang, J.H., et al.: Vertical osteotomy vs. sagittal split osteotomy of the mandibular ramus: comparison of operative and postoperative factors, J. Oral Surg. **33**:596, 1975.

Salivary Gland Disease

11

GENERAL CONSIDERATIONS

I. Swelling in the submandibular or preauricular area often is a patient's presenting complaint. It may or may not be accompanied by pain. The diagnosis and treatment of such patients often include diseases of the parotid and submaxillary salivary glands (Table 11-1).

   A. The major differential diagnostic problem is separating lymph node enlargement from salivary gland enlargement.

   B. Other general diagnostic considerations include odontogenic infections in cases of submandibular swelling and bony diseases of the ramus of the mandible in cases of preauricular swelling.

II. History is most important to the differential diagnosis. An acute enlargement in these areas, particularly when related to eating, suggests an obstruction to salivary flow; a progressive enlargement suggests a neoplastic process. Bilateral enlargement places the diagnosis in a different category of diseases, which includes Sjögren's syndrome, sarcoidosis, and other more esoteric metabolic problems.

DIAGNOSTIC PROCEDURES

I. Clinical examination is performed to determine whether any of the following pertain:

   Swelling is tender
   Enlargement is firm, soft, or rubbery
   Seventh nerve function is intact
   Salivary flow is adequate from Stensen's duct
   Fluctuant material can be milked from the duct
   A stone can be palpated in the duct

II. A history is taken to reveal the duration, any fluctuation in size, the presence of pain, etc.

III. Laboratory tests are performed to differentiate tumor from lymph node disease.

   A. Sialography is often helpful in demonstrating a filling defect.

   B. Computed tomography with contrast often shows enhance-

Table 11-1 SALIVARY GLAND DISEASES BY MAJOR CATEGORY

Disease	Location	Comments
Submaxillary sialadenitis	Submandibular	Acute enlargement, tender, fluctuates with meals; palpable stone in floor of mouth; pus from Wharton's duct; occlusal radiograph shows stone (rarely radiolucent); usually penicillin sensitive, but pus should be cultured
Parotitis	Preauricular	Acute enlargement, less common than sialadenitis; fluctuates with meals; pus from Stensen's duct; stone palpable in cheek or seen on periapical radiograph positioned over duct; frequently due to *Staphylococcus;* may not be associated with stone, but with decreased secretion as in Sjögren's syndrome; secondary ascending infection
Parotid tumor	Preauricular	Slow growth, usually painless; unilateral, but Warthin's may be bilateral; majority are benign; pain and seventh nerve involvement suggest malignancy
Submaxillary tumor	Submandibular	Less common; slow growth
Minor gland tumor	Any area of mucosa but palate and buccal mucosa usual	Slow growth; may appear as lump or ulcer; on palate it must be differentiated from maxillary sinus tumor and from necrotizing sialometaplasia

ment of a benign mixed tumor; it is most useful for assessing tumor involvement in both superficial and deep parotid portions.

  C. However, the status of CT with sialography is controversial.

IV. Parenchymal salivary gland disease must be differentiated from lymph node disease. Major considerations include parenchymal disorders (e.g., Sjögren's syndrome, sarcoidosis) and infiltrative processes that invade the periparotid lymph nodes (e.g., tuberculosis, leukemia, lymphoma). The latter fall in the group of diseases termed Mikulicz's syndrome. (See Table 11-2.)

MANAGEMENT PROCEDURES
Bacterial sialadenitis or parotitis

  I. Whether preauricular or submandibular, bacterial sialadenitis and parotitis have a rapid onset of a firm tender swelling. A history of

Table 11-2   LYMPH NODE DISEASE MIMICKING SALIVARY GLAND DISEASE

Disease	Location	Comments
Cat scratch disease	Submandibular	Matted nodes, history of cat scratch; no evidence of pus from Wharton's duct; skin test available
Lymphoma	Submandibular or preauricular	Progressive enlargement; may be localized disease; firm, nontender; may cause secondary gland obstruction; skin test for anergy
Leukemia	Submandibular	May be localized; WBC elevated
Metastatic tumor	Either	From fossa of Rosenmüller
Infectious diseases	Submandibular	Tuberculosis, coccidioidomycosis; skin tests available

swelling with meals is often elicited. Pus can usually be expressed from either Stensen's or Wharton's duct on the involved side.

   A. Both stricture and stone may contribute to the onset and must be searched for.

   B. Extensive probing of either duct and especially sialography are contraindicated in a sick patient with purulent drainage.

 II. Bacterial infections of the salivary glands usually occur in the debilitated, dehydrated, or postoperative patient. Any systemic condition like Sjögren's that leads to decreased flow of saliva also predisposes to retrograde glandular infection.

III. Prior to the advent of antibiotics and simple means of intravenous fluid administration, these conditions were life threatening.

IV. Before beginning treatment, the clinician must determine

   A. The patient's status in terms of toxicity—temperature, state of hydration, malaise

   B. Whether an obstruction present—palpation for stones in the ducts, periapical films of Stensen's duct and mandibular occlusal views to search for a stone in Wharton's duct

   C. The status of the gland secretion—purulent, inspissated (thick) or ropy saliva

 V. Appropriate culture of purulent material must be made, and laboratory tests (including WBC count) should be done.

Bacterial infections of the salivary glands

  I. If the patient with a bacterial infection is free of systemic signs or symptoms, is afebrile or has only a low-grade temperature, gives of history of recurrent swelling with meals, and now has a tender swelling, thick or purulent duct drainage, and a demonstrable stone in the duct, there are several considerations to be borne in mind:

A. Such a patient is best managed by

> Culture of saliva
> A prescription for dicloxacillin 500 mg q.i.d. × 7 da
> Instructions to drink plenty of fluids
> Use of sour lemon candies to promote saliva flow
> Application of moist heat to the swelling

B. Close follow-up is advised.

C. Attempts to remove the stone should be instituted once antibiotic treatment is underway.

II. If the patient feels sick, has a temperature of 101° F or above, has a very tender swelling, appears dehydrated, has pus in the salivary drainage with or without a demonstrable stone, and has an elevated WBC count, the following should be done:

A. The patient should be admitted for intravenous fluid therapy, antibiotics, and supportive care.

1. An IV is started with D5W at 100 ml/hr unless a cardiac or renal condition exists.

2. Oxacillin is given in standard IV dose since *Staphylococcus* is an important pathogen in many cases.

3. Sour lemon candies or swabs are used to promote saliva flow.

B. The usual course will be improvement in the systemic condition, defervescence, and a drop in the WBC count within 1-2 da. Failure to show improvement within 4 da should arouse a suspicion of abscess formation. (This would be unusual.)

III. Attempts to remove a stone surgically and/or perform sialography to locate a duct stricture when no stone is demonstrable should be deferred until infection is under control and the patient's general condition warrants it. Sialography may also be indicated as part of the work-up for a patient suspected of having Sjögren's syndrome, which may present as a secondary infection of the salivary gland.

Sjögren's syndrome

I. Currently several forms of Sjögren's syndrome are recognized (Table 11-3):

> A primary form
> A secondary form associated with rheumatoid arthritis or another connective tissue disease
> A form characterized by lymphocytic aggressive behavior, which in rare cases results in lymphoma

II. Classically xerostomia, keratoconjunctivitis sicca, and rheumatoid arthritis form the originally described triad. Lymphocytic infiltration of salivary gland and lacrimal gland tissue characterizes the

Table 11-3   PRIMARY AND SECONDARY FORMS OF SJÖGREN'S SYNDROME

Characteristics	Primary	Secondary
Rheumatoid arthritis or other connective tissue disease	No	Yes
Lymphocytic infiltration of organs	+++	+
Risk of lymphoma	++	+
Rheumatoid factor in serum	Yes	Yes
Antinuclear antibodies	Species-specific B	Rheumatoid arthritis precipitin
Histocompatibility typing	HLA-BB HLA-DR3	HLA-DR4

Code	+	Moderately likely
	++	Likely
	+++	Very likely

disease. Decreased salivary flow and/or tearing may be associated with enlarged parotid glands in one third of patients.

III. Work-up for a patient suspected of having Sjögren's will include the following:

LE prep
Antinuclear antibodies
Serum amylase
Rheumatoid factor
Ophthalmological examination for eye signs
 Schirmer's test for tearing
 Fluorescein
Sialography for sialectasia
Minor salivary gland biopsy (of the labial glands in the lower lip is most convenient)

Biopsy technique

A. In the lower lip a small anteroposterior incision is made, hemostasis being provided by the assistant (who holds both sides with a sponge).

B. Scissors are used for blunt dissection of several small glands, which are submitted to biopsy. Usually no bleeding requiring clamping is encountered. The incision must be away from any superficial vessels in the mucosal tissue.

C. The wound is closed with interrupted 3-0 catgut sutures.

D. The patient should apply pressure to the wound with a sponge for 5 min.

IV. Treatment of Sjögren's syndrome is generally supportive.

A. Artificial saliva and tears may be helpful.

B. Steroids have a beneficial effect on salivary gland enlargement but not on xerostomia.

C. Radiation of 400 cGy* has been implicated in the development of pseudolymphoma or true lymphoma and is contraindicated.

D. Only because of excessive enlargement of the salivary gland is parotidectomy indicated.

Sarcoidosis

 I. Sarcoidosis is a poorly understood disease characterized by Langhans' giant cell granulomatous inflammation. It is frequently brought to attention because of pulmonary symptoms or abnormalities in pulmonary function tests. It can be related to interstitial lung parenchymal involvement or to hilar adenopathy. Cutaneous and uveal tract manifestations are not uncommon. About 6% of patients have parotid involvement, characterized by enlargement, xerostomia, and often fever (Heerfordt's syndrome [uveoparotid fever]).

 II. A specific skin test (the Kveim test) is often used. However, it provides a diagnosis only of exclusion unless a biopsy of lymph node, liver, lung, or skin shows the characteristic histopathological features.

III. Laboratory findings of significance are hypercalcemia (often responsive to steroids), a mildly elevated alkaline phosphatase, an elevated serum gamma globulin, and possibly an elekated serum amylase. The xerostomia of sarcoidosis often responds to steroids, unlike that of Sjögren's syndrome.

IV. Open biopsy of the periparotid or parotid tissue is usually required for confirmation.

Salivary gland tumors

 I. Work-up of a suspected salivary gland tumor includes the following:

A. Major gland (parotid the most common site)

1. Clinical examination

a. Location and consistency are important. Benign mixed tumors are usually firm but rubbery. Suspicion of fluid may suggest Warthin's tumor, which is often cystlike. Lack of fixation suggests a benign lesion.

b. Examination for adenopathy is necessary.

c. The most critical differential point is distinguishing between a parenchymal and a nodal problem.

2. Laboratory examination. Blood work-up is virtually noncontributory unless there is a question of infection. Tumors almost never have associated infection, unlike Sjögren's syndrome, which has involved glands. Less common submaxil-

---

*The designation centigray (cGy) is used instead of rad.

Table 11-4   TUMORS OF THE SALIVARY GLANDS

Type	General	Clinical
Benign tumors		
Pleomorphic adenoma (benign mixed tumor)	90% of tumors of all salivary glands	Firm but rubbery; recurrent lesions may show subcutaneous growth; no seventh nerve signs; treatment includes superficial parotidectomy or excision
Warthin's tumor	Papillary cystadenoma lymphomatosum.	May be cystic; rarely seen in minor glands; males are involved more often than females; found especially in men over 55; treatment is excision or superficial parotidectomy
Oncocytoma	Small, rare, encapsulated	Rare
Malignant tumors		
Malignant mixed tumor	Relatively rare; due to transformation of benign tumor	Very firm, often with skin fixation, seventh nerve signs; parotidectomy with neck dissection indicated if adenopathy is present; postoperative radiation is useful in selected cases

lary gland tumors may be confused with infected submandibular nodes or an obstructed gland.

3. Radiological examination
   a. Plain films are used to rule out a stone, and sialography to determine parenchymal versus nodal disease.
   b. Computed tomography may replace sialography if the question of ductal pathology is unimportant or if there is a question of deep lobe involvement.

Table 11-4   TUMORS OF THE SALIVARY GLANDS—cont'd

Type	General	Clinical
Malignant tumors—cont'd		
Adenocarcinoma Acinic cell	Very rare	Hard; treatment includes wide excision of tissue if in minor gland; hemimaxillectomy may be necessary if neural invasion is suspected; treatment is total parotidectomy, with or without nerve sacrifice, with possibility of nerve grafting; postoperative radiation has definite place in management; one must consider maxillary sinus origin in palatal lesions; use of polytomes of palate and midface or CT scans can show extent
Adenoid cystic	Cylindroma; slow growing but with early neural invasion	
Mucoepidermoid carcinoma	Age of patient variable; low to high grade based upon mucous cell/epidermoid cell ratio	Treatment is based on age of patient, lesion location, histology; can infiltrate and metastasize; wide excision for mucosal lesions superficial to total parotidectomy based upon tumor extent; necrotizing sialometaplasia considered in a differential diagnosis

4. Special test
   a. Despite early interest and promise of the technique, radionuclide imaging is not helpful in diagnosis of major gland tumors.
   b. Ultrasound may be useful if a vascular or cystic lesion is suspected.
B. Minor gland (palate the most common site)
   1. Clinical examination. Benign mixed tumors of the palate rarely ulcerate, although adenoid cyst and mucoepidermoid often present in such a fashion. One must ascertain whether there is nasal obstruction or whether the sinus symptoms for palatal lesions may be coming from carcinoma of the maxillary sinus.
   2. Radiographic examination. Maxillary occlusal radiographs or, more commonly, tomograms of the hard palate are important in determining osseous involvement.
C. The most important part of the work-up is obtaining a tissue diagnosis. A sufficient index of suspicion for parotid or submaxillary gland tumor often is an indication for surgery with biopsy at the same time. Accessibility makes biopsy of minor gland lesions prior to definitive treatment possible.
II. A listing of salivary gland tumors is found in Table 11-4.
III. Lesions mimicking salivary gland tumors include the following:
A. Nasal fossa tumors. Those in the fossa of Rosenmüller may spread to the parotid lymph nodes and look like parotid tumors.
B. Antral carcinoma. This sometimes presents as a minor salivary gland tumor of the palate. Sinus radiographs and polytomes of the palate may show osseous changes or lesions. These radiographs are also helpful in planning treatment of palatal minor gland tumors.
C. Lymphadenopathy of the submaxillary area. Hodgkin's, leukemia.
D. Branchial cleft cyst. These are usually posterior to the submaxillary gland and are nontender; no history of enlargement with meals is reported.
E. Necrotizing sialometaplasia. This usually appears on the palate as an ulcerative lesion. It can be confused with a minor salivary gland tumor, especially a mucoepidermoid carcinoma, since it occurs in younger patients.

GENERAL REFERENCES

Gorlin, R.J., and Goldman, H.M., editors. Thoma's oral surgery, ed. 6, St. Louis, 1970, The C.V. Mosby Co.

Mason, D.K., and Chisholm, D.M.: Salivary glands in health and disease, Philadelphia, 1975, W.B. Saunders Co.

Moutsopoulos, H.M., et al.: Sjögren's syndrome: current issues, Ann. Intern. Med. 92:212, 1980.

Facial Trauma

12

GENERAL CONSIDERATIONS

I. The patient who sustains facial trauma should be evaluated for other potential injuries. These are often much more severe and certainly more life threatening. Attention to the general overall management of the trauma patient is thus a first objective of this review. Trauma management is a team effort.

II. The ABCs of trauma management must be followed: the *airway* is assessed and if found to be obstructed a passage secured; *breathing* must be adequate, and the *circulation* intact. Usually the adequacy of vital signs is ensured simultaneously with other assessments. For example, respiratory distress can be observed while the pulses are being checked and the the general condition of the patient can be noted after clothing has been removed. Any unnecessary movement of the neck should be avoided until the status of the cervical spine has been checked.

PRELIMINARY ASSESSMENTS
Airway and Breathing

I. One must establish the presence of respiration. If breathing is labored or stridorous, immediate intervention must eliminate the cause. Many of these actions are performed simultaneously.

II. The procedure for airway assessment is as follows:
   A. Inspection. Check the oral cavity for dentures, loose teeth, blood, bleeding from open mandibular fracture, etc.
   B. Debridement. Remove any obstructing bodies and/or suction the nasal and oral cavities.
   C. If these measures do not improve respiration, consider nasal obstruction and the use of head extension (keeping in mind the possibility of cervical spine injury) or soft rubber nasal airway.
   D. During examination of the chest, check for symmetrical chest movement and the presence of bilateral breath sounds on auscultation to rule out pneumothorax. Note any paradoxical motion since multiple rib fractures can cause a flail chest, which has dire hemodynamic consequences as well as marked respiratory importance.
   E. Placement of an oral airway may be helpful.

F. If the mandible has fallen posteriorly as a result of fracture, temporary stabilization with wire may bring the jaw and tongue forward, relieving obstruction.

G. If no measures improve the situation, intubation may be indicated. Oral endotracheal intubation is more rapid, but a nasal endotracheal tube may be more efficacious in the patient with facial trauma. There are few real contraindications to nasal endotracheal intubation in these patients. Nasal bone fracture and CSF rhinorrhea are often cited, but in fact they are not if one considers that the nasal tube runs posteriorly in a horizontal direction, not in a superior direction.

H. Tracheostomy is almost never indicated or required in an emergency room setting.

Pneumothorax

I. An injury that permits air to enter the space between the outer covering of the lungs and the inner lining of the chest wall creates a negative pressure that collapses the lung on the ipsilateral side.

A. This typical pneumothorax results in a hyperresonant chest because the entire pleural cavity, not just the lungs, is filled with air. Breath sounds are decreased or absent depending upon the extent of the collapse.

B. The chest film shows collapsed lung parenchyma and a lack of vascular markings out to the periphery of the lung field.

II. Treatment is directed at evacuating the air from the pleural space. In an emergency a needle may be placed just above the superior border of the second rib (to avoid the intercostal vessels at the inferior rib margin) so air can escape. If converted to a valve, the needle may prevent reentry of air until a regular chest tube is inserted and placed to water suction.

Flail chest

Fracture of several ribs or other bony chest wall components leads to paradoxical motion of the chest wall with inspiration and expiration. There are hemodynamic consequences since paradoxical chest motion impairs venous return, which in turn reduces cardiac output. Treatment is positive-pressure respiratory support, which maintains the ribs in position.

Hemothorax

I. Hemothorax usually occurs with collapse of lung parenchyma. Blood is found in the pleural cavity along with air.

II. Drainage is performed with a chest tube placed in the seventh intercostal space midaxillary line. This tube lies posteriorly and drains fluid and air when the patient is recumbent.

Cardiac tamponade

I. Blood in the pericardium prevents normal cardiac contractility, making the heart an ineffective pump. The heart is enlarged, heart sounds are soft, and there is a paradoxical pulse.

II. Treatment is evacuation of fluid from the pericardial space.

Hypotension

I. The trauma patient with decreased systolic and diastolic blood pressure and thready rapid pulse is a common diagnostic and management problem.

II. Management of the hypotensive patient is as follows:

A. Do the general appraisal and take a history if the patient is awake and alert. The patient's clothes must be removed for the examination. A family member may be the best source of information.

B. Airway patency is assured (see p. 259).

C. Start a secured peripheral IV and central line to monitor central venous pressure (see Chapter 4). Insert a Foley catheter to monitor urine output. A urine sample is sent for analysis, particularly for occult blood or hematuria.

D. Begin lactated Ringer's solution at full rate to provide a fluid challenge.

E. Draw blood samples for type and cross-match, electrolytes, amylase, and CBC simultaneously with line placement.

F. After the airway is secure and fluids are started, monitor vital signs frequently and begin the general physical examination of the patient.

1. Head—lacerations, contusions, Battle's sign (ecchymotic area behind the ear, significant of basilar skull fracture); great care must be exercised during examination of the neck until cervical spine injury can be adequately assessed radiographically

2. Chest—obvious injuries, rib fractures, and paradoxical chest motion; auscultate to assure adequacy and symmetry of breath sounds; auscultate the heart for abnormal sounds; the back should also be included in this examination

3. Abdomen—tenderness and guarding may indicate an injured viscus; if high suspicion of internal abdominal injury exists, do a paracentesis (insert an Intracath via a stab incision just below the umbilicus into the peritoneal cavity and run in 1L of Ringer's lactate, withdrawing the fluid via a large syringe; assess its redness visually or perform a hematocrit; if newspaper print cannot be viewed through the withdrawn fluid, significant internal bleeding is likely and the patient needs exploration)

4. Flank—tenderness may indicate renal injury or retroperitoneal bleeding; examination of the urine is important in this assessment

5. Extremities—lacerations, contusions, and fractures; pelvic and humerus injuries are particular causes of large blood loss; make sure that all pulses are present and symmetrical

G. When the physical examination is completed and the patient's condition permits, a proper radiographic examination can be performed. This will include a skull series, facial bone series, cervical spine films, chest films, abdominal (KUB) films, extremity films, and an intravenous pyelogram (to evaluate any hematuria).

H. Hypotension in a patient taking steroids raises the possibility of inappropriate adrenal stress response. Additional steroids should be given (e.g., 400 mg cortisone hemisuccinate IV).

MANAGEMENT PROCEDURES
Suspected head injury

I. All the aforementioned preliminary assessments should be followed for the patient with suspected head injury. Special attention must be given to differentiating the effects of alcohol from those of serious neurological injury.

II. The patient's level of responsiveness is assessed: Can he be aroused easily, or only with painful stimuli? Can he answer simple questions appropriately? Is he oriented to time and place? The Glascow coma scale is useful for this (see box).

A. The development of equipment for monitoring various functions in critically ill patients has not altered the need for assessing the level of consciousness.

B. The Glasgow coma scale evaluates three aspects of behavioral response: eye opening, verbal, and motor.

It provides a simple grading of arousal and functional capacity of the cerebral cortex.

It assesses brain stem function by observation of the pupil and ocular motility.

It is limited in localizing brain dysfunction on the basis of decorticate and decerebrate postures to the extent that posturing does not always mean brain stem damage.

It is not intended as a prognostic indicator; nevertheless, the level of responsiveness and the duration of a patient's remaining at a given point on the scale correlate closely with outcome.

III. A general examination is performed:
A. Pupils—for reactivity and symmetry; also gross vision
B. Any lateralizing signs—weakness or asymmetry of deep tendon reflexes
C. Abnormal reflexes—e.g., Babinski

IV. Frequent monitoring of neurovital signs is important. Increasing intracranial pressure may be seen as the Cushing reflex (with increasing blood pressure, bradycardia, and bradypnea).

V. A cranial nerve examination is performed. Normal findings, or tests needed in the unconscious patient, are as follows:

Nerve	Conscious patient	Unconscious patient
I	Gross vision	Consensual light reflex (optic nerve intact when light into right eye causes left pupil to constrict)
II	Gross smell	Not testable
III	Pupillary constriction to light	As above for CN I
IV	Upward and outward gaze	
V	Sensation in face	Corneal reflex
VI	Lateral gaze	Centralizing of eye when head turned to either side
VII	Facial expression	Changes with painful stimulus (grimace)
VIII	Hear finger snap	Vestibular portion tested by doll's head maneuver or caloric test (cold water placed in uninjured ear causes eyes to move toward side of test)
IX	Gag reflex	Gag reflex
X		
XI	Shoulder shrug	
XII	Tongue movement	

The Glasgow coma scale

Eye opening	
Spontaneous	4
To speech	3
To pain	2
None	1
Best verbal response	
Oriented	5
Confused (conversation)	4
Inappropriate (words)	3
Incomprehensible (sounds)	2
None	1
Best motor response	
Obeying (follows commands)	6
Localizing	5
Normal flexion	4
Flexing (abnormal posture)	3
Extending (abnormal)	2
None (no movement)	1

VI. Cerebrospinal fluid leaks should be sought. The facial trauma patient may exhibit either CSF rhinorrhea or CSF leak from the ear.

   A. Rhinorrhea is often found with LeFort injuries of the maxillo-facial complex. It is difficult to diagnose with certainty. Low sugar content of the CSF and the clarity of CSF on a piece of linen versus the cloudiness of mucus are often said to be helpful in the differentiation. In fact, the appearance of fluorescein dye in nasal secretions after its central injection (via lumbar puncture) is the best way of demonstrating CSF rhinorrhea. The vast majority of such injuries heal with reduction and fixation of the facial fractures. The presence of an aerosol on skull film in the area above the cribriform plate suggests a large dural tear, which may require more than facial fracture fixation for treatment.

   B. CSF leak from the ear is usually associated with condylar injuries often not resulting in fracture of the condyle itself. Blood from the ear may be an associated finding.

VII. Management of increased intracranial pressure includes

Drugs
  Diuretics
    Osmotic mannitol
    Furosemide (Lasix)
  Steroids—dexamethasone
  Ventilation
Intubation with rapid support—blows off carbon dioxide, which has a vasodilating effect on the cerebral vessels; induced respiratory alkalosis is thus helpful
Bur holes
Monitoring
  Subarachnoid bolt (measurement of ICP)
  Subdural catheter
  Intraventricular catheter

Facial fractures

I. Foreign bodies, dentures, tooth fragments, and bone fragments are removed from the oral cavity and upper airway.

II. Especially in the semiconscious or unconscious individual, care is taken to guarantee an adequate airway. This may involve use of oropharyngeal, nasopharyngeal, or endotracheal intubation or tracheostomy.

III. If there is active intraoral or extraoral bleeding, hemostasis is obtained by pressure or ligation first.

IV. Temporary stabilization of fractures, particularly in the mandible, with wires is helpful in reducing bleeding and providing comfort.

V. Severe nasal bleeding may be controlled by packing with petrolatum gauze. Uncommonly, anterior nasal packing may require additional posterior nasal packing. This is conveniently placed by means of gastric catheters threaded through the nose to the pharynx and led out through the mouth; gauze packs are attached by sutures through the perforations at the catheter tips; when the catheters are withdrawn through the nose, the packs are brought securely to the posterior nasopharynx; the sutures are tied externally at the nose so the packs will not be aspirated.

   A. CSF rhinorrhea is not a contraindication to anterior nasal packing, since the cribriform plate is superior to the pressure packs.

   B. Nasal endotracheal intubation, similarly, is not contraindicated since the nasal tube traverses the lower portion of the nasal cavity and will not block the leak. Obviously each case must be appropriately managed on an individual basis.

   VI. A thorough eye examination must be done in all patients, particularly those with suspected zygomatic and maxillary injuries.

VII. Teeth in the line of fracture must be checked. Any that are mobile or show evidence of root fracture or severe crown injury should not be maintained. If erupted, third molars in the area of angle fractures should be considered for removal since this will permit satisfactory intraoral open reduction to the performed.

Mandibular fractures

   I. Radiographic assessment of mandibular fractures utilizes

   Lateral oblique and PA views of the mandible—good for general appraisal

   Reverse Towne's view—particularly good for condylar fractures

   Panoramic view—best for overall diagnosis

   Base view or occlusal view—for judging the symphyseal region

   II. Treatment alternatives for mandibular fractures are

   A. Closed reduction

   1. In the dentulous patient alignment of teeth in proper occlusion and application of a "cast" via intermaxillary fixation are done. Niro arch bars are particularly good. If gaps in the dentition exist, firmer Erich arch bar material is helpful.

   2. In the edentulous patient, use of dentures or splints placed via circummandibular wires is appropriate. Overtreatment of the fracture in an edentulous atrophic mandible is to be avoided since the periosteal blood supply and consequent osteogenesis have increased importance to the repair process. In certain edentulous mandibles the Joe Hall Morris appliance is quite useful, permitting stabilization of the fracture without disruption of the tissue in the area of the injury.

B. Open reduction
1. Intraoral. Open reduction with upper border or circum-mandibular wiring is a useful technique, especially in the angle region. Some parasymphyseal fractures can be approached via an intraoral "degloving" technique (development of a mucoperiosteal flap to gain access to the area of fracture).
2. Extraoral. This is the most versatile approach to the majority of fractures. It allows lower border fixation by a variety of appliances:

Interosseous wires (direct, figure-8, four hole)
Bone plates and screws
Kirschner rod

3. Open reduction may be used with or without intermaxillary fixation.
III. Considerations in the choice of method include
A. Site of the fracture and its position relative to the teeth
1. A fracture through a dentulous area, especially if it is undisplaced, may be treated by closed reduction with arch bars and intermaxillary fixation (IMF) or with a splint and no IMF. If the fracture is displaced, the treatment of choice may be extraoral open reduction with arch bars and IMF or with a splint and no IMF.
2. If the fracture is distal to the last tooth and undisplaced, IMF with arch bars may suffice. Since there are no teeth distal to the fracture, a dental splint is useless. If the fracture is displaced, IMF may be combined with either intraoral or extraoral open reduction.
B. Degree of displacement and mobility. In general, the greater the displacement and/or mobility of the fracture segments the greater is the indication for an open as opposed to a closed technique of reduction.
C. Adequacy of the dentition and occlusion. Closed reduction requires adequate dentition and occlusion. In condylar fractures associated with inadequate posterior occlusion, it may be necessary to use posterior bite blocks to prevent collapse of the posterior facial vertical dimension, which may lead to anterior open bite if both condyles are fractured.
D. Type and duration of anesthesia demanded by a given procedure and the age, condition, and suitability of the patient for a general anesthetic
E. Requirements imposed by intercurrent acute problems, other injuries, or preexisting medical conditions
1. If a mandibular fracture accompanies extensive midface injuries, open reduction of the fracture may be indicated to establish and maintain the facial vertical dimension in treatment of the maxillary injuries.
2. Similarly, in a head injured patient treatment may be toward

more rigid fixation because of the lack of cooperation and abnormal movements often observed. In addition, the use of steroids and the frequent delay in onset of treatment in this group of patients can lead to a higher complication rate.

IV. Considerations in formulating a treatment plan include

A. Condylar fractures

1. Most condylar fractures are well treated by a conservative approach, closed reduction and immobilization with IMF, especially if there is malocclusion or pain at the time of initial examination. If the patient is comfortable and can occlude satisfactorily, a liquid to soft diet may be all the treatment needed.

2. If IMF is used, it is maintained for 10-14 da. Then, if the patient is comfortable and able to occlude, physiotherapy is instituted to rehabilitate joint function. Soft diet, analgesics, and local heat are prescribed. If the patient is unable to occlude, there is no contraindication to continued IMF for 4-6 wk. However, this is usually not needed and adds the problem of trismus to management.

3. In children a high condylar fracture can lead to excessive hematoma formation and ankylosis. Therefore prolonged IMF is contraindicated. In fact, ankylosis can result from involuntary splinting without IMF and thus physiotherapy must be encouraged.

4. Specific indications for open reduction of a condylar fracture are

   a. Trismus at the end of IMF that appears to be due to obstruction by a displaced condylar fragment

   b. Laterally displaced condyle in children—open reduction may be indicated to provide bony contact for healing

   c. Bilateral fracture with severe midface injuries—open reduction is done to reestablish facial vertical dimension

   d. Bilateral fracture in the presence of cervical spine injury requiring brace treatment—the brace may force the mandible posteriorly, and thus open reduction can maintain the jaw position

B. Multiple fractures

1. Body plus condyle. Since early mobilization is desirable for the condyle, the body fracture should be repaired with a fixation method that does not depend entirely upon IMF. Thus condylar fracture may be an indication for open reduction of a body fracture that, alone, would have been treated by closed reduction and longer IMF.

2. Bilateral body and body plus angle. In such multiple fractures there can be a tendency toward a "bucket-handle" deformity because the anterior fracture segment is distracted downward by the infrahyoid muscles. In horizontally unfavorable parasymphyseal fractures there can be inward

collapse of the anterior segment with loss of anterior anchorage of the tongue, leading to airway obstruction. In these instances extraoral open reduction and rigid intraosseous fixation at the lower border are indicated to resist muscle pull.

   C. Comminuted fractures. Open reduction may involve the risk of detaching fragments of bone from their blood supply. Careful closed reduction is desirable if possible. No formula can be given, but each comminuted fracture should be considered in light of this basic principle.

V. Postoperative orders for the patient with mandibular fracture(s) include

   A. Drugs

     1. Meperidine (Demerol) 50 mg q. 4 h. IM p.r.n. for pain

     2. Prochlorperazine (Compazine) 10 mg IM stat and q. 6 h. p.r.n. for nausea

     3. Aspirin 0.6 g p.r. q. 4 h. p.r.n.; for temperature greater than 101° F, the house officer should be called

     4. IV orders

> 1 L Normal (balanced) saline
> 1 L D5W
> 1 L Normal saline and D5W (50:50)
> Rate 100 ml/hr
> Piggyback 3 million units of penicillin in 300 ml of D5W; give 50 ml q. 4 h.

     5. Oxymetazoline (Afrin) nasal spray in each nostril q.i.d.

     6. Pentobarbital (Nembutal) 120 mg p.r. q.h.s. p.r.n.; codeine elixir 30 mg/5 ml and penicillin elixir 250 mg/5 ml may be substituted when p.o. intake permits

   B. Nursing orders for the patient after open reduction of a fractured mandible (condition satisfactory, no allergies) include the following:

     1. Head of bed elevated 30 degrees

     2. Petrolatum to lips

     3. Scissors taped to the bedside

     4. Bed rest with bathroom privileges; ambulation is begun the morning after surgery

     5. High-protein high-calorie liquid diet; dietary consultation

     6. Cold vapor humidifier

     7. Deep breathing and coughing exercises

     8. Water-Pik for oral cleansing

     9. Suction setup at bedside

   C. Postoperative radiographs should be obtained before discharge.

   D. The patient is discharged when his condition is stable, he is afebrile and taking adequate fluid and nourishment by mouth, and it is determined that home environment is adequate for care.

E. Fear of vomiting is unwarranted after the initial postoperative period, but the patient should be instructed in how to cut and release elastic band fixation. A wire cutter should be at the bedside and with the patient if wire ligatures were needed for IMF.

F. Follow-up should be within 1 wk. Elastics should be checked, sutures removed, medications reviewed, and the patient reinstructed in hygiene and nutrition.

G. In general, most mandibular fractures show clinical union at 3 wk and should be tested clinically. If the fracture area is firm, a soft diet should be continued through 6 wk with maintenance of arch bars across fracture sites for at least 1 wk after IMF is removed.

Zygomaticomaxillary fractures

I. General considerations include all those listed earlier.
   A. In addition, a thorough eye examination is a necessity.
      1. Pupils—traumatic mydriasis or pupillary dilation most common finding
      2. Diplopia, especially in upward gaze—usually caused by edema; a proper ophthalmological examination, with the red and green glass test, may be necessary
      3. Full extraocular motions
      4. Subconjunctival hemorrhage
      5. Lacrimal drainage system—epiphora
      6. Fundus—to rule out hemorrhage and papilledema; the latter not an acute finding of increased intracranial pressure
      7. Enophthalmos
      8. Gross vision
   B. Palpation for bony injuries, including nasal fractures, is performed.
   C. The palate is checked for anteroposterior fractures.
   D. A search is made for infraorbital paresthesia.
II. Radiographic assessment includes
   A. Skull films (PA and lateral) for general appraisal
   B. Waters' views to check the antrum and zygomas
   C. "Jug-handle" (submentovertex) views for the zygomatic arches
   D. Tomograms, particularly for blowout orbital fractures
III. Treatment is, realistically, a clinical judgment based upon experience and the problem at hand.
   A. Most fractures of the middle third of the facial skeleton can be managed by internal fixation.
   B. Occasionally marked mobility of a LeFort II or III fracture will benefit from external rigid fixation in addition to internal wiring. Recent advances in craniofacial surgery have been applied to the treatment of LeFort injuries. Frontal flaps and other direct-access incisions permit improved results in wiring of nasal, supraorbital, and glabellar injuries.

C. Treatment alternatives for zygomatic fractures include the following:

1. Gillies method—based upon the anatomical location of the temporalis fascia, this is an excellent technique for reduction of a fractured zygomatic arch and also for reducing a stable fracture of the body of the zygoma. In the latter instance an additional incision is required to stabilize the zygoma. Although the radiographic appearance of rotation or displacement on a Waters view may be of value in determining stability preoperatively, this is not always possible.

2. Eyebrow approach—this technique permits access to the medial aspect of the zygoma, with excellent leverage for reduction. A Gillies (malar) elevator or urethral sound is placed medial to the zygomatic arch. This approach also permits wiring at the zygomaticofrontal suture for stability.

3. Infraorbital approach—this provides direct access for transosseous wiring of the fractured infraorbital rim. It has largely been displaced by the blepharoplasty approach, which is more cosmetic. The infraorbital approach is used when a laceration already exists in the skin beneath the eye. It is a good approach to use when Silastic sheet is needed for an orbital defect. (See discussion under blow-out fractures.)

4. Infraciliary approach—this is a conjunctival approach that is very cosmetic, but it has limited access for placement of wires.

5. Intraoral approach—with this technique the incision is placed in the buccal sulcus and the instrument remains beneath the zygoma and/or arch; it must not enter the sinus. This approach is limited for wiring.

6. Caldwell-Luc approach—with the Caldwell-Luc, elevation of the zygoma is accomplished through the antrum. This approach also can be used for assessment of the orbit. Antral packing may support the reduced zygoma, or an inflated Foley catheter balloon can be used. Again, there is limited access for direct wiring of an unstable fracture.

D. Unstable fractures of the zygoma are treated by the following:

1. Tranosseous wiring—this can be achieved by the eyebrow or blepharoplasty approach.

2. Kirschner rod—this has limited usefulness since other, more precise, methods are available; but it may have a place in certain instances. The rod is inserted from the contralateral antrum into the medial cortical bone of the fractured zygoma. The bone must be held in proper position so as not to cause an overreduction.

3. Cranial fixation—this is rarely needed, but the pin apparatus may be useful in exceptional cases requiring lateral traction.

4. Packing support—rarely will a reduced fractured zygomatic arch be unstable. In that instance a stab incision over the

arch permits placement of a rubber or gauze packing for lateral stabilization.

E. Blow-out fractures of the orbital floor, which commonly occur with fractures of the middle third of the facial skeleton, are controversial in terms of the need for and timing of repair.

1. A so-called pure blow-out fracture of the orbit is an isolated injury. Although the majority of orbital floor injuries occurring in conjunction with other fractures do very well when treated as part of the other injuries, a pure blow-out injury deserves special attention.

2. Relative indications for exploration of the blow-out injury are as follows:

   a. It is not an emergency, unless there is retrobulbar hemorrhage or emerging proptosis and pain.

   b. Clinical examination shows limitation of upward gaze and diplopia.

   c. Observation alone may show resolution of the diplopia.

   d. Entrapment of the globe can be demonstrated at forced duction testing after local anesthesia of the globe. The tendon of the inferior rectus is grasped with forceps, and attempts to rotate the globe superiorly encounter resistance.

   e. There is radiographic (tomographic) evidence of herniation of the orbital contents.

   f. Enophthalmos of greater than 2 mm is often directly observable and not amenable to reconstruction later.

3. Studies show that such signs and symptoms of blow-out fracture may result from edema and not from true entrapment of the inferior rectus muscle. Usually such edema resolves within 5-7 da, and the patient should be reevaluated at that time.

   a. If indications for exploration still exist, a blepharoplasty approach permits adequate exposure and insertion of a 1 mm Silastic sheet cut to size. This is not sutured to bone but is maintained in position by closure of the overlying periosteum as part of the septum orbitale.

   b. Intraoperative steroids are recommended, and care should be taken not to place too much pressure on the globe during the procedure.

F. Treatment alternatives in maxillary fractures include:

1. No fixation—usually done only for minimum injuries or in elderly patients considered to be poor risks who are without gross bony displacements

2. Intraoral fixation alone—for alveolar fractures and unilateral fractures; may be by means of arch bars and IMF or an equivalent; IMF is usually part of the treatment for all injuries.

3. External fixation—the Royal Berkshire halo or equivalent

   a. Craniomaxillary (rigid direct suspension of the detached middle third of the facial skeleton by a rod)

    b. Craniomandibular (indirect support of the fractured middle third between the mandible and an intact area of the skeleton above the maxillary fracture line)

   4. Internal fixation

    a. Transosseous wiring at various sites (e.g., the zygomaticofrontal suture)

    b. Direct suspension (wires from the zygomatic process of the frontal bone or the infraorbital or piriform area to a maxillary or mandibular splint)

    c. Direct support (antral pack)

    d. Transfixation (Kirschner wire from the contralateral antrum to the fractured zygoma for support; care must be taken with an endotracheal tube)

IV. Postoperative care of the patient is as follows:

  A. When there are no other injuries, the same orders as for mandibular fractures apply to zygomaticomaxillary injuries. In addition, the use of oxymetazoline (Afrin) nasal spray, pseudoephedrine (Sudafed) tablets, and sinus precautions will reduce sinus symptoms. Sinus precautions consist of no nose blowing, no use of straws, and no smoking, all of which can place a negative pressure on the maxillary sinus.

  B. The use of iced saline sponges is most effective in limiting periorbital edema and ecchymosis.

  C. A tongue blade taped over the injured side is most effective in reminding the patient and the nursing staff that the patient should not lie on the side of the treated fracture.

  D. If Silastic or Ash metal splints are used for nasal reduction and fixation, they should be checked for pressure necrosis regularly and removed within 10 da.

GENERAL REFERENCES

Andreasen, J.O.: Traumatic injuries of the teeth, Copenhagen, 1972, Munksgaard.

Champy, M., et al.: Mandibular osteosynthesis by miniature screw plates via a buccal approach, J. Maxillofac. Surg. **6**:14, 1978.

Chuong, R., et al.: A retrospective analysis of 327 mandibular fractures, J. Oral Maxillofac. Surg. **41**:305, 1983.

Juniper, R.P., and Awty, M.D.: The immobilization period for fractures of the mandibular body, Oral Surg. **36**:157, 1973.

Knight, J.S., and North. J.F.: The classification of malar fractures: an analyses of displacement as a gude to treatment, Br. J. Plast. Surg. **13**:325, 1961.

Pozatek, Z.W., et al.: Fractures of the zygomatic complex. An evaluation of surgical management with special emphasis on the eyebrow approach, J. Oral Surg. **31**:141, 1973.

Rowe, N.L., and Williams, J.L.: Maxillofacial injuries, Edinburgh, 1985, Churchill Livingstone.

Seldin, E.B., et al.: Mandibular fracture fixation and reconstruction using the lower border threaded rod: an eleven year follow-up study, J. Oral Maxillofac. Surg. **43**:115, 1985.

Stranc, M.F.: A classification of injuries of the nasal skeleton, Ann. Plast. Surg. **2**:468, 1979.

Odontogenic Infection

13

GENERAL CONSIDERATIONS

I. The extension of dental decay to the pulp chamber of a tooth or the presence of periodontal disease may give rise to signs and symptoms of infection. Most commonly toothache, pain upon mastication, or sensitivity to hot and cold are the presenting complaints and are usually treatable in the outpatient setting.

II. Another common odontogenic infection is pericoronitis, a purulent inflammation associated with a partially impacted wisdom tooth.

III. Management of these problems becomes complicated when the signs of generalized infection occur. This chapter will discuss the management of localized dental infection but emphasize the care of the patient who has a more serious odontogenic infection occurring with generalized symptoms. The bacteriology, use of antibiotics, and management of patients with specialized infections is also discussed.

INFECTIOUS PROCESSES
Localized abscess

I. Pain associated with a decayed tooth or a tooth involved by periodontal disease may be associated with swelling. Radiographs usually demonstrate either a periapical lucency or a deep pocket. The tooth may or may not be mobile but will be sensitive to percussion in an apical direction.

II. The basic principles of management include obtaining drainage and controlling the bacterial infection with antibiotics. A most important clinical determination is the presence of fluctuant swelling.

A. In the absence of a fluctuant swelling, local measures (e.g., pulpectomy or curettage of a pocket) usually provide adequate drainage. Removal of the offending tooth may be indicated on clinical or radiographic grounds because of inability to rebuild the tooth or the degree of bony destruction. Judicious use of the proper antibiotic is called for to prevent sequelae due to the presence of infection.

B. If a fluctuant swelling is present, all the above options exist plus the possible need to perform an incision and drainage of the swelling. Abscesses presenting as intraoral swellings usually are found on the buccal aspect of the offending tooth. Incision and drainage with a blade and insertion of a ¼ in gauze drain are a simple technical procedure. However, patient comfort may be improved by the use of nitrous oxide or diazepam (Valium) for sedation along with the local anesthetic. Such adjuncts are recommended because the sole use of local anesthetic in any surgical procedure in the presence of infection often will be inadequate.

C. The antibiotic of choice in the nonallergic patient is penicillin. Penicillin V is suggested since its use is less affected by the need for patient compliance in terms of schedule related to meals. Erythromycin, coated to reduce gastrointestinal upset, is used in the allergic patient. Doses required for adequate coverage of localized infections as described are 250 mg q.i.d., and treatment for 1 wk is suggested.

D. Controlling a localized infection with antibiotic use alone is inadequate and fails to follow the basic tenets of treatment detailed in A and B above (i.e., the establishment of drainage).

III. Any infection that results in swelling beyond simple buccal or mucosal enlargement or swelling that affects the soft palate, floor of the mouth, or tongue may be quite serious. Constitutional symptoms of fever, malaise, or chills must also arouse clinical suspicion of a more serious problem.

A. The most important clinical decision to be made is whether the patient's swelling represents an abscess or a cellulitis. An abscess demands surgical intervention whereas cellulitis is best managed medically, at least until signs of abscess formation occur.

B. A conservative approach to the management of the sick patient with odontogenic infection is most rewarding. Infections are no less serious because they arise from the teeth and supporting structures.

C. The decision to admit such a patient to hospital must be based upon an assessment of systemic toxicity and the adequacy of hydration. Although a temperature of 100° F is not worrisome, fever to 102° and higher may be observed and warrants direct attention.

D. Indications for hospitalization include
   1. Signs of severity

   Fever
   Dehydration
   Rapid progression of swelling
   Trismus
   Marked pain
   Quality or location of swelling

Elevation of tongue
Swelling of soft palate
Bilateral submandibular swelling—possibility of Ludwig's angina

2. Symptoms of severity

Marked pain
Malaise
Chills
Difficulty swallowing
Difficulty breathing

3. Laboratory test

Elevated temperature (over 101° F)
Elevated WBC count (over 10,000)
Shift to the left on differential count (increase in immature leuko-
cytes)

4. Associated problems

Diabetes mellitus
Patient taking steroids or other immunosuppresive drugs
Prosthetic valve or other prosthesis

E. Reasons for hospitalization are to provide

An antibiotic dosage impossible to achieve orally with patient com-
fort
Adequate hydration
Relief of pain
Extraoral surgical drainage if indicated
Appropriate monitoring of life-threatening symptoms

F. Admitting orders for the patient include the following:
1. Medications

5% D5W, 1000 ml at 100 ml/hr
Piggyback 6 million units aqueous penicillin in 500 ml D5W; give
83 ml q. 6 h.
Meperidine (Demerol) 50 mg p.o. or IM q. 4 h. p.r.n.

2. Procedures

Routine vital signs
Head of bed elevated 30 degrees
Nothing by mouth
Moist heat to facial swelling

Actinomycosis

I. Infection by *Actinomyces israelii* occurs in the head and neck
region. The clinician must always be alert to the finding of "sulfur
granules" on incision and drainage. Appropriate cultures must be
ordered. The organisms are extremely fastidious, and growth usually takes 4 wk. Clinical suspicion is thus very important. Penicillin
is required in a dose of 20 million units per day for an extended
time (4-6 mo).

II. Clinically the term "lumpy jaw" is used for this condition. The patient usually has a tender facial swelling that is difficult to distinguish from the swelling of any other odontogenic infection. Chronicity by history will guide the astute clinician to search for the organisms on culture.

Osteomyelitis

I. Infection of bone secondary to odontogenic infection is, fortunately, uncommon. In children the cause is often difficult to determine. Osteomyelitis is a chronic infection, and therefore patients usually do not have acute pain or swelling but rather insidious discomfort.

II. The diagnosis is made by finding osteolytic areas of sequestrum formation. In the jaws the use of tomography is very helpful in defining the full extent of disease; bone scanning may be helpful in the edentuous patient, but often periodontal disease limits its applicability. This is particularly important in planning the area of surgical debridement.

III. Decortication of the mandible is the treatment of choice. The maxilla is rarely involved. The proper use of antibiotics requires determination of bactericidal levels based upon culture and sensitivity testing. Although high-dose intravenous treatment for 1 mo is suggested, testing often permits such levels to be maintained by combinations of IM and p.o. penicillin and probenecid (Benemid) to limit renal excretion. The use of external irrigation with antibiotics has neither scientific nor clinical merit.

IV. Work-up of suspected osteomyelitis includes the following:
   A. Clinical examination for exposed bone, the causal tooth, or other disease
   B. Radiographic examination, including tomography, to define the extent of disease properly
   C. Appropriate culture of purulent material and bone from debridement; previous antibiotic treatment may affect results

ODONTOGENIC INFECTION IN THE COMPROMISED HOST

I. Although the vast majority are usually mixed infections sensitive to penicillin, odontogenic infections in the patient compromised by chemotherapy often present unusual bacterial and fungal indications.

II. A number of studies of patients receiving chemotherapy for leukemia have shown that gram-negative infections occur in this group. Such patients are usually immunosupressed by steroids or other antimetabolites, and under these circumstances *Pseudomonas* and *Proteus* infections occur. A higher than usual rate of *Candida* infections also occurs in these patients.

III. The clinician must be astute in recognizing an infection that is completely altered in its presentation because of leukopenia. In a patient whose WBC count is 1000, pericoronitis may appear with-

Table 13-1 ODONTOGENIC INFECTIONS

Examination	Normal	Compromised host
Bacteriological	Mixed infection, rarely gram-negative	Increased presence of gram-negative organisms
Clinical	Swelling, pain, pus, fever	Innocuous findings, no pus, often little swelling; may have dark papules of gingiva in *Proteus* infections
Laboratory	Elevated WBC count, fever	Depressed WBC count, often no fever

out opercular swelling or purulence. Careful attention to the response of the patient to any prescribed antimicrobial is a must. (See Chapter 4.)

IV. Comparison of odontogenic infections in the normal and the compromised host is given in Table 13-1.

TREATMENT PROCEDURES
Antibiotics (see Table 13-2)

I. General considerations
   A. Selection of an antibiotic is based on the following considerations:
      1. Antibiotics treat infections, not fever.
      2. One must identify the nature of the infection.
         a. What organ system—history, physical examination, laboratory findings
         b. What organism—Gram stain, culture
      3. The choice of antibiotic depends upon
         a. Need to treat specifically—i.e., antibiotic sensitivity testing
         b. Host factors

            Hypersensitivity
            Organ dysfunction—renal, hepatic
            Immunosuppression

         c. Drug pharmacology

            Route and dose
            Tissue distribution
            Toxicity
            Cost

      4. Reevaluation is needed to look for alteration of flora and superinfection
   B. Disadvantages of antibiotics include the following:
      1. Antibiotics do not prevent infection.
      2. There is inherent drug toxicity.

Text continued on p. 282.

Table 13-2 ANTIBIOTICS USEFUL IN TREATING ODONTOGENIC INFECTIONS

	Dose	Clinical considerations and toxicity
Penicillins		
Penicillin	250 mg p.o. q.6h. for 7 da	Adequate for most infections
	500 mg p.o. q.6h. for 7 da	For more severe infections and infections in patients without toxemia, with diabetes, etc.
	500,000 units IM aqueous, 600,000 units IM procaine, 6-10 million units IV aqueous	For immediate coverage if needed, followed by oral dose schedule; used for severe infections in hospitalized patients; side effects include GI upset with oral treatment; possibility of allergic reaction, urticaria being most common; aqueous penicillin contains 1.7 mEq of K per million units; in cardiac patients volume and dose may be important
Methicillin	1 g IM (1 g diluted in 50 ml sterile saline injected over 15 min q.4h.)	Penicillinase resistant; used only against penicillinase-producing staphylococci; better agents are available
Oxacillin	0.5-2 g q.4-6h. IV, 0.5-2 g q.6h. IM, 0.25-1 g q.4-6h. p.o.	Oral absorption unpredictable; oxacillin, dicloxacillin, and nafcillin all more effective than methicillin against nonstaphylococcal gram-positive organisms
Dicloxacillin	0.125-1 g q.4-6h. p.o.	Oral drug of choice because of its good absorption; good also for sialadenitis of suspected staphylococcal origin
Extended-spectrum penicillins		
Amoxicillin	0.25-1 g q.8h. p.o.	Amoxicillin is similar to ampicillin but has superior GI tract absorption; potential advantages are in situations requiring high peak levels or when t.i.d. schedule is preferred; amoxicillin equal to ampicillin for pneumococci, streptococci, staphylococci (nonpenicillinase producers), *Neisseria, Hemophilus influenzae, Escherichia coli, Proteus mirabilis;* slightly more effective than ampicillin against enterococci and *Salmonella*
Ampicillin	0.5-2 g q.4-6h. IV, 0.5-2 g q.6h. IM, 0.25-1 g q.6h. p.o.	

Carbenicillin	20-40 g/da in 6 doses IV, 0.5-1 g q.6h. IM, 0.5-1 g q.6h. p.o.; IM and p.o. for urinary tract infections	Generally effective against ampicillin-sensitive organisms but less active on per weight basis; unlike ampicillin, it resists degradation by beta-lactamases of many gram-negative bacteria; thus it is active against strains of *Pseudomonas*, enterococci, and indole-positive *Proteus* species; also more effective than other penicillins against many anaerobes, especially *B. fragilis*; inactive against penicillinase-producing staphylococci; use with an aminoglycoside (e.g., gentamicin) for *Pseudomonas*; good in immunosuppressed patients; never mix drugs in same IV bottle
Ticarcillin	12-24 g/da in 6-8 doses IV, 1 g q.6h. IM	Similar to carbenicillin, often acting like it; synergistic with aminoglycosides against many gram-negative bacteria
Metronidazole		Presumably an anaerobic-specific antimicrobial

Penicillin alternatives

| Erythromycin | 250 mg p.o. q.6h, 500 mg p.o. q.6h. for 7 da | Adequate for most infections; larger dose for more severe infections or sick patients; not recommended for IM or IV use because of local tissue irritation |
| Clindamycin | 0.6-2.7 g/da IV in 2-4 doses, 300 mg q.6-8h. IM, 150-300 mg q.6h. p.o. | Spectrum similar to that of lincomycin and erythromycin; useful against nonenterococcal gram-postive organisms and most anaerobes (including *Bacteroides fragilis*, which is often resistant to penicillin); diarrhea may occur in 1-10% of patients and may progress to pseudomembranous colitis due to toxic product of *Clostridium difficile* |

Cephalosporins and cephamycins

| Cephalothin | 4-12 g/da IM or IV | Main advantage is its activity against gram-positive cocci, including penicillinase-producing staphylococci, about 95% of *E. coli*, most *Salmonella* and *Shigella*, and many *Proteus mirabilis* and *Klebsiella pneumoniae*; *Enterobacter* and indole-positive *Proteus* species are not sensitive to first-generation cephalosporins but are sensitive to cefamandole and cefoxitin; cephapirin and cephacetrile are similar new drugs |

Continued.

Table 13-2 ANTIBIOTICS USEFUL IN TREATING ODONTOGENIC INFECTIONS—cont'd

	Dose	Clinical considerations and toxicity
Cephalosporins and cephamycins—cont'd		
Cefazolin	1-4 g/da IM or IV	More effective against *E. coli*, less effective against staphylococci; main advantages are its higher blood levels, longer half-life, and relative lack of pain with IM use
Cephalexin	0.25-1 g q.6h. p.o.	Oral drug of choice; cephradine and cefadroxil are similar but more expensive
Cefamandole	1-3 g. q. 4-6h. IV, 0.5-1 g q. 4-6h. IM	Newer drug with enhanced spectrum against gram-negative organisms, primarily *H. influenzae, Enterobacter*, and indole-positive *Proteus*; less effective against staphylococci and streptococci; unlikely drug for usual odontogenic infections
Cefoxitin	1-2 g q. 4-8h. IV, 1 g q. 6h. IM	New semisynthetic cephamycin; more resistant to beta-lactamases of gram-negative organisms; not more effective against *Pseudomonas* or most *Enterobacter*; also active in vitro against most anaerobes, including *B. fragilis*; because of its higher cost, its recent use as prophylactic drug in major head and neck surgery does not appear justified

Tetracyclines

Tetracycline	250-500 mg q.6h. p.o.	GI toxicity
Oxytetracycline	250-500 mg q.6h. p.o.	GI toxicity
Chlortetracycline	25-500 mg q.6h. p.o.	GI toxicity
Doxycycline	100 mg q. 12 h. p.o. or IM	Excellent absorption; does not accumulate in serum of patients with renal failure
Minocycline	200 mg initially, 100 mg q.12h. p.o.	Long acting, but little use in odontogenic infections; main use is in *Nocardia* infections
Chloramphenicol	0.5-1 g q.6h. IV, 0.25-1 g q.6h. p.o.	Bacteriostatic, effective against wide variety of gram-positive and gram-negative bacteria; drug of choice for *Salmonella* and ampicillin-resistant *H. influenzae*; no use in odontogenic infection but often useful combined with penicillin for prophylactic coverage in facial trauma patient; used intravenously; main toxic effect, aplastic anemia

Aminoglycosides

Streptomycin	0.5-1 g q.12h. IM	Rarely used alone because of rapid development of resistance; based upon its synergistic effect, it was earlier used with penicillin against staphylococci
Kanamycin		Because of its ototoxicity and nephrotoxicity, this agent has been largely supplanted by gentamicin
Gentamicin	1-2 mg/kg q.8h. IV, IM	Effective for *Proteus* and *Pseudomonas* infections resistant to other drugs; reduced dose necessary with impaired renal function
Tobramycin	1-2 mg/kg q.8h. IV, IM	Less expensive; *Pseudomonas* more sensitive to it; thus should be reserved for serious infections with *Pseudomonas* or gentamicin-resistant organisms
Amikacin	15 mg/kg/da in 3 divided doses	Similar to kanamycin

3. Patient sensitization may occur.
4. Selection may result in resistant organisms, causing

Superinfection
Alteration of microbial world

II. Penicillins
   A. Numerous studies of the bacteriology of odontogenic infection suggest that better than 95% of the offending organisms are appropriately treated with penicillin. Routine culture and sensitivity is not recommended unless there is clinical suspicion of an unusual causal bacterium. Such situations exist for all extraoral incision and drainage procedures, any compromised host, and any clinically resistant infection.
   B. In general, penicillin, erythromycin, cephalosporin, and clindamycin are most useful. The specific application of each is based on the clinical setting, need for an intravenous or intramuscular route of administration, and potential toxicity.

III. Cephalosporins and cephamycins
   A. Cephalosporins and cephamycins are comparable to the extended-spectrum penicillins. Their advantage lies in their resistance to inactivation by the beta-lactamases produced by staphylococci and many enteric bacteria. There is some cross-reaction (10-20%) in penicillin-allergic patients.
   B. The major use of cephalosporins and cephamycins in odontogenic infection is when it is suspected that an infection, particularly of the salivary glands, is staphylococcal.

IV. Tetracyclines
   A. The tetracyclines were the first true broad-spectrum antibiotic. They are bacteriostatic and active against a wide range of gram-positive and gram-negative organisms, being most valuable in treating mixed infections.
   B. Tetracyclines are the most widely prescribed drug for odontogenic infections and are as good a choice as penicillin.

V. Aminoglycosides
   A. Streptomycin, kanamycin, gentamicin, tobramycin, and amikacin will be discussed only briefly because of their limited need in the treatment of odontogenic infections and other infectious diseases treated by the oral and maxillofacial surgeon. Some knowledge of these drugs will be useful because of the use of streptomycin in prophylaxis of infectious endocarditis.
   B. These drugs share several pharmacological and therapeutic properties:

They are bactericidal.
They have wide-spectrum activity.
Development of bacterial resistance to them is slow, except for streptomycin.
They have poor GI absorption.
They are nephrotoxic.
They are ototoxic.

Table 13-3 ANTIBIOTIC SENSITIVITY TESTING

Cocci	Rods
Gram positive	
Streptococcus—penicillin	*Actinomyces*—penicillin
Staphylococcus (penicillinase resistant)—penicillins	*Clostridium* (anaerobic)—penicillin
Peptostreptococcus (anaerobic)—penicillin	
Gram negative	
Neisseria—penicillin	*Pseudomonas*—gentamicin, carbenicillin
Veillonella (anaerobic)—penicillin	
	Hemophilus—ampicillin
	Enterobacteriaceae—aminoglycosides or ampicillin
	Bacteroides (anaerobic)—clindamycin, penicillin

VI. Antibiotic sensitivity testing. Table 13-3 presents the usual organisms of odontogenic infection grouped according to their appearance by Gram stain.
   A. Anaerobic culture method. Special tubes are available and are far better than culturing plates in an atmosphere free of oxygen. Two tubes are used; thus the first swab is placed in a second special tube containing materials, ensuring anaerobic conditions.
   B. The method of Gram staining material is as follows:
      1. Smear the material as a thin transparent film on a clean slide.
      2. Gently heat the slide in a flame to fix.
      3. Flood the slide with an alcoholic solution of crystal violet for 5-10 sec; pour off.
      4. Flood the slide with Lugol's iodine solution for 5-10 sec.
      5. Wash with acetone or acetone-alcohol solution rapidly until the color comes off.
      6. Pass briefly (2-3 sec) under water to wash.
      7. Counterstain with safranin for 5-10 sec and rinse with water.
      8. Dry.
VII. Summary of antibiotics
   A. Standard (narrow-spectrum) antibiotics for penicillin-susceptible organisms.

   Penicillin G
   Penicillin V

B. Standard (narrow-spectrum) antibiotics for penicillin-resistant organisms:

Methicillin
Oxacillin
Cloxacillin
Dicloxacillin
Nafcillin

C. Extended-spectrum antibiotics for penicillin-susceptible organisms:

Amoxicillin
Ampicillin
Carbenicillin

D. Extended-spectrum antibiotics for penicillin-resistant organisms:

Cephalosporins
Cephamycins

Incision and drainage

I. The important clinical decisions to be made revolve around when to drain and what to drain. Since an abscess represents dead white blood cells, antibiotics do not penetrate this hypoxic area and surgical drainage is a must.
II. Fluctuance of a swelling (a soft spot within the swelling) is the most reliable physical sign.
III. Appropriate aerobic and anaerobic cultures should be obtained. Culture and sensitivity is requested, as should be also cultures for fungi and tuberculous organisms.

Follow-up studies

I. In a retrospective review of 175 admissions for facial infection (158 patients), clinical signs, daily temperature course and WBC count, and all culture data were compiled and analyzed by computer. Follow-up of more than 1 wk was obtained in 103 patients; in most of the remainder the dental infection resolved completely and there was no need for follow-up appointments.
   A. The average patient age was 36.9 yr (SD 17.1, range 7-95), and the male to female ratio was 1.3:1.
   B. The average hospital stay was 9.7 da (SD 9.0, range 1-46).
   C. The majority of infections (60%) were odontogenic. Others were related to soft tissues (including salivary glands) (17%), trauma (10%), and irradiation for tumor (8%). Only three followed major elective surgery.
II. Of the 302 cultures taken, 101 were reported as mixed flora and there were 398 bacterial strains identified.
   A. Sensitivity testing was performed in 64 cases. Most infections were composed of mixed aerobic and anaerobic flora.

B. Penicillin (or clindamycin) was the antibiotic of choice in most cases except those confined exclusively to soft tissues, where coverage against *Staphylococcus aureus* was necessary. This was true even when sensitivity testing in vitro showed penicillin resistance.

C. Aerobic gram-negative organisms were uncommon in dental infections (2 of 90 patients) and were best correlated with a long hospital stay (average 21 da). No cases of *Bacteroides fragilis* were identified.

III. The presence of fever (over 99.5° F), when combined with clinical suspicion, was the most accurate predictor of both the need for incision and drainage and the success of antibiotic treatment. In clinically similar groups, febrile patients had an 88% chance (71 of 81 patients) of having undergone a productive incision and drainage whereas afebrile patients had only a 30% chance (7 of 23).

A. After successful incision and drainage most patients (41 of 45) defervesced within 36 hr and remained afebrile until discharge. There was no difference in short-term follow-up between patients discharged at 12-36 hr and those discharged more than 2 da after becoming afebrile. Nine out of eleven patients who required readmission had osteomyelitis. There was no difference in clinical course during follow-up of 40 patients changed to oral antibiotics on the day before discharge as compared to other patients in the study.

B. The policy is thus reinforced: early admission, incision and drainage for febrile patients with significant clinical signs, discharge of patients after an afebrile period of 24-48 hr.

IV. Although some reports of *Bacteroides melaninogenicus* resistant to penicillin have appeared, this has not been found in our institution. Furthermore, the possible occurrence of *B. fragilis* has not been a problem.

GENERAL REFERENCES

Chow, A.W., et al.: Orofacial odontogenic infections, Ann. Intern. Med. **88:**392, 1978.

Sabiston, C.B., et al.: Bacterial study of pyogenic infections of dental origin, Oral Surg. **41:**430, 1976.

Socransky, S.S., and Gibbons, R.J.: Required role of *Bacteroides melaninogenicus* in mixed anaerobic infections, J. Infect. Dis. **115:**247, 1965.

Dental Considerations in Cancer of the Oral Cavity and Oropharynx

14

GENERAL CONSIDERATIONS

I. The oral cavity consists of the lips, floor of the mouth, oral portion of the tongue, buccal mucosa, upper and lower gingivae, hard palate, and retromolar trigone. The oropharynx includes four areas: the base of the tongue, the tonsillar region, the soft palate, and that portion of the pharyngeal wall between the epiglottic fold and the nasopharynx. Cancer can affect any of these areas.

II. Epidemiology

   A. Incidence

   1. Statistics for the U.S. in 1981 showed 815,000 new cancer cases: 27,710 of these were oral cancers, or 3.4%.

   2. Estimates for 1984 were that 870,000 new cancer cases would be diagnosed, of which 27,500 would be oral cancer: 4900 of the lip, 4900 of the tongue, 7900 of the pharynx, and the remainder of the buccal mucosa, salivary glands, etc. Some 4% would occur in men, and 2% in women.

   B. Histological types

   1. Squamous cell carcinoma. In general, the less-differentiated tumors have a higher incidence of positive lymph nodes and a higher risk of distant metastasis than do low-grade lesions of comparable size and from similar anatomical sites.

      a. The local and regional control of squamous cell carcinoma by radiation therapy is not much affected by grade, but the survival rate is lower for a high-grade tumor because of the increased rate of distant metastasis. Although during a course of radiation therapy the response rate or disappearance rate of high-grade lesions is usually more rapid than that of low-grade tumors, the rate of disappearance does not correlate with radiocurability.

      b. Tumors that grow in an exophytic pattern usually have a lower rate of lymph node metastasis and are more readily encompassed by an operation or by interstitial irradiation because their borders are well defined and the chance of missing the margins is lower. These lesions respond better to all treatments.

    c. Some carcinomas, generally poorly differentiated, tend to be infiltrative, with fingers of tumor cells beyond the visible or palpable lesion. This pattern is associated with a higher rate of regional lymph node metastasis and is often more difficult to eradicate surgically. Since irradiation portals usually have a generous margin around the obvious lesion, it is less likely that the margins will be missed with radiation therapy; however, control by radiation therapy alone is also less likely to be achieved for this growth pattern than for the more discrete lesions.

    d. Another point of importance is differentiating radiation necrosis from recurrent tumor histologically and identifying necrotizing sialometaplasia of the minor salivary glands in irradiated tissue. An expert pathological opinion is a must.

2. Lymphoepithelioma is a carcinoma with a lymphoid stroma. It occurs at an anatomical site that has lymphoid aggregates in the submucosa (e.g., the nasopharynx, tonsil, or base of the tongue). It also has a higher rate of cure by radiation therapy than does squamous cell carcinoma.

3. Verrucous carcinoma is often a confusing histological diagnosis, being described as hyperkeratosis or pseudoepitheliomatous hyperplasia. An exophytic lesion with an indolent growth pattern, it resembles a wart. Despite reports in the literature of its poor response to radiation therapy, our experience with this modality has been good over long periods of follow-up. If the morbidity of surgery is minimal, surgery remains a first choice of treatment; but radiation is a satisfactory alternative.

4. Spindle cell carcinoma, a squamous cell lesion with intermixed spindle cells resembling sarcoma, occurs in an estimated 2-5% of malignant specimens taken from the upper digestive tract. The degree of spindle cell component varies. Most important, there are no data to suggest that this histological type is important in treatment decisions.

5. Leukemias and lymphomas

    Leukemias
    Hodgkin's disease
    Non-Hodgkin's lymphoma
    Multiple myeloma
    Burkitt's lymphoma
    Midline granuloma

6. Other cancers of the head and neck

    Malignant salivary gland tumors
      Major glands
      Minor glands

Malignancies involving the jaw bones

Carcinoma	Metastases
Sarcoma	Ameloblastoma
Maxillary sinus cancer	Giant cell tumors

Laryngeal carcinoma
Nasopharyngeal carcinoma
Malignant melanoma
Skin and lip cancers

C. Age and sex (see Tables 14-1 and 14-2)
D. Sites of distribution of oral cancer include the following*:

Location	Percentage
Lip	44.9
Oral tongue	16.5
Floor of mouth	12.1
Mandiblular gingiva	12.1
Palate and maxillary gingiva	4.7
Buccal mucosa	9.7

E. Mortality. Cancer is the second major cause of death, behind heart disease, nationwide. The age-adjusted mortality rate per 100,000 population during 1978-1979 from all cancers was 216.9 for men and 132.7 for women, and from oral cancers alone was 5.8 for men and 1.9 for women.

III. Etiology and predisposing factors
   A. Tobacco
   B. Alcohol and cirrhosis
   C. Leukoplakia. Although hyperkeratotic lesions have traditionally been thought of as clinically suspicious, recent reviews (Tables 14-3 to 14-6) suggest some association with carcinoma, but not an overwhelming one. Based upon these data, management of white lesions should be observation and periodic biopsy, not aggressive surgery.

---

*Data from M.D. Anderson Hospital.

Table 14-1   AGE AND SEX DISTRIBUTION OF ORAL CANCER*

Years	Male	Female
<19	1	1
20-39	3	5
40-49	12	14
50-59	29	27
60-69	30	24
>70	25	29

*Based on cancers diagnosed and/or treated during the period 1969-1971 in seven metropolitan areas and two states.

Table 14-2   AGE AND SEX INCIDENCE OF ORAL CANCER PER 100,000 POPULATION

Years	Male	Female
40-49	11	4
50-59	29	9
60-69	43	11
70-79	49	12
>80	59	20

Same basis as in Table 14-1.

Table 14-3   LEUKOPLAKIA ASSOCIATED WITH CARCINOMA

Site of carcinoma	Patients	No. with leukoplakia (%)
Buccal mucosa	35	8 (23)
Gingival (alveolar) mucosa	43	9 (21)
Lip	249	38 (15)
Tongue	261	37 (14)
Floor of mouth	126	17 (13)
Oropharynx	160	18 (11)
Total	874	127 (15)

From Chierici, G., et al.: J. Oral Med. **23:**91, 1968.

Table 14-4   MALIGNANCIES AND PREMALIGNANT CHANGES IN BIOPSY SPECIMENS CLINICALLY DIAGNOSED AS LEUKOPLAKIA

Source (country), year	Patients	Findings (%)
Renstrup (Denmark), 1963	185	Carcinoma (3) Dysplasia (12)
Waldron (U.S.A.), 1975	3256	Carcinoma (3) Dysplasia (17)
Banoczy (Hungary), 1976	500	Carcinoma (10) Dysplasia (24)
Hahn (Germany), 1961	152	Carcinoma (10)
Silverman (U.S.A.), 1968	117	Carcinoma (10)

Table 14-5   MALIGNANT TRANSFORMATION IN ORAL LEUKOPLAKIAS OBSERVED OVER TIME

Source (country), year	Patients	Incidence (%)	Observation period (yr)
Einhorn (Sweden), 1967	782	4.0	1-44
Pindborg (Denmark), 1968	248	4.4	1-9
Kramer (England), 1969	187	4.8	—
Banoczy (Hungary), 1977	670	5.9	1-30
Silverman (U.S.A.), 1968	117	6.0	1-11

Table 14-6   PROGRESSION IN CLINICAL LEUKOPLAKIA FROM DYSPLASIA TO CARCINOMA

Source(country), year	Patients	Cancers (%)	Time (yr)
Mincer (U.S.A.), 1972	45*	5(11)	1-8
Banoczy (Hungary), 1976	69+	9(13)	1-20
Pindborg (Denmark), 1977	21‡	3(14)	7

*Of these lesions, 38% persisted, 7% disappeared spontaneously, and 44% were excised (about half recurring).

+Of these, 45% were excised (8 of the 9 malignant changes were in the 23 lesions not subjected to surgery).

‡In a control group of 40 dysplasias not associated with leukoplakia, only 1 became malignant.

TNM system of classification and staging

T   = Primary tumor
N   = Lymph node involvement
M   = Distant metastasis
TIS = Carcinoma in situ
T1 = Greatest diameter <2 cm
T2 = Greatest diameter 2-4 cm
T3 = Greatest diameter >4 cm
T4 = Massive tumor >4 cm with deep invasion
N0 = No clinically massive nodes
N1 = Single clinically positive homolateral node <3 cm
N2 = Single clinically positive homolateral node 3-6 cm (N2a) or multiple clinically positive homolateral nodes <6 cm (N2b)
N3 = Massive homolateral node(s), bilateral nodes, or contralateral node(s)
M0 = No evident metastasis
M1 = Distant metastasis present

    D. Erythroplasia (erythroplakia)
       1. The red, or red and white, oral mucosal lesion is far more likely than the solely white lesion to manifest a dysplastic or malignant change or to transform itself into one of these pathological states.
       2. Additionally, the differential diagnosis broadens to include candidal and other infections, traumatic ulcerations, and inflammatory disease.
    E. Oral lichen planus. Erosive chronic lichen planus has been associated with carcinoma.
    F. Syphilis
    G. Herpes simplex virus
    H. Dentures. Denture irritation can at most be only a carcinogenic cofactor in specifically predisposed individuals. This supposition is based upon the fact that more than 35 million Americans over 30 yr of age wear one or two complete dentures and yet carcinoma of the palate and alveolar mucosa accounts for less than 11% of all oral cancers. Still, the frequently observed denture sore spot must be observed carefully and all attempts made to minimize denture irritation.
    I. Dental radiation
    J. Fluoridated water

IV. Diagnosis
    A. Delay in diagnosis
    B. Signs and symptoms

Ulceration or erosion	Chronicity
Erythema	Lymphadenopathy
Induration	Leukoplakia
Fixation	

    C. Biopsy
    D. Exfoliative cytology
    E. Fine needle biopsy
    F. Toluidine blue

V. Spread of tumor (see Tables 14-7 and 14-8)
    A. Local extension
    B. Lymphatic spread
    C. Hematogenous spread
    D. Metastases to the mouth

VI. Prognosis
    A. Staging and reporting of end results. The TNM classification is used as the basis for staging:

Stage I	T1, N0, M0
Stage II	T2, N0, M0
Stage III	T3, N0, M0; T1 or T2 or T3, N1, M0
Stage IV	T4, N0 or N1, M0; any T, N2 or N3, M0; any T, any N, M1

Table 14-7 LYMPH NODE PALPATION GUIDELINES

Cause	Texture	Sensitivity	Mobility
Acute infection or inflammation	Soft	Tender	Movable
Malignancy	Firm	Nontender	Movable or fixed

Table 14-8 DISTRIBUTION OF CERVICAL LYMPH NODE METASTASES IN 1155 PATIENTS WITH OROPHARYNGEAL SQUAMOUS CARCINOMA

Site of primary tumor	Percent of regional lymph nodes involved	Nodal regions most commonly involved	
		First	Second
Nasopharynx	87	Subdigastric	Postcervical
Base of tongue	78	Subdigastric	Midjugular
Tonsillar fossa	76	Subdigastric	Midjugular
Oropharynx	59	Subdigastric	Midjugular
Retromolar pillar	45	Subdigastric	Submaxillary
Soft palate	44	Subdigastric	Midjugular
Oral tongue	35	Subdigastric	Submaxillary
Floor of mouth	31	Submaxillary	Subdigastric

Table 14-9 ORAL CANCER END RESULTS IN 1570 CASES (% OF 5 YR SURVIVALS)

Tumor site	Stages			
	I	II	III	IV
Hard palate	93	40	16	8
Oral tongue	90	64	34	6
Soft palate	73	48	32	5
Buccal mucosa	72	61	42	0
Floor of mouth	68	70	50	9
Mandibular gingiva	64	49	37	10
Maxillary gingiva	62	64	36	29
Posterior tongue	50	44	26	1

B. Cause of death
1. In a study of 94 deaths at M.D. Anderson Hospital from head and neck cancer, 43 (46%) were due to infection and 12 (12%) to hemorrhage.
2. Hypercalcemia may occur in advanced head and neck cancers and complicates management by causing gastrointestinal complaints, confusion, and dehydration.
3. Carcinomatosis is an infrequent cause of death.
4. Distant spread occurs in over 10% of patients.

C. Table 14-9 demonstrates the importance of detection at an early stage in reducing mortality. These data further document an improved survival rate for localized as compared to advanced metastatic disease. Increased survival was noted when the figures for 1969-1973 were compared to those for 1942-1966 and reflected advances in treatment techniques rather than increases in detection at an early stage.

MANAGEMENT PROCEDURES

I. Surgery and radiation are the only curative treatment for carcinoma arising in the head and neck. Chemotherapy used alone is not curative, and its role as an adjunct to surgery or radiation or both is under investigation. The decision as to which modality to use rests upon such factors as the functional and cosmetic result, the general stage of the patient's health, and the preference of the patient and his family.

II. Primary lesion
A. Surgery. Given comparable cure rates, the following represent advantages of surgical intervention:
1. A limited amount of tissue is exposed to treatment.
2. Treatment time is shorter.
3. The risk of immediate and late radiation complications is avoided.
4. Irradiation can be reserved for a subsequent head and neck primary tumor that may not be treatable by surgery. (The need for irradiation in this situation is quite low.)
5. Pathological examination may show more extensive involvement, which may then be treated by immediate irradiation.

B. Radiation. Following are the advantages of radiation treatment (assuming comparable cure rates):
1. The threat of a major operation can be avoided. Even though operative mortality is only 1-2%, this may appear high since there is no immediate threat from radiation therapy.
2. No tissues are removed.
3. Elective irradiation of the lymph nodes can be included with little added morbidity whereas if surgery is the primary modality one must either follow the neck for disease or perform an elective neck dissection.

4. The salvage of an irradiation failure by surgery is more likely to succeed than the salvage of a surgical failure by operation, irradiation, or both.

5. Multiple primary lesions can be treated simultaneously.

III. Cervical lymph nodes

A. The incidence of subclinical disease in the regional lymphatics when the neck is clinically negative ranges from 16-54%, and the risk of subclinical disease for any single primary lesion may be estimated by the size (or T stage) and the differentiation of the lesion. Nasopharyngeal and supraglottic lesions are exceptions to this rule of thumb.

B. To avoid unnecessary intervention, a policy of "wait and see" may be followed for the N0 neck and treatment started later (often successfully) if clinically positive nodes appear. However, even though such a policy may be judged successful, these patients are at an increased risk of distant metastasis and have a poorer prognosis. Elective neck treatment is therefore indicated when the associated morbidity is low; and it has the added advantage, because of its high success rate, of eradicating the lesion initially and thereby simplifying follow-up examinations.

C. Management of the clinically negative neck is as follows:

1. Radiation treatment

a. There is a large volume of data supporting the success of radiation therapy in eradicating subclinical diseases of the regional lymphatics. Given the presumed 25% overall risk of subclinical disease in the regional lymph nodes, the efficiency of neck irradiation is 90%.

b. If the primary lesion is to be treated by irradiation, then elective neck irradiation incurs little or no added cost and little added morbidity. Elective neck irradiation is usually not recommended for small superficial T1 lesions, however, in which the risk of subclinical disease in the lymph nodes is small, since the portals required for this include a large amount of normal mucosa and the majority of both parotid glands.

2. Elective neck dissection

a. It is a difficult decision to recommend full radical neck dissection, with the resulting cosmetic and functional losses, unless the potential benefit is considerable. Recent operative modifications reduce this morbidity.

b. The Bocca operation (or functional neck dissection) preserves the spinal accessory nerve, jugular vein, and sternocleidomastoid muscle and works as well as radical neck dissection for subclinical (N0) disease.

c. The supraomohyoid neck dissection differs from the Bocca procedure in that the lower internal jugular nodes below the omohyoid muscle are not removed because of the insignificant risk of metastasis to them in certain oral cavity lesions.

d. An elective supraomohyoid neck dissection on one or both sides may be better thought of practically as a staging procedure. If the nodes are negative, no further treatment is given. If the nodes are positive, the neck dissection is completed or postoperative radiation therapy is used.

e. Functional supraomohyoid neck dissection is not sufficient treatment for lesions of the oropharynx because it will miss tumor in the lower neck. It is a more difficult and longer procedure than the standard radical neck dissection.

D. Management of the clinically positive neck is as follows:

1. Radical neck dissection is satisfactory treatment for the ipsilateral nodes in a patient with N1 or N2a disease.

2. Radiation therapy is added for other N stages and/or for control of contralateral subclinical disease. Radiation therapy alone is sufficient for lower-limit N1 disease but should usually be combined with a neck dissection for upper-limit N1, N2a, or N3 disease. In practice it is always safer to add a neck dissection immediately after radiation therapy, since the detection of neck node recurrence after high-dose irradiation is difficult because of fibrosis and salvage is generally unsatisfactory.

IV. Combined surgical and radiation treatment

A. The cure rates for early carcinomas of the oral cavity and oropharynx, T1 and T2, are good. The rates for advanced tumors, T3 and T4, are less satisfactory whether treatment is by surgery alone or radiation therapy alone. At our institution twice-a-day radiation therapy is used. Early results suggest improvement in T3 tumors. In these more extensive lesions, failures of surgical treatment are usually due to marginal recurrences whereas failures of radiation therapy are primarily the result of inability to control either the radioresistant nidus at the primary site or the nodal disease. Therefore a combined program of surgery and radiation therapy is frequently employed. This permits surgical resection of gross disease, even when the resection margins are inadequate, followed by irradiation for subclinical or occult disease. Such an approach also allows effective palliation and even occasional cure of many patients who are not otherwise salvageable or who are faced with functionally and cosmetically crippling alternatives.

B. Preoperative radiation therapy

1. The aims of preoperative radiotherapy are to

a. Prevent marginal recurrences

b. Control subclinical disease in the primary site or in the nodes

c. Convert technically inoperable tumors into operable ones

2. Preoperative irradiation has the theoretical advantage of treating cancer cells in their maximum state of oxygenation.

3. The disadvantages of preoperative radiation therapy are that
   a. The extent of tumor is obscured at the time of surgery.
   b. There is a delay in the surgery.
   c. There is an increased risk of postoperative complications.

4. Conventional protocol. The dosage used is subcancericidal, consisting of 4500 cGy* in 1 mo. Radical surgery follows 1 mo later and is performed as if radiation therapy had not been given. Such an approach is applicable to medium or advanced tumors, which have poor radiotherapeutic or surgical cure rates and are not associated with significant postoperative function and cosmetic morbidity.

5. Preoperative or sequential postradiation resection. Dosage is cancericidal, 6000 to 6500 cGy in 6-7 wk delivered to the primary site as well as to the first-echelon lymph nodes. In contradistinction to the conventional protocol, radiation therapy is followed by limited surgical resection with only the residual nidus of the primary lesion in the muscles and bone excised. This method assumes that the peripheral superficial disease has been controlled by the high-dose irradiation.

C. Postoperative radiation therapy
1. The advantages of postoperative radiation therapy are that a higher dosage of radiation can be delivered and the clinician has a better understanding of the known sites of residual disease as well as the extent of pathological involvement. The aim of such treatment is to eradicate residual cancer at the resection margin and any subclinical disease implanted in the wound or in the neck nodes.

2. Postoperative radiation therapy is usually performed about 3-4 wk after surgery, when the wound is healed. A dose of 5500 cGy in 6 wk is used if the surgery was radical. If the surgery was primarily a debulking procedure, high-dose radiotherapy for gross residual disease must be given.

D. Radiation effects
1. Mucocutaneous changes
2. Loss of taste
3. Loss of salivary function
4. Nutritional deficiencies
5. Dental caries
6. Candidiasis
7. Osteoradionecrosis (Table 14-10)

---

*Centigrays (rads).

Table 14-10 REPORTED INCIDENCES OF OSTEONECROSIS IN PATIENTS IRRADIATED FOR HEAD AND NECK CANCER

Hospital	Patients	Years	Dose (cGy)	Cases (%)
M. D. Anderson	381	1966-1971	6000-7500	54(14)
Geisenberger	108	1948-1960	5000-9500	10(9)
Swedish	104	1939-1951	4000-8500	6(6)
Westfield	491	1940-1957	4000-18,000	26(5)
University of California	278	1961-1969	5000-7000	10(4)
Roswell Park	47	1968-1972	3600-12,900	2(4)

      a. The incidence of osteoradionecrosis varies depending upon the reporting institution, aggressiveness of radiotherapy, and follow-up time.

      b. The risk of spontaneous osteoradionecrosis is somewhat unpredictable but is related to the dose of radiation delivered. The risk is increased even more in dentulous patients if teeth within the treatment field are removed after therapy.

      c. Careful attention to the teeth in the line of proposed therapy is most important, but extractions are not the only method of preventing sequelae. (See "Dental management of the oral cancer patient," p. 302.)

    8. Soft tissue necrosis

V. Chemotherapy

  A. Carcinoma of the oral cavity and oropharynx represents a continuing challenge to and frustration for the medical oncologist. At present the role of chemotherapy remains to be defined; its impact on long-term survival is negligible. There is a need to find ways of improving local and regional control, avoiding deforming surgical procedures, reducing the incidence of distant metastases, treating recurrences when surgery and radiation therapy are no longer an option, and reducing the dose of radiation and risk of complications. The medical oncologist is referred patients who have advanced cancer on initial presentation or who have received surgery, radiation therapy, or both. They are elderly, cachectic, depressed, and desperate. Accordingly, data on the use of single agents and combination treatments are difficult to interpret.

  B. Drugs. Some studies of single agents suggest a modicum of success. There is no evidence that long-term survival is affected. Drugs most often used are

    Methotrexate
    Bleomycin
    Cisplatin

  C. Combination chemotherapy. The response rates to combination regimens are better than those to single-agent regimens, especially in previously untreated patients. It is unclear, however, what impact these improved response rates will have on survival.

  D. Combined modality treatment. Theoretically the use of chemotherapy as a first treatment might control the primary site and downgrade the primary lesion, sensitize the tumor to radiation effects, create a situation in which a less extensive operation was required, and reduce the risk of distant metastases. Studies to date have failed to substantiate any of these in humans. Currently better-designed trials using more potent agents (e.g., cisplatin) are underway.

VI. Specific considerations
 A. Lip
  1. Since radiation therapy and surgery yield equally high cure rates for small limited cancers, the selection of treatment depends upon the cosmetic result following the procedure. Surgery is also preferred for extensive cancer associated with bone involvement and for significant soft tissue involvement that will require major reconstructive surgery.
  2. Radiation therapy is best for

   Superficial lip cancer involving more than one third of the entire lip
   Cancer involving the commissure and upper and lower lips
   Recurrent tumor
   The patient who refuses surgery

  3. Radical neck dissection with adjuvant radiation therapy is needed for metastatic nodes, but prophylactic or elective neck dissection or irradiation for the N0 neck is not indicated. Low-grade lip cancers rarely metastasize, and subsequent nodal metastases are also rare. Therapeutic neck dissection results are comparable to prophylactic dissection results for occult nodes. Thus the small group of patients in whom metastases develop can still be cured and the majority spared an operation.
 B. Oral tongue
  1. Management of carcinoma of the oral tongue is controversial and depends upon the size, location, and growth pattern as well as the nodal status.
  2. For T1 and T2 lesions, both surgery and radiotherapy are effective.
   a. Small lesions can be satisfactorily treated by transoral resection, without resulting functional morbidity. This is particularly true in older patients, who tolerate prolonged curative radiation therapy less well. Radiation therapy is preferred for small, posteriorly situated, poorly defined lesions, which are more difficult to approach for surgical excision.
   b. Large, superficial, exophytic T1 and T2 lesions without much muscle involvement can be treated by radiation therapy, with high control rates and excellent cosmetic results.
   c. Medium-sized tumors with involvement of the adjacent floor of the mouth are well treated by comprehensive radiation therapy to the primary site and neck nodes, with surgery reserved for salvage of residual or recurrent disease. Primary surgical treatment in these cases would have to include partial glossectomy, partial mandibulectomy, and radical neck dissection.

3. For T3 and T4 lesions with deep muscular invasion and often associated nodal metastases, treatment is best a combination of radiation therapy and surgery.

C. Floor of the mouth
   1. Obstruction of Wharton's duct may cause enlargement of the submaxillary gland, which can mimic nodal involvement. In T1 lesions nodal metastases are low; but T3 and T4 lesions are associated with a high incidence of node involvement, which may be bilateral. Evaluation of the extent must include inspection for involvement of the undersurface of the tongue and adjacent gingiva. Normal mucosa over the mandible without fixation almost always precludes mandibular involvement. Dental radiographs are best for showing bone involvement.
   2. Small tumors limited to the mucosa are highly curable by radiation therapy alone. T2 and early exophytic T3 lesions may receive a trial course of radiation. If a good response is obtained, treatment should be completed and salvage surgery may be considered for residual disease at the primary site and neck nodes.
   3. When the adjacent mandible is thought to be involved, surgical excision with a rim of normal inner border of the mandible is indicated followed by postoperative radiation therapy. Large T3 and T4 lesions with marked involvement of adjacent tissue require combined radiation therapy and surgery as a composite resection. The irradiation may be preoperative or postoperative.

D. Retromolar trigone and anterior pillar. Treatment can be by either radical surgery or radiation therapy.
   1. Superficial T1 and T2 lesions are treated by radiation therapy, with surgery reserved for salvage.
   2. Large infiltrating lesions (T3 and T4) with or without metastatic nodes are treated by combined high-dose limited-field irradiation and composite resection.

E. Buccal mucosa
   1. Small T1 lesions with well-defined margins can be treated by surgical removal. The lesion as well as adjacent suspicious tissue will be eradicated.
   2. T2 lesions are well treated by radiotherapy, with good functional and cosmetic results.
   3. T3 and T4 lesions with deep muscular invasion are poorly treated by radiation therapy. En bloc excision of the primary and regional lymph nodes is the treatment of choice.
   4. Verrucous carcinoma has been discussed previously.

F. Gingivae. Treatment depends upon the extent of the lesion, the status of the lymph nodes, and the presence or absence of bone involvement. Panorex or polytomes of the mandible are a minimal work-up for bone involvement.

1. Small T1 exophytic lesions without bone involvement can be treated by radiotherapy alone.
2. Large lesions, T2 and T3, require high-dose radiation, and local control of disease is poor. The risk of osteoradionecrosis is high. Therefore advanced lesions associated with destruction of the mandible with or without metastases should be treated by radical surgery. Good survival rates are obtained with partial mandibulectomy and radical neck dissection.

G. Soft palate
   1. Surgical resection of carcinoma of the soft palate is unsatisfactory and often results in marginal recurrences. Even when surgery is succesful, the effects on swallowing and speech are unacceptable.
   2. T1 and T2 exophytic mucosal tumors should be treated by radiation therapy.
   3. Advanced T2 and T3 lesions are often associated with nodal involvement, and radiation therapy is given first for cure, with residual disease treated by local resection. Surgical resection for nodal involvement, even if bilateral, is indicated if control of the primary can be achieved by irradiation. Chemotherapy with or without radiation therapy may offer some degree of palliation.

H. Hard palate
   1. The hard palate is the most common site of occurrence of minor salivary gland tumors. Squamous cell carcinoma is rare and generally ulcerative with invasion of bone. There is a low incidence of nodal involvement.
   2. Early lesions without bony involvement can be treated by radiation therapy, with surgery reserved for salvage.
   3. Advanced, deeply ulcerated, infiltrative lesions with bone destruction are best treated by combined radiation therapy and surgery, with prosthetic rehabilitation of the defect.

I. Tonsil
   1. Radiotherapy gives excellent results for T1 and T2 lesions, with far less functional and cosmetic morbidity than results from surgery.
   2. Advanced tumors of the tonsil (T3 and T4) with invasion of the base of the tongue are rarely curable by either radiation therapy or surgery alone and should be managed by combined methods.

J. Base of tongue
   1. A high percentage of these patients have nodal involvement. Agressive primary surgery is extremely mutilating and often followed by marginal recurrence and nodal disease.
   2. T1 and T2 lesions are radiosensitive and curable by radiation therapy alone, with results comparable to those achieved by surgery.

3. Large infiltrative (T3 and T4) lesions are rarely curable by single-modality treatment. Combined high-dose radiation therapy and limited surgery offer the best treatment.
4. For totally inoperable lesions palliative irradiation or chemotherapy is all that can be offered.

K. Pharyngeal wall
1. Early lesions are extremely rare and can be controlled by either surgery or radiation therapy.
2. Advanced tumors with nodal disease require combined therapies. Surgical procedures usually require laryngopharyngectomy with or without esophagectomy and radical neck dissection. Despite aggressive approaches, the ultimate prognosis is poor.

Dental management of the oral cancer patient

I. Problems arising in the dental management of oral cancer patients are most often related to needed treatment procedures rather than to the malignancy itself.
II. Radiotherapy and chemotherapy are the modalities most often associated with dental and oral complications, which can include

Mucositis
Xerostomia
Radiation caries
Osteoradionecrosis

Management of the irradiated patient

I. Radiation-induced oral complications can occur in
A. Mucosa. A transient mucositis results from the direct effect of radiation on mucosa; however, xerostomia resulting from radiation-damaged salivary glands and direct injury of bone tend to be more permanent complications.
B. Enamel. Radiation caries is thought to be not so much a direct effect of radiation on enamel as the result of a lack of natural cleaning activity associated with a dry mouth.
C. Bone. Because of its high mineral content, bone absorbs more energy than do soft tissues. This phenomenon may account for the osseous damage that occurs when soft tissue malignancies are irradiated and also is responsible for the most severe dental complication arising from radiotherapy, osteonecrosis.
II. Osteoradionecrosis is an infection of irradiated bone that leads to pain, bone loss, functional disability, and cosmetic disfigurement.
A. The chief features are exposed bone and pain arising either from the bone itself or from adjacent soft tissues that have been irritated by contact with devitalized bone. Radiation parameters that influence the occurrence of osteoradionecrosis are
1. Quality and quantity of radiation. Before the 1960s orthovoltages were generally used in the treatment of oral malignan-

cy. Such radiation was associated with a 17-37% incidence of osteoradionecrosis. With the advent of megavoltage units, the incidence of osteoradionecrosis declined to 2-5%. As a result, megavoltages have come to be perceived as "bone sparing." Doses in excess of 5000 cGy are not uncommon, yet at this level of exposure death of bone cells and a progressive obliterative arteritis (endarteritis, periarteritis, hyalinization, fibrosis, and thrombosis of vessels) result. The consequences of cellular death are an aseptic necrosis of the portion of bone directly in the beam of radiation with compromised vascularity in the adjacent bone. Although the irradiated bone may function normally, when microorganisms gain entry via mucosal ulcerations the result is lacerations, scaling of teeth, compound fractures, periodontal disease, and infection necessitating endodontics or exodontics.

2. Size of portals. Portal size, dose fractionation, meticulous collimation, and shielding of normal tissues are now recognized as variables that are important in defining the risk of radiation-related oral complications. The use of intraoral cone delivery of radiation minimizes exposure of normal tissues and permits greater conservation of teeth.

3. Location and extent of lesion. The mandible is associated with a higher incidence of osteoradionecrosis than is any other bone. This is probably explained by the fact that most oral tumors are perimandibular and susceptibility is increased by the dense mandibular cortical plates, with less extensive vascular network than exists in the maxilla.

4. Condition of the teeth and periodontium. Establishing and maintaining the health of the dentition dramatically diminish the likelihood of radiation-induced complications. Guidelines for establishing and maintaining dental health are discussed later.

B. Methods for managing the patient with osteoradionecrosis are beyond the scope of this presentation; instead, we will limit ourselves to methods of preirradiation and postirradiation dental care that minimize the possibility of developing osteoradionecrosis. The following guidelines have been promulgated on the basis of collected clinical documentation and clinical and basic research; however, it should be recognized that the subject remains controversial.

1. Guidelines for preirradiation dental care are as follows:
   a. All nonrestorable teeth and teeth with significant periodontal disease in the direct beam of radiation should be extracted before radiation therapy begins.
   b. In patients with poor oral health and poor motivation to maintain oral hygiene, complete extractions are recommended.

   c. Extensive alveoloplasty should be performed to permit a primary mucoperiosteal closure. All sharp bony margins should be smoothed (since irradiated bone will not remodel spontaneously).

   d. To allow initial healing and required restorative treatment, radiation should be delayed 10-14 da.

   e. All remaining teeth should be restored and periodontal treatment completed within this 2 wk interval. Instructions and an opportunity to practice oral hygiene should be provided.

   f. A custom tray is used for application of a 0.4% stannous fluoride gel, a 1% sodium fluoride gel, or 1% acidulated fluorophosphate gel. After flossing, fluoride treatment should be performed for 15 min twice a day.

2. Guidelines for postirradiation care are the following:

   a. Dentures should not be used for 1 yr after treatment.

   b. The need for the patient to continue oral hygiene and fluoride therapy should be emphasized.

   c. Saliva substitute can be provided (VA Oralube or Orex) if xerostomia-induced soft tissue disorders arise. Such saliva substitutes contain minerals and fluoride and may help to reharden tooth surfaces.

   d. If postirradiation pulpitis develops and the tooth is restorable, endodontics with antibiotic prophylaxis should be instituted.

   e. Necessary extractions should be limited to one or two per sitting. Removal should be as atraumatic as possible with trimming only of sharp bone margins and without raising extensive flaps or attempting to obtain a linear closure. Antibiotic prophylaxis is important. Specific antibiotic recommendations are as follows:

     (1) Aqueous penicillin, 1 million units, is given intravenously 15 min before surgery, and then oral doses of penicillin-V, 500 mg q.i.d. for 10 da. The initial oral dose should be given 1 hr after the parenteral dose.

     (2) Alternatively, 1 g penicillin-V given orally 1 hr before the procedure and then the same postsurgical regimen as above.

     (3) In patients allergic to penicillin, give 1 g erythromycin 1 hr before surgery and then 500 mg q.i.d. for 10 da.

Management of patients receiving chemotherapy

I. In recent years, the use of chemotherapy in managing malignant oral disease has expanded dramatically. Unfortunately, complications arising from such treatment have also increased. Oral morbidity resulting from malignant disease and its chemotherapeutic treatment are a significant and challenging problem, without completely satisfactory solutions.

II. Pretreatment evaluation

A. Ideally patients planned for chemotherapy should be completely evaluated by a general dentist. After chemotherapy has begun, it may not be possible to obtain radiographs or perform other diagnostic procedures, so this initial evaluation provides an important baseline.

B. The circumstances under which chemotherapy patients are evaluated may not be optimal since such persons may be debilitated even prior to the initation of chemotherapy. Typically the patient may have severe oral pain, limited opening, and accumulated debris or other obstructions. The use of topical anesthetic agents may be helpful in examination.

1. Baseline and subsequent visits should include both intraoral and extraoral examinations, radiographs if possible, and selected laboratory studies

2. The most important laboratory values are total WBC count, differential analysis (i.e., PMNs, lymphocytes, and blast forms), platelet count, bleeding time, PT, and PTT. These and other clotting parameters may be required if contemplated dental treatment will elicit bleeding.

C. After collection of an adequate data base, difficult decisions need to be made regarding the type, timing, and aggressiveness of proposed treatment. An important factor in such planning appears to be the patient's bone marrow status and predicted effects on peripheral blood counts over the next 7-10 da.

D. The need to extract all teeth in patients undergoing chemotherapy is no longer accepted; however, hopelessly nonrestorable teeth should be removed, the remaining teeth cleaned of both supragingival and subgingival deposits, and periodontal therapy instituted for periodontal pockets that the patient will not be able to keep plaque-free. Additional dental treatment can then be completed to help assure an aesthetic, functional, comfortable, and disease-free mouth.

III. Preventive therapy

A. The basic concepts involved in preventing oral complications arising from chemotherapy (i.e., bleeding, infection, pain) are similar to those outlined for the irradiated patient.

1. Patient education is the first step in any preventive regimen. Meticulous oral hygiene resulting from both the patient's and the dentist's (or hygienist's) efforts greatly minimizes the likelihood of complications.

2. The patient's blood count will begin to fall following chemotherapy, and professional hygiene measures must be adjusted accordingly. In general, moderately aggressive hygiene measures are appropriate if the patient is not severely myelosuppressed (WBC $>2000/mm^3$, with $>20\%$ PMNs and platelets $>20,000/mm^3$).

3. Brushing (using a soft brush), flossing, and thorough scaling are desirable. Frequent rinsing also helps to remove debris and bacteria. The patient's dental appliances can be worn as usual if they fit well and if he is closely observed for ulcer formation.

B. Active myelosuppression complicates the situation. Based upon clinical impression, it seems that when the patient's total WBC count drops below $1500\text{-}2000/mm^3$ with less than 10% PMNs brushing and flossing should be stopped. This is a subject of controversy, however, since there are no absolute guidelines for assessing safe peripheral blood count levels.

1. The risk of bacteremia resulting from attempts at hygiene must be evaluated in the context of bacteremias resulting from florid oral disease. In such patients, mouth rinsing and tooth cleansing using a wet 2×2 in sponge can usually be continued.

2. Because of their ability to provoke bacteremias in an immunosuppressed patient, oral irrigation devices are not advised.

C. Oral bleeding is commonly associated with immunosuppression. Management of the underlying causes for such bleeding is the province of the hematologist; however, the dentist may be consulted on local measures to control bleeding and adjust existing appliances to minimize oral trauma. The incidence of oral bleeding increases exponentially with platelet counts below $20,000/mm^3$.

D. As observed for irradiated patients, fluoride is of significant benefit in preventing caries. Excellent oral hygiene, low sugar intake, and fluoride rinses can do much to minimize caries experience.

Management of patients receiving both radiation and chemotherapy

I. It is not uncommon to encounter a patient receiving both of these treatment modalities. Increasingly, patients are seen who have been treated with surgery as well as with radiation and chemotherapy. The basic concepts in management are essentially the same as outlined previously.

II. Some treatment regimens that have proved successful are as follows:

A. Individualized fluoride treatment programs can include either of the following:

1. Brushing at bedtime with a stabilized 0.4% stannous fluoride gel.

2. Nightly rinsing with freshly prepared 0.1% aqueous stannous fluoride.

B. Control of intraoral soft tissue problems
    1. Pain. Dyclonine with diphenhydramine rinses or 2% viscous lidocaine solution
    2. Decreased salivary flow. A specific preparation (e.g., VA Ora-lube)

GENERAL REFERENCES

M.D. Anderson Hospital and Tumor Institute: Neoplasia of the head and neck, Chicago, 1974, Year Book Medical Publishers, Inc.

Million, R.R., and Cassisi, N.J.: Management of head and neck cancer. A multidisciplinary approach, Philadelphia, 1984, J.B. Lippincott Co.

Randolph, V.L., et al.: Combination therapy of advanced head and neck cancer, Cancer **41:**460, 1978.

Shillitoe, E.J., et al.: Immunoglobulin class of antibody to herpes simplex virus in patients with oral cancer, Cancer **51:**67, 1983.

Silverman, S., editor: Oral cancer, New York, 1981, American Cancer Society.

Wang, C.C.: Radiation therapy for head and neck neoplasms, Hertfordshire, England, 1983, John Wright & Sons, Ltd.

Cysts and Tumors

15

GENERAL CONSIDERATIONS

I. Cysts and neoplasms of the maxilla and mandible include a variety of odontogenic and nonodontogenic, epithelial, and mesenchymal lesions. These lesions will be discussed according to their tissues of origin and will be separated into odontogenic and nonodontogenic categories.

II. Clinical features that may be of assistance in the differential diagnosis of jaw lesions include

A. History—signs and symptoms, mode of onset, rate of progression

B. Radiographic features—relative lucency or opacity, definition of borders, unilocular or multilocular outline

C. Relationship to teeth—contiguity, tooth vitality, tooth displacement, root erosion

D. Relationship to bony cortex—central or peripheral or both, cortical expansion or perforation

E. Location within the jaw—maxilla or mandible or both; anterior or posterior jaw, inferior or superior to the inferior alveolar canal

F. Coexistence with other diseases—e.g., giant cell lesions of the jaws with hyperparathyroidism

III. Odontogenic cysts, fissural cysts, odontogenic tumors, and nonodontogenic tumors will be discussed. Emphasis will be on differential diagnosis and treatment planning based upon biological behavior.

JAW CYSTS

I. Odontogenic cysts

A. Apical and residual cysts

1. These cysts derive from epithelial rests within the periodontal ligament, which may be stimulated to proliferate by chronic inflammation initiated by pulpal necrosis.

2. The apical cyst is the most common odontogenic cyst. It is attached to the apex of a pulpally compromised tooth and is also known as a radicular cyst.

3. The residual cyst is essentially the same process that is dis-

Osseous Lesions and Related Clinical Findings

	Pain	Paresthesias	Growth rate	Mucosa	Palpation	Radiograph	Special tests and features
Cysts	− (unless infected)	−	Slow	−	Firm to springy	Circumscribed	Tooth vitality, impacted teeth, multiple Gorlin's
Odontogenic tumors	−	−	Slow	−	Firm to springy	Circumscribed	Ameloblastoma, root resorption
Benign nonodontogenic tumors	−	−	Slow (GCRG is exception)	−	Firm to springy	Circumscribed	Central giant cell reparative granuloma, AV malformation (bruit-thrill), systemic intravascular coagulopathy, myxoma (no root resorption)
Malignant tumors	+	+ (especially lymphoma)	Rapid	− (but can be fixed or ulcerated)	Firm, spongy, crepitant	Diffuse (cortical perforation)	CT scan (to show extent of bone perforation)
Inflammatory bone disease	+	−	Days, weeks	−/+	Firm to spongy	Diffuse	WBC count, skin tests, tomograms (to show extent of osteomyelitis)
Primary bone diseases	−	−	Slow	−	Firm	Generalized	Paget's (alkaline phosphatase), hyperparathyroidism (calcium or phosphate radioimmunoassay)

Code: + Present or involved
− Not involved

covered after a tooth has been removed. Distinction between a residual cyst and a primordial cyst of a supernumerary tooth may be impossible.

4. Radiographic appearance of these lesions is typically a well-defined unilocular radiolucency within the alveolar bone.

5. Treatment is enucleation. Endodontic therapy alone may allow involution of a small apical cyst. Recurrence is rare.

B. Dentigerous (follicular) cyst
   1. This is an odontogenic cyst that
      a. Derives from cells of the reduced enamel epithelium after the crown of the tooth has been completely formed
      b. Is always associated with an unerupted tooth
      c. Is generally unilocular radiographically; when multiple cysts are encountered, the basal cell nevus syndrome should be considered
      d. May cause cortical expansion although not perforation
      e. Is usually associated with impacted mandibular third molars or maxillary canines, since these are the most commonly impacted teeth
      f. Is a potential site for development of an ameloblastoma; multiple cases of ameloblastoma have been reported arising in the wall of dentigerous cysts; fewer cases of mural squamous cell carcinoma have been reported; all dentigerous cysts should be carefully examined microscopically for associated neoplastic processes
   2. Treatment includes enucleation and removal of the associated tooth. One must rule out keratocyst. Marsupialization is rarely indicated. Recurrence rates vary with the size and location of the cyst but are usually less than 5% in most series.

C. Primordial cyst and odontogenic keratocyst
   1. The primordial cyst (PC) derives from undifferentiated dental lamina and therefore is not associated with a tooth crown. It has a keratinizing squamous lining. All such cysts are keratocysts, but not all keratocysts are primordial.
   2. The odontogenic keratocyst (OKC)
      a. Derives from dental lamina
      b. Occurs predominantly in the posterior (molar, ramus) areas of the jaws
      c. Is often multilocular, often grows rapidly, and can induce paresthesia and cortical perforation
      d. Recurs at a high rate; reported recurrence rates vary (range 10-65%) depending upon size and location of the cyst, treatment, and duration of follow-up; recurrences may be discovered 10 yr or more after treatment; a high recurrence rate may be related to satellite cysts or to the higher mitotic index seen among the lining cells; recurrences have been reported in bone grafts

e. Contains fluid with lower protein content than serum; aspiration may therefore be helpful in preoperative assessment of suspected jaw cysts

3. The basal cell nevus syndrome should be considered when multiple keratocysts of the jaws are detected. This is an autosomal dominant disease characterized by

Jaw cysts
Multiple early-onset basal cell carcinomas
Palmar and plantar pitting
Skeletal abnormalities (bifid ribs, vertebral anomalies, pectus excavatum, hypertelorism)

4. Treatment is enucleation. Large or recurrent lesions may require en bloc resection with immediate bone graft reconstruction. Lesions that display aggressive clinical behavior may be best approached as a neoplasm rather than as a typical odontogenic cyst. Use of cauterizing solutions (Carnoy's solution) or excision of the overlying mucosa to minimize the possibility of recurrence has been suggested. Marsupialization is rarely indicated. Close long-term follow-up is essential since recurrences may arise 10 yr or more after initial treatment.

D. Calcifying odontogenic cyst (Gorlin cyst)
1. This lesion is similar to the calcifying epithelioma of Malherbe and is thought to be of epithelial origin. It has characteristics of both a cyst and a solid tumor.
2. The lesion most commonly affects the mandible (70% of cases). It grows slowly and may involve soft tissue. The large majority (75%) have been central, with the remainder either entirely peripheral or accompanied by superficial bone erosion.
3. It appears typically as a radiolucency containing radiopaque foci.
4. Treatment is enucleation. Recurrence may be due to soft tissue spread.

II. Nonodontogenic cysts (fissural)
A. General features
1. Fissural cysts form at the junction between developing structures of the face as a result of incomplete involution of epithelial cells. This aberration can result in so-called fissural cysts, which may be either laterally or medially situated. Such lesions occur within bone, soft tissue, or both.
2. Any fissural cyst in the maxilla may contain oral and/or nasal respiratory epithelium.
3. Adjacent teeth are vital and often displaced.
4. Treatment in all cases is enucleation. Recurrence is virtually unknown.
B. Lateral fissural cysts of the maxilla
1. These cysts develop at the point of fusion of the globular

portion of the median nasal process and the maxillary process.

2. They occur at the junction of the primary palate (lip and premaxilla) with the secondary palate (posterior to the lateral incisor).

    a. When within bone, they are called globulomaxillary cysts.

    b. When in the lip or lateral nose, they are nasolabial cysts.

    c. When eroding through labial cortex, they are nasoalveolar cysts.

3. They usually present as a swelling of the upper lip or nasal base, including the nasal floor. The differential diagnosis of swelling within the nasal floor (most commonly in blacks and females) should include the lateral fissural cyst.

C. Median fissural cysts of the maxilla

1. Nasopalatine cysts develop from paired nasopalatine ducts, which enter the mouth just posterior to the incisive papilla. They are the most common fissural cyst. Within this group are the incisive canal cyst and the cyst of the papilla incisiva. These designations are determined by location, the latter being entirely within soft tissue.

2. Median palatine cysts derive from epithelial remnants at the median palatine fissure (as a midline palatal swelling).

D. Fissural cyst of the mandible

1. This extremely rare cyst is located in the symphysis. Fewer than 10 cases have been reported.

2. The surrounding teeth are vital and may be displaced, an important feature in distinguishing this lesion from apical cysts.

III. Diagnosis and treatment of jaw cysts

A. Several clinical and radiographic features of a radiolucent lesion of the jaw that may be of assistance in diagnosis and treatment planning include

1. Association with teeth. Are the teeth vital? If so, the apical cyst can be ruled out.

2. Composition of the cyst. Is the lesion unilocular or multilocular? The latter may suggest a keratocyst or noncystic neoplasm (e.g., myxoma).

3. Cyst fluid aspirate. Keratocysts have a relatively low protein concentration compared to serum. Blood that can be aspirated easily is consistent with a central vascular malformation or an aneurysmal bone cyst.

4. Location. Noting whether a lesion is medially or laterally situated and determining its proximity to the teeth can aid in distinguishing fissural cysts from odontogenic cysts. Lesions that appear in non–tooth-bearing areas of the jaws (e.g., the proximal ramus or inferior to the mandibular canal) are probably nonodontogenic.

B. Two general modes of treatment are employed for the various cysts of the jaws:
   1. Enucleation of the cyst in its entirety
   2. Marsupialization, a process of exteriorizing the cyst, thus decompressing it, by making its lining continuous with the lining of the oral cavity

C. In general, enucleation is preferred since the cyst is completely removed and entirely available for histological evaluation. In practice, marsupialization is rarely necessary but may be indicated when a cyst is extremely large and enucleation might be incomplete or when injury to contiguous neurovascular, dental, and sinus structures is likely. Advocates of marsupialization claim that this technique is less likely to devitalize teeth and induce oroantral fistulas. When this method is chosen, consideration should be given to eventual enucleation once the cyst has contracted over time.

D. The decision to carry out primary closure of a bony cavity after removal of a cyst is a matter of clinical judgment. The incision must be planned to allow the suture line to be supported as much as possible by bone. Consideration should also be given to creating an osteoperiosteal flap (i.e., reflection of the bony cortex overlying the cyst while it remains attached to the mucoperiosteal flap). In general, the size and location of the cyst determine whether to place a dressing and thus commit the wound to healing by secondary intention.

E. Cysts up to 20 mm in size will usually heal primarily, particularly in the maxilla, where dependent drainage is advantageous. In the mandible the tendency toward blood clot liquefaction and delayed healing is exaggerated by the unfavorable influence of gravity. Trimming the bone margins of residual defect (saucerization) will help limit dead space by allowing the reapproximated flap to partially collapse into the cavity.

F. Relative indications for placement of a dressing are
   1. A large bony defect with unfavorable drainage
   2. A previously infected cyst
   3. When significant bleeding has been encountered

G. It is arguable that even when a large bony defect is encountered primary closure is still indicated; if the original lesion is uninfected, there is a good chance of successful healing. Should the wound break down because of premature blood clot liquefaction and dehiscence of the incision, the argument continues, one can then place a dressing and proceed in a fashion similar to the planned method of healing by secondary intention.

H. If a dressing is indicated, we usually employ ½-1 in gauze impregnated with balsam of Peru. The pack is withdrawn either partially or totally, usually on the fifth or seventh day, and is changed regularly until the residual defect has contracted enough that the wound can be readily managed by irrigations.

1. Autogenous bone may be placed in large cavities to promote healing by stabilizing clot and promoting osteogenesis. However, this is rarely indicated with jaw cysts.
2. Demineralized bone has been advocated for speeding osteoinduction. Its obvious advantage lies in the avoidance of potential donor site morbidity.

JAW TUMORS

I. Odontogenic tumors
   A. General features
      1. Odontogenic tumors result from the misdirection of cellular activity involved in odontogenesis.
      2. They are classified according to the embryological process of induction (i.e., the process of change brought about by the action of one tissue type upon another, specifically epithelium and mesenchyme).
      3. In the U.S. they comprise about 9% of all tumors of the oral cavity.
   B. Epithelial tumors with minimum induction
      1. Ameloblastoma
         a. This tumor derives from cell rests of the enamel organ (dental lamina) or from the epithelium of odontogenic cysts, primarily dentigerous cysts. Ameloblastoma accounts for 1% of all jaw cysts and tumors.
         b. Eighty percent occur in the mandible, 75% of these in the molar-ramus area. Most patients are in their third to fifth decades of life.
         c. The ameloblastoma grows by slow and persistent expansion. It rarely causes nerve compromise or pain. Its behavior in the maxilla may differ from that in the mandible because of the greater cortical density of the latter, which tends to confine the tumor.
         d. Radiographically the lesion is classically multilocular (multicystic, MC) although unilocular (unicystic, UC) lesions are encountered.
         e. A peripheral ameloblastoma has been described and has a more innocuous biological pattern than the UC or MC forms. Most reported cases have involved the gingiva.
         f. Treatment is controversial, although there is general agreement that the peripheral form can be excised conservatively without removing contiguous bone and the UC form can be enucleated. The MC form should be excised with a margin of uninvolved bone. Immediate bone graft reconstruction is appropriate.
         g. Recurrence rates have been reported to be 30%, probably reflecting the tumor's ability to penetrate bone. A small number of instances of distant metastases have been reported.

2. Adenomatoid odontogenic tumor (adenoameloblastoma)
   a. This lesion is not related to ameloblastoma.
   b. Its pathogenesis is uncertain, but it may arise from cell rests of the enamel organ, from odontogenic cysts, or from disturbances of the developing enamel organ.
   c. It usually presents as a painless swelling of the jaw.
   d. It is often associated with an impacted tooth, particularly a mandibular canine.
   e. It may contain areas of calcified material of the dystrophic type.
   f. The majority of patients are in their second decade; 65% have been female.
   g. Treatment is conservative excision. Recurrences have not been reported, even after incomplete removal.
3. Calcifying odontogenic tumor (Pindborg tumor)
   a. This is a benign neoplasm that arises from reduced enamel epithelium. It has been found to
      (1) Occur frequently in middle age, similar to the ameloblastoma
      (2) Affect the mandible most commonly (3:1 relative to the maxilla), usually in the premolar-molar area
      (3) Often present as a painless swelling
      (4) Be associated with an unerupted tooth (in perhaps 50% of cases)
      (5) Invade locally, behaving similarly to an ameloblastoma
      (6) Appear as a radiolucency with radiopaque foci of either unilocular or multilocular configuration; its early radiographic appearance may be indistinguishable from that of a dentigerous cyst
   b. Treatment should be similar to that for the ameloblastoma, (i.e., conservative surgical excision with a margin of uninvolved bone).
C. Epithelial tumors with induction. Clinically benign behavior is expected with induction. All tumors in this category behave accordingly, and conservative excision is appropriate management.
   1. Ameloblastic fibroma
      a. This odontogenic tumor is characterized by slow progression with possible cortical expansion but not invasion.
      b. Patients are generally in the 5-20 yr age group.
      c. Painless swelling, usually in the premolar-molar area, is the commonest presentation. The mandible is affected more often than the maxilla.
      d. Histologically there is encapsulation around cords and islands of epithelial cells in a connective tissue stroma. Thus it is a true mixed tumor. The stroma, which strongly

resembles the embryonal connective tissue of the primitive dental pulp, allows distinction from ameloblastoma.

   e. It presents usually as a well-defined unilocular radiolucency not associated with an impacted tooth. Occasionally it is multilocular.

   f. Treatment is enucleation. Recurrence is rare.

2. Squamous odontogenic tumor. This recently described lesion may be characterized as follows:

   a. Benign mixed tumor consisting of squamous odontogenic epithelial islands in a mature fibrous connective tissue stroma

   b. Probably arises from rests of Malassez in the periodontal ligament or from gingival mucosa.

   c. Appears as a painless swelling or loosening of teeth

   d. Occurs most commonly in the second and third decades, with no sex predilection

   e. Usually discovered in the anterior maxilla and posterior mandible

   f. In the maxilla, displays a more aggressive behavior than in the the mandible; this is presumably related to the lesser density of bone in the maxilla

   g. A discrete radiolucency adjacent to one or more teeth

   h. Treated generally by enucleation or curettage; more aggressive maxillary lesions may best be managed by en bloc excision; recurrences have not been reported

D. Mesenchymal odontogenic tumors

1. Myxoma

   a. This benign swelling is not clearly odontogenic but is found virtually exclusively in the jaws.

   b. It is a slow-growing and persistent tumor that is locally invasive with periods of rapid expansion. It does not metastasize. Variations in rates of expansion are often not readily explained by histology.

   c. Peak incidence is in the second and third decades. Both jaws are affected.

   d. Histologically the tumor is characterized by stellate cells with long anastomosing cytoplasmic processes in a mucinous matrix. It is important to distinguish this pattern from the myxoid features of other tumors.

   e. Typically a multilocular radiolucency is seen. Distinction from ameloblastoma or central giant cell lesions may be impossible.

   f. Treatment is controversial, but generally en bloc excision is recommended since local invasiveness is a feature of this lesion. Small lesions may be aggressively curetted. Large ones displaying aggressive behavior (cortical perfortion, rapid expansion) should be resected. Reported recurrence rates average 25%.

2. Odontoma
   a. The odontomas constitute a group of solid odontogenic tumors containing both enamel and dentin. Mature ones contain cementum as well.
   b. Odontomas may be classified as compound, complex, and ameloblastic.
      (1) Compound odontomas are the most highly differentiated variety. Essentially, when a calcified lesion of the jaws manifests morphological similarity to a tooth, this designation is appropriate. Such tumors display a predilection for the incisor-canine region, and if they interfere with eruption of contiguous teeth this may be an indication for their removal. Simple excision is proper therapy.
      (2) Complex odontomas are a type of hamartoma that is intermediate in prevalence between the compound and the ameloblastic types. Their morphology is less similar to that of a tooth, and they often are associated with an unerupted tooth. They demonstrate slow growth, affecting females more often than males (2:1), and approximately 70% occur in the second and third molar areas. Conservative excision is appropriate.
      (3) Ameloblastic forms include the ameloblastic odontoma and the ameloblastic fibroodontoma, which are tumors consisting essentially of a compound or complex odontoma with an associated soft tissue component of ameloblastic tissue or ameloblastic epithelial islands scattered in a fibromyxoid stroma. Correspondingly they may show a cystlike radiolucency around the calcified component. Sarcomatous transformation of ameloblastic fibroodontoma has been reported. Nevertheless, conservative treatment (curettage) is appropriate with close long-term follow-up.
3. Cementoma
   a. The term *cementoma* is applied by clinicians to the lesion perhaps more appropriately called periapical cemental dysplasia, PCD.
   b. It describes a group of lesions that contain cementum, including PCD, cementifying fibroma, and cementoblastoma.
      (1) Periapical cemental dysplasia (PCD) is the most common lesion in the cementoma group, appearing mainly in blacks and females, rarely among patients younger than 25 yr of age. It is usually discovered at routine examination as a periapical radiolucency continuous with the periodontal ligament (in its early stages) or as a mixed radiolucent-radiopaque

irregular lesion (in later stages). In its mature stage, fully calcified osteocementum is found. Surgery is not indicated except in the rare instances of chronic gingival ulceration and secondary infection. Conservative excision is then appropriate.

(2) Cementifying fibroma is difficult to separate from ossifying fibroma and will be discussed in the next section (nonodontogenic tumors).

(3) Cementoblastoma is a benign tumor that is self-limiting, attached to the root of a tooth (most commonly a mandibular premolar or molar), and composed of globules of cementum. It does not recur after simple enucleation.

II. Nonodontogenic tumors

   A. General features

   1. Benign nonodontogenic mesenchymal tumors make up the majority of jaw tumors in children.

   2. Odontogenic epithelial tumors are relatively more common in adults—e.g., ameloblastoma occurs overwhelmingly in middle-aged persons.

   3. Nonodontogenic tumors may be classified according to their presumed tissue of origin.

   Benign mesenchymal
   Malignant mesenchymal
   Vascular
   Hematopoietic-reticuloendothelial
   Neurogenic
   Malignant epithelial

   4. Some lesions are difficult to classify in this fashion and are thus placed in conceptually convenient groups. For example, the aneurysmal bone cyst is included in the vascular group. The present discussion will consider only the *benign* categories. Malignant jaw tumors are discussed elsewhere in this text.

   B. Benign mesenchymal tumors

   1. Giant cell lesions. These tumors fall into three groups—giant cell reparative granuloma (GCRG), brown tumor of hyperparathyroidism, and giant cell tumor (GCT). Distinction among them by histological criteria may be impossible. Therefore, clinical features must be employed to categorize the lesions and determine treatment. Clinically aggressive tumors (rapid expansion, perforation of the bony cortex, tooth erosion) are considered giant cell. There remains significant controversy, however, over whether a true giant cell tumor of the jaws can even be said to exist since such lesions of the jaws do not undergo malignant conversion, as is relatively common with GCTs of the long bones.

a. Giant cell reparative granuloma (GCRG)

   (1) This tumor is clinically quiescent, affecting the mandible more often than the maxilla and females more often than males (2:1). It occurs usually in children and young adults.

   (2) It is generally located in the premolar area, rarely if ever posterior to the 6 yr molar. It is the most common central jaw tumor to cross the midline.

   (3) The patient usually has no symptoms. The lesion often is discovered as an incidental radiographic abnormality. It may be of either unilocular or multilocular configuration, sometimes with faint central trabeculations. Cortical expansion, occasionally with perforation, is common. Teeth are typically displaced rather than eroded.

   (4) Differential diagnosis of these radiographic changes should include GCRG, myxoma, central vascular malformation, central mucoepidermoid carcinoma, odontogenic keratocyst, and ameloblastoma. When the GCRG presents because of swelling or pain, the symptoms are usually slight.

   (5) Curettage or conservative excision is appropriate. Recurrences are uncommon; but when they arise and/or if the aggressive clinical features described accompany reappearance of the lesion, consideration should be given to revision of the diagnosis to GCT (and more aggressive resection may be indicated).

b. Brown tumor of hyperparathyroidism

   (1) This tumor is characterized by histological, clinical, and radiographic features indistinguishable from those of GCRG.

   (2) There are central jaw changes occurring with both primary (parathyroid adenoma or hyperplasia) and secondary (chronic renal failure) hyperparathyroidism.

   (3) Diagnosis is made from biopsy findings consistent with those in GCRG and elevated serum parathyroid hormone (PTH). Radiographs demonstrate resorption lacunae in the phalanges and loss of the lamina dura. Histological findings interpreted as consistent with GCRG should always lead to consideration of hyperparathyroidism.

   (4) Treatment principally concerns the primary disease. Primary hyperparathyroidism requires excision of the autonomous focus of PTH production. The secondary form requires management of the renal disease, including calcium and vitamin D supplements.

        (5) Brown tumors may require resection if they are large and/or if the associated cortical expansion causes functional problems. Small lesions may involute once the primary disease has been controlled.

    c. Giant cell tumor (GCT)

        (1) True GCT of the jaws is rare. We employ clinical criteria to make the designation when biopsy shows histology consistent with GCRG. Rapid expansion inducing significant pain, root resorption, rapid cortical perforation, and multiple recurrences of early onset indicate an aggressive although benign lesion that should be designated GCT.

        (2) There has been only one well-documented case of malignant GCT of the jaw. Distinction from osteosarcoma, which may contain many giant cells, is essential.

        (3) GCT of the jaws seems to be intermediate in aggressiveness between the innocuous GCRG of the jaws and the aggressive sometimes malignant GCT of the long bones.

        (4) Treatment is controversial. En bloc resection with immediate reconstruction is appropriate for very aggressive tumors and for those that have recurred several times after curettage or simple excision.

2. Myxoma. This benign tumor was discussed in the odontogenic category, although some experts place it in the non-odontogenic groups since many occur in non–tooth-bearing parts of the jaws.

3. Fibrous dysplasia

    a. This lesion of the jaws is usually monostotic, although it may be part of a generalized disease with or without endocrine abnormalities. It frequently presents as a painless slowly progressive swelling in the first and second decades. Periods of rapid expansion may be seen—e.g., during the pubertal growth spurt or during pregnancy. The lesion rarely changes significantly after age 25 yr. When expansion of the bones of the craniofacial skeleton is significant, functional deficits may occur, particularly interference with vision and mandibular hypomobility.

    b. Other important features of fibrous dysplasia include the following:

        (1) The maxilla is involved more commonly than the mandible and, by extension into the orbit, the process may cause proptosis or obstruct vision.

        (2) Radiographic changes vary according to the age of the patient and the activity of the disease. In very young patients with rapidly expanding fibrous dysplasia, radiographs demonstrate a multilocular or unilocular radiolucent lesion with cortical thinning.

In older patients with clinically quiescent lesions, radiographs demonstrate a mixed radiolucent-radiopaque or simply a radiopaque mass.

(3) Serum calcium, phosphorus, and alkaline phosphatase are normal (Appendix II, p. 339).

(4) Histology is characterized by a mixture of fibrous tissue, bone, giant cells, blood vessels, and mast cells. There appears to be a direct correlation between clinical disease activity and cellularity of the connective tissue as well as with the numbers of mast cells.

(5) Treatment is indicated when there is interference with vision, nasal breathing, and jaw function as well as to improve appearance, since fibrous dysplasia may markedly distort facial skeletal form and symmetry. Surgical recontouring by excision and burring is the usual treatment and is most predictable once the patient has reached skeletal maturity. Long-term follow-up is important since rare instances of spontaneous sarcomatous change have been reported, although most of these occurred subsequent to radiation therapy, which (it is now clear) plays no role in management of this disease.

4. Ossifying fibroma
   a. This tumor is considered a variant of fibrous dysplasia and is included in the general category of fibroosseous lesions. It is characterized by
      (1) Slow expansion, rarely causing pain or paresthesia
      (2) Occurrence more commonly in the mandible than the maxilla, in contrast to fibrous dysplasia
      (3) Peak incidence in the third and fourth decades
   b. A well-defined radiolucency is seen in early stages. The lesion progressively calcifies and, as it does so, its borders become less distinct.
   c. The ossifying fibroma may not be separable clinically, radiographically, or histologically from a cementifying fibroma.
   d. Treatment consists of local excision or enucleation. The tumor separates readily from surrounding bone. Rare instances of aggressive behavior have been described, features not explained histologically. Such lesions warrant more extensive excision.

5. Cherubism
   a. This tumor has histological features that make it inseparable from the GCRG. However, its historical and clinical features allow easy diagnosis. These include
      (1) Autosomal dominant inheritance with 50-70% penetrance in females and 100% penetrance in males—expressivity is variable but usually bilateral and sym-

metrical; sporadic spontaneous mutations may occur

(2) Evident usually by 3-4 yr of age, presenting as a slowly progressive painless swelling—the mandible is affected more often and to a greater extent than the maxilla; disease progression slows by about 10 yr of age and the lesions may regress at puberty

(3) Association with firm nontender cervical lymphadenopathy common—increased skin pigmentation is less common

(4) Deciduous teeth that exfoliate prematurely—multiple missing and impacted secondary teeth ("floating teeth") occur

b. Radiographically a multilocular, usually bilaterally symmetric, expansion of the jaws is seen. The cortex is thinned. The posterior mandible is most commonly involved, although the condyles are always spared. Teeth seem to be floating within the tumor and may be malformed.

c. Treatment must be individualized. Surgical contouring is appropriate when expansion is severe, leading to functional jaw or airway disturbances, or when the disease causes social problems in the older child. If possible, intervention is delayed until growth has ceased.

6. Osteoblastoma and osteoid osteoma. These lesions are histologically indistinguishable. Both display trabeculae of woven bone and osteoid in a vascular fibrous stroma. Separation is based upon growth potential.

a. The osteoblastoma may be significantly larger than 1 cm in diameter whereas the osteoid osteoma is rarely larger. In addition, the latter classically causes severe pain that is most intense at night.

b. The osteoblastoma is a solitary radiolucency. The osteoid osteoma has a distinct sclerotic border around an otherwise similar lesion.

c. Treatment of both lesions is en bloc excision. Recurrence after curettage is common. Because the calvarium is the usual site of osteoblastoma in the craniofacial skeleton and may cause trismus if the temporal bone is involved, a combined maxillofacial and neurosurgical approach may be required for excising this tumor.

C. Vascular lesions. Central vascular lesions of the jaws are uncommon. Distinction between hemangioma and vascular malformation is important in the understanding of these lesions. The aneurysmal bone cyst will also be discussed.

1. The hemangioma is a true tumor of endothelium and is the most common benign tumor of childhood. It is usually not present at birth, exhibits a period of rapid postnatal growth, and typically involutes slowly until age 5-7 yr. Central hem-

angioma of the facial bones is rare (fewer than 100 cases). Most have occurred in the mandible. Less than 1% of hemangiomas of the maxillofacial region in one large series were of the central type.

2. Vascular malformations are morphogenetic abnormalities of vascular channels that are present at birth and grow proportionately with the host. Expansion may occur secondary to trauma, infection, and bleeding. Isolated central vascular malformations of the jaws are rare; over one third of lesions affecting the maxillofacial region directly involve the underlying bone as well.

   a. Central vascular lesions may display a multilocular appearance radiographically. Hypertrophy and distortion of bone occur with lymphatic malformations. Destructive changes of bone are common with arterial malformations.

   b. Treatment must be individualized. Central jaw hemangiomas rarely bleed spontaneously and usually do not require treatment. If bleeding is a problem, selective embolization and en bloc resection may be required. Evaluation for potential chronic coagulopathies is essential in the management of vascular malformations (chronic consumption coagulopathy). Total resection of vascular malformations is often not possible. Partial resection with the assistance of selective embolization may allow control of hemorrhage.

3. Aneurysmal bone cyst consists of blood-filled spaces lined by spindle cells. Multiple giant cells are also seen. Some areas may be histologically indistinguishable from giant cell reparative granuloma. There is no true epithelial lining. This is a slow-growing tumor, usually of the mandible, affecting females most commonly. Painless swelling is the general presentation, which appears as a multilocular radiolucency on further examination. Treatment is curettage. Recurrence is rare.

D. Hematopoietic-reticuloendothelial tumors. Histiocytosis X is a spectrum of diseases of unknown etiology characterized by the accumulation of cholesterol-laden histiocytes in hard and/or soft tissues. The histiocytosis group includes eosinophilic granuloma, Hand-Schüller-Christian disease, and Letterer-Siwe disease. (Burkitt's lymphoma is discussed with this group although it is not a true histiocytosis X.)

1. Eosinophilic granuloma is the localized form of histiocytosis, usually affecting the craniofacial skeleton (particularly the jaws). The posterior body and angle regions of the mandible are most often involved. Dental symptoms may lead to discovery of the lesions and can include loose teeth, delayed healing of extractions sites, and chronic gingival ulcers.

   a. Radiographically the teeth appear to be floating, simulating severe periodontal disease. The cortex is usually thinned and expanded. The lesion is typically well demarcated, although usually with an irregular outline.

  b. Treatment is enucleation and curettage and/or low-dose radiation (600-1000 cGy*).

2. Hand-Schüller-Christian disease is the disseminated chronic form of histiocytosis, affecting multiple organ systems. Diabetes insipidus, proptosis, and dental malocclusion may be caused by tumor infiltration of the pituitary gland, orbit, and jaws. Hepatosplenomegaly, eczematoid skin changes, and deafness may be associated findings.

  a. Radiographically the individual lesions are similar to those found in eosinophilic granuloma. Jaw lesions tend to be more diffuse. Teeth are displaced as the alveolar bone is destroyed.

  b. Treatment is variable. Individual lesions may be improved by curettage and/or radiation. Various chemotherapy regimens have been tried, with variable success. The disease is slowly progressive.

3. Letterer-Siwe disease is the acute, often fulminating, form of histiocytosis. It usually affects children 2 yr of age or less. The disease is relentless as massive invasion of liver, spleen, and marrow occurs. Generalized lymphadenopathy, constitutional disturbance, pulmonary and gastrointestinal involvement, and skin changes are inevitable. Bone lesions are less prominent in this form, although central jaw involvement may lead to changes simulating severe periodontal disease. Treatment is by various chemotherapy protocols. Further discussion is beyond the scope of this chapter.

4. Burkitts's lymphoma is a disease of unclear etiology, predominantly affecting males, that may involve many organ systems—including the facial and long bones, nervous system, salivary glands, pelvic and abdominal viscera, and retroperitoneum.

  a. Jaw involvement is most common in the African form of this disease. The maxilla is affected more commonly than the mandible (2:1), and bimaxillary disease is not infrequent. Jaw presentations include premature loss of teeth and swelling.

  b. In the early stages this disease may present radiographically as a loss of lamina dura around adjacent teeth.

  c. Treatment consists of surgical debulking and high-dose administration of alkylating agents. Remission occurs in over 90% of cases.

E. Neurogenic tumors. Benign neurogenic tumors involving the jaws include the traumatic neuroma, neurofibroma, neurilem-

---

*Centigrays (rads).

moma, and melanotic neuroectodermal tumor of infancy. We will not discuss the traumatic neuroma since it is not a true neoplasm.

1. Neurofibroma is a tumor derived from Schwann cells. Approximately one third of persons afflicted with neurofibromatosis have abnormalities of the underlying bone such as cystic change with cortical expansion, subperiosteal erosion, or bony hypoplasia. The latter may occur without apparent central involvement. Central lesions are usually solitary rather than as one of many in a person with neurofibromatosis.

    a. Central neurofibromas usually cause dull discomfort and paresthesia. Most are found in the mandible.

    b. Radiographic findings may include a fusiform expansion of the inferior alveolar canal or multilocular radiolucent changes in areas contiguous to overlying soft tissue lesions.

    c. In contrast to the neurilemmoma, neurofibromas are not encapsulated. In addition, they are known to undergo sarcomatous change in a significant number of cases, although there has been little experience with central jaw lesions. Long-term follow-up must be stressed.

    d. Treatment is local excision. Since the involved bone is very vascular, resection may result in significant blood loss. The mandibular nerve is sacrificed if involved. Immediate bone and/or nerve grafting should be considered.

2. Neurilemmoma (schwannoma) also derives from Schwann cells. The affected person usually experiences pain, swelling, and often paresthesia. The mandible is most commonly involved.

    a. This tumor is encapsulated and, consistent with this feature, appears radiographically as a unilocular or multilocular lucency with well-defined borders.

    b. Treatment is enucleation. Recurrence is rare.

3. Melanotic neuroectodermal tumor of infancy

    a. This tumor, of neural crest origin, presents in children during the first year. Although reported in extragnathic sites, the canine area of the anterior maxilla is most commonly involved. Characteristic findings are swelling of the upper lip, usually without pain, and displacement of adjacent tooth buds.

    b. The tumor has infiltrating projections within a vascular fibrous stroma. Granules of melanin are seen.

    c. Treatment is conservative local excision. Recurrence rates of about 15% have been reported. There appears to be no malignant potential.

III. Diagnosis and treatment of jaw tumors

    A. Diagnosis is based largely upon history, physical examination, radiographic and laboratory investigations, and biopsy. The mature surgeon will be aware that histological designations are sometimes ambiguous and must be carefully correlated with the clinical features that essentially summarize the biological behavior of the tumor. The central giant cell lesions and the various forms of ameloblastoma highlight the importance of such correlations.

B. Aggressive but histologically benign lesions (characterized by rapid expansion, root resorption, paresthesias, cortical perforation, and invasion of soft tissue as well as recurrences of early onset) may require deviation from "standard" treatment protocols. Wider resection may be appropriate. Treatment must be determined by histology and biological behavior of the tumor.

C. Radiolucent jaw lesions warrant routine assessment of serum calcium, phosphorus, and alkaline phosphatase.

D. Any central jaw tumor characterized by the pathologist as "giant cell reparative granuloma" warrants consideration of hyperparathyroidism, since the brown tumor is histologically indistinguishable from the reparative granuloma. Appropriate laboratory studies would include those just listed as well as serum parathyroid hormone levels (perhaps serum BUN and creatinine) and screening radiographs of the jaws and hand.

E. Tumors discussed in this chapter do not metastasize, although local recurrences may arise. When discontinuity defects result from resection, immediate bone graft reconstruction is indicated. When the sensory branches of the trigeminal nerve are sacrificed, immediate interpositional nerve grafting using the sural or greater auricular nerve is indicated.

F. When children are affected by these tumors, treatment must not be compromised because of fears of interfering with subsequent facial growth. Although essential to consider, growth disturbances can be minimized by early functional rehabilitation—achieved by early jaw reconstruction and, in selected instances, the aid of dental prostheses.

GENERAL REFERENCES

Batsakis, J.G.: Tumors of the head and neck, ed. 2, Baltimore, 1979, The Williams & Wilkens Co.

Chuong, R., et al.: The odontogenic keratocyst—an update, J. Oral Maxillofac. Surg. **40**:797, 1982.

Gorlin, R.J., and Goldman, H.M., editors: Thoma's oral pathology, ed. 6, St. Louis, 1970, The C.V. Mosby Co.

Gorlin R.J., et al.: Odontogenic tumors in man and animals: pathological classification and clinical behavior. A review, Ann. N.Y. Acad. Sci. **108**:722, 1963.

Mehlisch, D.R., et al.: Amelobalstoma: a clinicopathologic report, J. Oral Surg. **30**:9, 1972.

APPENDIX I

Oral Manifestations
of Systemic Disease

CHRONIC INFECTIOUS DISEASES

	Clinical features	Diagnosis	Oral manifestations	Treatment
Leprosy (*Mycobacterium leprae*)	Slightly contagious granulomatous disease Skin most commonly involved	Histological exam acid-fast bacilli	Nodular lesions on mucous membranes Facial paralysis bilaterally if CN VII involved	
Fungus Actinomycosis (*Actinomyces israelii*)	Chronic noncontagious suppurative infection	Immunofluorescent antibody stains of drainage or necrotic debris *Actinomyces israelii* or anaerobic culture	Hard, circumscribed, inflammatory masses (chronic); multiple fistulas (chronic)	I & D; large long-term doses of penicillin
Histoplasmosis (*Histoplasma capsulatum*)	Septic fever; pulmonary involvement; enlargement of spleen, liver, lymph nodes; contaminated soil in semi-Tropics	Histoplasmin skin test; serological tests Cultures	Ulcerations, nodular lesions	
Blastomycosis (*Blastomyces dermatidis*)	Skin papules; sometimes fatal pulmonary involvement; contaminated soil		Ulcerative papules	0.02% amphotericin-B ointment for oral lesions

Tuberculosis (*Mycobacterium tuberculosis*)	Droplet spread; fatigue, decrease in weight, fevers	Chest radiograph Ziehl-Neelsen stain; Mantoux skin test Caseous avascular necrotic nodule surrounded by multinucleated giant cells	Oral lesions rare; painless nodule ulcerates; osteomyelitis with tubercle bacilli on histology	Dental rehabilitation after sputum becomes negative Ethambutol, isoniazid, streptomycin, aminosalicylic acid
Syphilis (*Treponema pallidum*)	Spread by sexual intercourse and through oral cavity	Physical examination, dark-field examination of chancre, serological examination of blood; dark field examinations of oral lesions difficult due to presence of other acquired spirochetes	Congenital (linear scars at angles of lips; hypoplasia of permanent incisors and molars, deafness [CN VIII], interstitial keratitis, increased corneal opacity) Acquired (indurated nodule ulcerates, often painful; mucous patch, painful raised gray lesion with erythematous base, ulcerates; gumma, indurated, ulcerated, enlarging lesion; loss of taste, paresthesias, neurological involvement)	Penicillin, follow-up with physical and serological examinations

CONNECTIVE TISSUE DISEASES

Collagen diseases	Clinical features and diagnostics	Oral manifestations	Treatment
Lupus erythematosus			
Chronic (discoid)	Reddish macular skin lesions with yellow scales, "butterfly pattern" in malar area Histological Hyperparakeratosis Perivascular lymphocytes Hyaline degeneration of connective tissue LE prep	Mucocutaneous disease; 25% have oral lesions; erythematous keratinized lesions on buccal mucosa and lower lip	Antimalarials suppress but do not cure
Systemic	Especially affects heart and kidneys; altered immune reactivity; hemolytic anemia; fever, weakness, decreased weight, anorexia LE prep	Similar to those of discoid lupus, particularly in acute form; hyperemia, edema, and extension of lesions more pronounced	Antimalarials, steroids, therapies of specific organ involvement-failure

Dermatomyositis	Degenerative disease of connective tissue, skin, skeletal muscles; 25% associated with malignancy	Muscles of tongue and deglutition degenerate, may undergo necrosis and hyaline degeneration; mucosal lesions similar to lupus; painful tongue involvement with swelling, degeneration, atrophy, diffuse mucosal erosion	Systemic steroids suppress but do not cure; may end spontaneously or progress to fatality
Scleroderma	Disease of collagenous connective tissue; results in hardening of skin and subcutaneous tissues, atrophy, and pigmentation; indurated lesions of neck, trunk, extremities following distribution of peripheral nerves; osteoporosis, soft tissue calcifications, especially at joints; collagen fibers atrophy and compress into compact masses histologically; decreased elastic tissue; dissappearance of most skin appendages (e.g., hair) in affected areas	Indurations of mucosa and submucosa, atrophy, pigmentation, false ankylosis of TMJ, painful induration of tongue and gingiva, thickening of periodontal ligament at radiography	Physiotherapy; systemic steroids may repress but not cure

ANEMIAS

Type	Causes and diagnostic	Oral manifestations	Treatment
Microcytic hypochromic (iron deficiency)	Blood loss resulting in iron deficiency (GI bleeding); rarely from dietary deficiency of iron; decreased HCT, decreased Hgb; small faint RBCs on smear	Plummer-Vinson syndrome (glossitis with dry indurated tongue and dysphagia, atrophy of mucous membrane of mouth and pharynx)	Oral ferrous salts; identify and correct any acute or chronic blood loss
Megaloblastic (pernicious)	Decreased vitamin B_{12} because of decreased absorption due to lack of gastric intrinsic factor; arrest of erythrocyte maturation; megaloblasts and macrocytes on smear	Smooth tongue, painful, atrophy of papillae, pale oral mucosa, petechiae	Vitamin B_{12} injections
Aplastic	Aplasia of bone marrow shown at needle biopsy; leukopenia occurs first because of shorter life-span of leukocytes; caused by extrinsic chemicals, antibiotics, radiation	Pallor, petechiae, opportunistic infections	Control infections (because of leukopenia)

Normocytic	Toxins inhibit RBC formation and decrease life-span of RBCs; may be secondary to chronic inflammatory disease or renal failure	Pallor, mucositis	Remove etiological factors; hygiene; improved diet
Polycythemia vera	Absolute increase in number of circulating RBCs; etiology unknown; splenomegaly most constant feature	Gingiva deep purplish red, often swollen; tongue may also be involved as well as all mucosa; cyanosis due to presence of reduced hemoglobin in excess of 5 g/100 ml	Symptoms relieved by phlebotomy
Thalassemia	Hereditary, especially in people of Mediterranean descent; thalassemia major (impaired hemoglobin synthesis, hemolipids), thalassemia minor (mild chronic anemia)	Pallor; few if any oral symptoms	Patients with thalassemia major may need frequent transfusion
Sickle cell	Hereditary hemolytic type; misshapen RBCs can cause embolism and thrombosis; happens when hemoglobin reduces during decreased oxygen tension	Pallor and icterus, petechiae, osteoporotic changes on jaw radiographs and periapical films	Avoid hypoxia; in acute crisis, administer oxygen by nasal cannula and IV fluids

HEMATOLOGICAL LESIONS

Type	Oral manifestations
Infectious mononucleosis (Epstein-Barr virus)	Palatal petechiae, lymphadenopathy
Agranulocytosis (arrested maturation of granulocytes in marrow)	Gangrenous stomatitis, sore throat
Hodgkin's disease (lymphoma)	Cervical (and other) adenopathy
Hemophilia	Spontaneous bleeding, excessive continuous bleeding after minor mucosal trauma
Thrombocytopenic purpura	Spontaneous bleeding, mucosa bleeds easily and excessively from minimum trauma, petechiae
Acute leukemia	Ulcerative stomatitis, progressively worsening; gangrenous necrosis of gingiva; swollen, edematous, painful gingiva; frequent, chronic herpetic lesions; bleeding, petechiae; lymphadenopathy
Chronic lymphocytic leukemia	As above, marked tonsillar enlargement with hard cervical lymphadenopathy
Chronic myelogenous leukemia	Gingival bleeding and enlargement, toothache, ulcerative lesions, petechiae

RETICULOENDOTHELIOSES (HISTIOCYTOSIS X)

	Oral manifestations	Other considerations
Eosinophilic granuloma	Oval or round, irregular, sharply demarcated radiolucencies of maxilla and mandible; extrabony lesions may occur as tender swelling	Usually solitary granuloma (usually) of bone consisting of histiocytes and eosinophils
Hand-Schüller-Christian	Swelling of gingiva, early necrosis, maxillary and mandibular osseous xanthomatosis, tooth extrusion	Reticuloendothelial cell proliferation infiltrates and replaces bone and soft tissue; exophthalmos, diabetes insipidus, defects of membranous bones; histiocytes are lipid laden
Letterer-Siwe	Hemorrhage and ulceration of gingiva; lytic destruction of alveolar bone	Progressive, acute, disseminated proliferation of histiocytes

COMMON ENDOCRINE AND STORAGE DISEASES

Type	Oral manifestations	Other considerations
Diabetes mellitus	In uncontrolled or poorly controlled patient, exaggerated periodontal response to common irritants (plaque), producing fulminant suppurative periodontitis and acetone breath; xerostomia results in mucositis In controlled diabetic, no special oral manifestations; periodontium reacts to irritants same as in nondiabetic	Maintain dentition to avoid infections
Amyloidosis	Nodules of gingiva (50%), tongue (50%), pharynx, respiratory and GI tracts; tongue purpura	Diagnosis by biopsy
Lipidoses (Gaucher's disease)	Osteoporosis of mandible with large radiolucencies, yellowish patches on mucosa (histiocytes engorged with cerebroside lesions)	Cerebroside accumulation in spleen, liver, bone marrow, lymph nodes causing portal cirrhosis
Niemann-Pick disease	Jaws infiltrated with lipid-containing cells; large radiolucencies	Sphingomyelin accumulates in RE system
Mucopolysaccharidoses (Hurler syndrome, Hunter syndrome, etc.)	Broad mandible; localized areas of destruction in jaws may be seen	Primarily genetically determined disturbance of mucopolysaccharide metabolism; a range of diseases

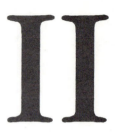
HEMATOLOGY

Hematocrit (HCT)
  42-53%, males
  37-48%, females
Hemoglobin (Hgb)
  13-18 g/100 ml, males
  12-16 g/100 ml, females

Methemoglobin — 0.4-1.5% of total hemoglobin

Erythrocyte (RBC) count — 4.2-5.9 million/mm^3

Mean corpuscular hemoglobin (MCH) — 28-30 μμg

Mean corpuscular hemoglobin concentration (MCHC) — 32-36%

Mean corpuscular volume (MCV) — 86-98 mμ^3

Serum hemoglobin — 2-3 mg/100 ml

White blood (WBC) count, normal differential screen
  Granulocytes — 52-79%
  Lymphocytes — 11-39%
  Monocytes — 4-15%
  Differential leukocyte count (adults)
    PMNs — 40-75%
    Bands — 0-4%
    Lymphocytes — 20-45%
    Monocytes — 2-10%
    Eosinophils — 1-6%
    Basophils — <1%

Eosinophil count — 70-440/mm^3

Reticulocyte count — 0.5-2.5%

Erythrocyte sedimentation rate (ESR)
  1-13 mm/hr, males
  1-20 mm/hr, females

Special hematology studies

Vitamin B$_{12}$	205-876 pg/ml
Folic acid (serum)	>3.3 ng/ml
Serum ferritin	0-12 ng/ml (iron deficiency) 13-20 ng/ml (borderline iron deficiency) 21-50 ng/ml (normal range; however, could be consistent with iron deficiency if liver disease or inflammation is present) >400 ng/ml (iron excess)
Iron	50-150 µg/100 ml (higher in males)
Iron-binding capacity	250-410 µg/100 ml

Coagulation studies

Prothrombin time (PT)	±2 sec of control value (normal 11 sec)
Partial thromboplastin time (PTT)	25-40 sec
Platelet count	150,000-350,000/mm^3
Thrombin time	±5 sec of control value
Bleeding time test	2-9.5 min
Fibrin split products (FSP)	1:4 or less
Protamine sulfate	1:20 or less
Circulating platelet aggregates (CPA)	0.8 or greater
Ristocetin cofactor	>40%

Hepatitis-related studies

Antibody to hepatitis-A virus (anti-HAv)

IgG detectable	Infection with hepatitis-A in remote past
IgM detectable	Infection with hepatitis-A currently or recently

Antibody to hepatitis-B core antigen (anti-HBc)

Detectable	Current or past hepatitis-B infection

Hepatitis-Be

  Antigen (HBe Ag)   Detectable: High infectivity

  Antibody to HBe   Detectable: Low infectivity

Blood plasma and serum chemistries

Electrolytes

Calcium	8.5-10.5 mg/100 ml (children slightly higher)
Chloride	100-106 mEq/L
Lithium	0.5-1.5 mEq/L
Magnesium	1.5-2.0 mEq/L
Potassium	3.5-5.0 mEq/L
Sodium	135-145 mEq/L
Phosphorus	3.0-4.5 mg/100 ml (infants up to 6 mg/100 ml)

Carbon dioxide content   24-30 mEq/L (infants 20-26 mEq/L)

Osmolality   280-296 mOsm/kg H_2O

Protein

Total	6.0-8.4 g/100 ml
Albumin	3.5-5.0 g/100 ml
Globulin	2.3-3.5 g/100 ml

Electrophoresis   Percent of total protein

Albumin	52-68
Globulins	
Alpha-1	4.2-7.2
Alpha-2	6.8-12
Beta	9.3-15
Gamma	13-23

Bilirubin   Direct up to 0.4 mg/100 ml
                    Total up to 1.0 mg/100 ml

Glucose   70-110 mg/100 ml (fasting)

Triglycerides   40-150 mg/100 ml

Cholesterol   120-220 mg/100 ml

Lipoproteins (as cholesterol)

HDL	30-65 mg/100 ml, males
	35-80 mg/100 ml, females
LDL	70-190 mg/100 ml

Cardiac enzymes
    CPK (creatine phosphokinase)   17-148 U/L, males
                                      10-79 U/L, females
    CPK isoenzymes   5% MB band or less
    LDH (lactic dehydrogenase)   45-90 U/L
    SGOT (aspartate aminotransfer-   7-27 U/L
        ase)
    SGPT (alanine aminotransfer-   1-21 U/L
        ase)

Renal-related studies

Urea nitrogen (BUN)   8-25 mg/100 ml
Creatinine   0.6-1.5 mg/100 ml
Uric acid   3.0-7.0 mg/100 ml
Acid phosphatase   0-0.5   Fishman-Lerner · unit/100
                                        ml
Alkaline phosphatase   13-39 U/L (infants and adoles-
                                        cents up to 104 U/L)
Carbon monoxide   Less than 5% total hemoglobin
                                        (symptoms with over 20% sat-
                                        uration)
Copper   70-150 μg/100 ml
Lead   Up to 50 μg/100 ml
Ammonia   12-55 μmol/L

Medications and drugs

Carbamazepine (Tegretol)   2.0-8.0 μg/ml
Chloramphenicol   10-20 μg/ml
Ethosuximide (Zarontin)   40-100 μg/ml
Phenobarbital   15-50 μg/ml
Phenytoin (Dilantin)   5-20 μg/ml
Procainamide (Pronestyl)   4.0-10.0 μg/ml
Propranolol   100-300 μg/ml
Quinidine   1.2-4.0 μg/ml
Salicylate   Therapeutic 20-25 mg/100 ml
                                       (25-30 mg/100 ml to age 10
                                       yr)
                                     Toxic over 30 mg/100 ml (over
                                       20 mg/100 ml after age 60 yr)
Serum digoxin   1.2-1.7 ng/ml
Serum digitalis   17 ± 6 ng/ml
Sulfonamide   5-15 mg/100 ml
Valproic acid   50-100 μg/ml
Vitamin A   0.15-0.6 μg/ml

APPENDIX III

Guidelines for Prophylactic Antibiotic Coverage*

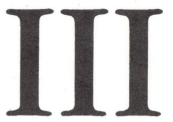

Endocarditis prophylaxis recommended:
  Prosthetic cardiac valves (including biosynthetic valves)
  Most congenital cardiac malformations
  Surgically constructed systemic-pulmonary shunts
  Rheumatic and other acquired valvular dysfunction
  Idiopathic hypertrophic subaortic stenosis (IHSS)
  Previous history of bacterial endocarditis
  Mitral valve prolapse with insufficiency*
Endocarditis prophylaxis not recommended:
  Isolated secundum atrial septal defect
  Secundum atrial septal defect repaired without a patch 6
      or more mo earlier
  Patent ductus arteriosus ligated and divided 6 or more
      mo earlier
  Postoperative coronary artery bypass graft (CABG)

This list gives just the common conditions. It is not meant to be all-inclusive.

*Definitive data to provide guidance in managing patients with mitral valve prolapse are particularly limited. It is clear that in general such patients are at low risk of contracting endocarditis, but the risk-benefit ratio of prophylaxis in mitral valve prolapse is uncertain.

*Modified from Shulman, S.T., et al.: Circulation **70**:6, 1984.

SUMMARY OF RECOMMENDED ANTIBIOTIC REGIMENS FOR DENTAL OR RESPIRATORY TRACT PROCEDURES

Standard regimen

For dental procedures that cause gingival bleeding, and oral–respiratory tract surgery	Penicillin-V 2.0 g orally 1 hr before, then 1.0 g 6 hr after initial dose; for patient unable to take oral medications, 2 million units of aqueous penicillin-G IV or IM 30-60 min before procedure and 1 million units 6 hr after initial dose may be substituted

Special regimens

Parenteral regimen for use when maximum protection desired (e.g., for patients with prosthetic valves)	Ampicillin 1.0-2.0 g IM or IV plus gentamicin 1.5 mg/kg IM or IV, ½ hr before procedure, followed by 1.0 g oral penicillin-V 6 hr after initial dose; alternatively, parenteral regimen may be repeated once 8 hr after initial dose
Oral regimen for penicillin-allergic patients	Erythromycin 1.0 g orally 1 hr before, then 500 mg 6 hr after initial dose
Parenteral regimen for penicillin-allergic patients	Vancomycin 1.0 g IV slowly over 1 hr, starting 1 hr before; no repeat dose is necessary

Pediatric doses: Ampicillin 50 mg/kg per dose; erythromycin 20 mg/kg for first dose, then 10 mg/kg: gentamicin 2.0 mg/kg per dose; penicillin-V full adult dose if greater than 60 lb (27 kg), one-half adult dose if less than 60 lb (27 kg); aqueous penicillin-G 50,000 units/kg (25,000 units/kg for follow-up); vancomycin 20 mg/kg per dose. The intervals between doses are the same as for adults. Total doses should not exceed adult doses.

PROPHYLAXIS RECOMMENDATIONS FOR DENTAL PROCEDURES AND SURGERY OF THE UPPER RESPIRATORY TRACT

Standard regimen

Oral penicillin. For adults and children over 60 lb (27 kg), penicillin-V 2.0 g 1 hr prior to the procedure and then 1.0 g 6 hr after the initial dose. For children less than 60 lb, 1.0 g 1 hr prior to the procedure and then 500 mg 6 hr after the initial dose.

For the patient unable to take oral antibiotics prior to a procedure, 2 million units of aqueous penicillin-G (50,000 units/kg for children) IV or IM 30-60 min before the procedure and 1 million units (25,000 units/kg for children) 6 hr after the initial dose may be substituted.*

---

*Children's antibiotic doses should not exceed the maximum adult doses.

For patients with prosthetic valves and others with highest risk of endocarditis

Parenteral ampicillin and gentamicin. Ampicillin 1.0 to 2.0 g (50 mg/kg for children) plus gentamicin 1.5 mg/kg (2.0 mg/kg for children) both IM or IV ½ hr prior to the procedure, followed by 1 g oral penicillin-V (500 mg for children under 60 lb) 6 hr after the initial dose. Alternatively, the parenteral regimen should be repeated once 8 hr after the initial dose.*

Standard regimen for patients allergic to penicillin

Oral erythromycin. Erythromycin 1.0 g (20 mg/kg for children) 1 hr prior to the procedure and then 500 mg (10 mg/kg for children) 6 hr after the initial dose.*

For the patient unable to tolerate oral erythromycin, changing to a different erythromycin preparation may be beneficial. For the patient who cannot tolerate either penicillin or erythromycin, an oral cephalosporin (1.0 g 1 hr before the procedure plus 500 mg 6 hr after the initial dose) may be useful; but data are lacking to allow specific recommendation of this regimen. Tetracyclines *cannot* be recommended for this purpose.

Regimen for high-risk patients allergic to penicillin

IV vancomycin. Vancomycin 1 g (20 mg/kg for children) IV *slowly* over 1 hr starting 1 hr before the procedure.* Because of the long half-life of vancomycin, a repeat dose should not be necessary.

Notes

In unusual circumstances or in the case of delayed healing, it may be necessary to provide additional doses of antibiotic even though bacteremia rarely persists longer than 15 min after the procedure. Penicillin-V is the preferred form of oral penicillin because it is relatively resistant to gastric acid.

In the mouth of a patient who is taking oral penicillin for secondary prevention of rheumatic fever or other purpose, viridans streptococci may be present that are relatively resistant to penicillin. In these cases the physician or dentist should select erythromycin or one of the parenteral regimens.

The patient with a prosthetic heart valve in whom a high level of oral health is being maintained may be offered oral antibiotic prophylaxis for routine dental procedures. Parenteral antibiotics are recommended, however, for the patient with a prosthetic valve who require extensive dental procedures, especially extractions, or oral or gingival surgical procedures.

---

*Children's antibiotic doses should not exceed the maximum adult doses.

Index